FEL Apt

ACH - 4888

# WITHDRAWN

| DATE |  |  |  |
|---|---|---|---|
|  |  |  |  |
|  |  |  |  |
|  |  |  |  |
|  |  |  |  |
|  |  |  |  |
|  |  |  |  |
|  |  |  |  |
|  |  |  |  |
|  |  |  |  |
|  |  |  |  |
|  |  |  |  |
|  |  |  |  |
|  |  |  |  |

# THE STRANG COOKBOOK
## FOR
## CANCER PREVENTION

Laura Pensiero, R.D.,

*and*

Susan Oliveria, Sc.D., M.P.H.,

*with*

Michael Osborne, M.D.

———————

*Foreword by Jacques Pépin*

# THE STRANG COOKBOOK FOR CANCER PREVENTION

## A COMPLETE NUTRITION AND LIFESTYLE PLAN TO DRAMATICALLY LOWER YOUR CANCER RISK

A DUTTON BOOK

DUTTON
Published by the Penguin Group
Penguin Putnam Inc., 375 Hudson Street, New York, New York 10014, U.S.A.
Penguin Books Ltd, 27 Wrights Lane, London W8 5TZ, England
Penguin Books Australia Ltd, Ringwood, Victoria, Australia
Penguin Books Canada Ltd, 10 Alcorn Avenue, Toronto, Ontario, Canada M4V 3B2
Penguin Books (N.Z.) Ltd, 182–190 Wairau Road, Auckland 10, New Zealand

Penguin Books Ltd, Registered Offices: Harmondsworth, Middlesex, England

First published by Dutton, an imprint of Dutton Signet, a member of Penguin Putnam Inc.

First Printing, April, 1998
1   3   5   7   9   10   8   6   4   2

 REGISTERED TRADEMARK — MARCA REGISTRADA

LIBRARY OF CONGRESS CATALOGING-IN-PUBLICATION DATA:

Pensiero, Laura J.
The Strang cookbook for cancer prevention : a complete nutrition and lifestyle plan to dramatically lower
your cancer risk / Laura J. Pensiero and Susan A. Oliveria ; with Michael P. Osborne.
p.    cm.
ISBN 0-525-94313-7
1. Cancer—Nutritional aspects.   2. Cancer—Risk factors.   3. Cancer—Prevention.   4. Lifestyles—
Health aspects.   I. Oliveria, Susan A.   II. Osborne, Michael P.   III. Title.
RC268.P46   1998
616.99'4052—dc21        97-34933
CIP

Printed in the United States of America
Set in Goudy
Designed by Eve L. Kirch

PUBLISHER'S NOTE

This book is printed on acid-free paper. ∞

Dedicated to the patients
and benefactors of the
Strang Cancer Prevention Center.

In close affiliation with The New York Hospital-Cornell Medical Center since 1991, Strang has established the Strang-Cornell Cancer Research Laboratory dedicated to the prevention of cancer; the Strang-Cornell Breast Center, the first of its kind in New York City, and the Strang-Cornell Gastrointestinal Cancer Prevention Center.

Building on the past 65 years, the dedicated scientists and medical staff at Strang are determined more than ever to fulfill Strang's mission of interdisciplinary research to prevent cancer and promote care through early detection.

# ACKNOWLEDGMENTS

We are especially grateful to all the chefs who took time from their busy schedules to create beautiful and delicious recipes; without their help this book would not have been possible. We are particularly fortunate to have had one-on-one contact with Gianni Scappin, a contributing chef, during recipe testing. A special thank-you to Steven DeBrocky for his support and encouragement, as well as his help in promoting the idea for this book during its early stages of development.

We are grateful to Dr. Andrew Dannenberg for his enthusiasm. A colleague and friend, he provided the strong mentoring and support needed to complete this book. Comments on the first draft from Paul Christos, Deborah Plutzer, Ivan Rico, and Rachel Weiss improved the book considerably and we appreciate their help. Many thanks to our colleague Dr. Barbara Levine for her nutrition expertise. Harold Newmark's guidance and insightful comments during the writing of the section on phytochemicals helped to produce a concise and understandable chapter on this complex topic. Our colleagues Dr. Edward Giovannucci at the Harvard School of Public Health and Dr. Arline Salbe at the National Institutes of Health provided invaluable guidance for the science and applied nutrition sections, and we appreciate their help.

Sincere appreciation to our editor, Deirdre Mullane, who had the insight and creativity to help us present complex and diverse topics in an easy to understand manner.

Thanks also to All-Clad Metal Crafters Inc., who generously provided premium-quality cookware to complete the testing of each recipe.

Finally, we would like to thank Anne Fisher for her generous financial support to Strang Cancer Prevention Center and the Anne Fisher Nutrition Center. We are also grateful to all the donors who have generously contributed to Strang.

# ✧ CONTENTS ✧

# ⬧ FOREWORD ⬧

## Jacques Pépin

It is only in recent years that doctors and cooks have tried to understand one another and have started to work together to integrate our eating habits and lifestyles into a regimen intended to keep us healthy and long-lived. Not that this is a new premise. The ancient Greek and Roman doctors, poets, and philosophers—from Hippocrates, Seneca, and Archestratus to the School of Salerno's humoral theory in the Middle Ages—incorporated food and medicine in a literature that taught cooking as well as medicine.

The yin and yang of the Chinese places great emphasis on food habits and well-being, just as French gastronome Brillat-Savarin's aphorism "Tell me what you eat, and I will tell you what you are" encompasses today's notion that health is tightly interwoven with our consumption of food.

Thomas Edison unknowingly defined the goal of the Strang Cancer Prevention Center better than anyone when he said that "The doctor of the future will give no medicine but will educate his patients in the care of the human frame, in diet, and in the cause and prevention of disease."

Based on the latest nutritional research, there is no question that the quality of our food, the percentage of fat, and the amount of fiber from fruits and vegetables in our diet are all factors directly related to our physical health. The phytochemicals or "vegetable chemicals," which are the natural substances present in many fruits and vegetables, may be the plentiful and inexpensive pharmacy that we turn toward tomorrow.

The fusion of the cook and the doctor will be essential to comprehend that new source of health. Wouldn't it be great if we could make sense of the mass of nutritional information, often contradictory, that bombards us nowadays? Think of how invaluable it would be to have basic distinct guidelines that explain how eating fruits and vegetables can help to prevent disease and show us how to incorporate them without fuss into our daily fare.

This is precisely what the Strang Cancer Prevention Center provides in this book, and as a chef, home cook, and someone interested in good food and health, I am indebted to Laura Pensiero, Dr. Susan Oliveria, and Dr. Michael Osborne for providing us with the essential tools to better our lives and the lives of our family members and friends.

# ⇟ PREFACE ⇟

*Michael Osborne, M.D.*

The majority of cancer is related to lifestyle and therefore may be preventable. Good nutrition and exercise are of paramount importance. Strang Cancer Prevention Center is dedicated to interdisciplinary research into cancer prevention and promotion of cure through early detection. Worldwide it is estimated that approximately 7.6 million people will develop cancer and 5 million will die of the disease annually. In the United States, more than 2 million develop cancer each year and about 560,000 die of the disease. One in two men and one in three women develop cancer in their lifetime. For the first time it is projected that more people will develop cancer than heart disease in the next millennium. Research studies over the past fifty years have clearly shown that exercise and healthy nutrition are key factors in the prevention of cancer as well as cardiovascular disease. It is estimated that diet and obesity are responsible for about 30 percent of all cancer deaths while sedentary lifestyle is responsible for about 5 percent. Thirty-three percent of cancer deaths would be prevented by cessation of smoking and reduction in alcohol intake.

Understanding of the risk factors and modification of lifestyle will do a great deal to lessen the individual risk of disease. The last half of the nineteenth century and first half of the twentieth century have seen the conquest of a major scourge of the human race, infection, by prevention and treatment. Today the challenge is prevention of cancer and heart disease.

This book will show you how nutrition and lifestyle changes can give you the maximum benefit for prevention of cancer and other serious diseases. A healthy lifestyle will not only prolong life but will increase its enjoyment by enhancing its quality and quantity. A healthy diet and exercise leads to reduced stress, greater stamina, less fatigue, and better general well-being. I urge you to use the information here to stay healthy and get the most out of life.

# ✦ INTRODUCTION ✦

If healthy eating can improve both the quality and duration of our lives, why is it that we often do not follow fundamental nutrition guidelines? In some cases a lack of information may be the problem. Although some of us are aware of the role that nutrition can play in keeping us healthy, far too many others do not have this knowledge. In other cases conflicting information has left many people frustrated and confused about what foods are good for them and which ones should be limited in their diets. In *The Strang Program for Cancer Prevention* we have attempted to explain the complex relationship between diet and health in a thorough but easy-to-understand manner. At the same time we have made great efforts to separate facts from misconceptions or gimmicks that can be misleading.

As an epidemiologist at the Strang Cancer Prevention Center, I try to determine what lifestyle or behaviors affect the risk of developing cancer. The writing of this book has been motivated by a strong desire to educate individuals about the importance of nutrition in cancer prevention. Communicating the importance that diet can have in promoting cancer, as well as the notion that people can modify their behaviors and lifestyle, is paramount. Individuals can reduce their risks of not only cancer, but also other chronic diseases like obesity, diabetes, and cardiovascular disease if they maintain a healthy diet made up of lots of fruits and vegetables, whole grains, and foods low in fat. I believe it is important for people to understand where these recommendations come from and the research studies that support them.

The public has many misconceptions about the role of diet in protecting against disease. Almost on a weekly basis there is at least one article appearing in a newspaper or on television dealing with nutrition. The public has been overwhelmed with the results of dozens of studies often in disagreement with one another. I have taken this opportunity to clarify these misconceptions by giving the reader the current valid scientific knowledge on the role of diet in promoting and preventative cancer, including the strengths and limitations of different types of studies. I hope that from the information included here, you can learn how to evaluate the studies that are reported and understand how they apply to your everyday food choices and reduce your own risk of cancer.

SUSAN OLIVERIA, Sc.D., M.P.H.

My early counseling experiences as a clinical nutritionist brought me to the realization that if people are to make real and lasting changes in their diets, they need, in addition to just theoretical knowledge, practical tools they can use when shopping, cooking, and dining out. This recognition, along with a love of cooking, led me to enroll in The French Culinary Institute. To my clinical colleagues as well as many of my chef instructors, it was a source of good-natured amusement that a registered dietitian would choose to study classical French cuisine. After graduating in 1992 I founded Nutrition Source, a nutrition and culinary consulting company. This has provided me with the extraordinary opportunity to serve as a liaison between the two worlds of the culinary arts and health care.

Many notable chefs have graciously contributed recipes to this book, but "hands-on" work with two of them has enhanced my own recipe development skills tremendously. Jacques Pépin, Dean of Special Studies at The French Culinary Institute, has been a great source of inspiration to me, exemplifying that a well-balanced marriage between health and cooking is possible without sacrificing the many pleasures of dining. His talent is deliciously displayed in his recipes for Red Onion, Grapefruit, and Tomato Salad (page 152) and Turkey Steaks with Grape and Currant Sauce (page 248).

The innate healthy balance that exists in the Mediterranean style of cooking I have learned from my husband, Gianni Scappin, a chef of Italian origin and training. Although the recipes in this book represent many ethnic cuisines, the Mediterranean influence is perhaps the most profound. This is because of the naturally healthy ingredients, the simplicity of cooking methods, and the appeal that this cooking style holds for many people. Gianni's knack for achieving tremendous flavor with fresh ingredients and sparing use of fat (almost always olive oil!) along with his recognition that simplicity is important to the home cook make his recipes tasty, healthy, and pragmatic. These recipes will become part of your regular repertoire.

My clients at the Anne Fisher Nutrition Center, a research and clinical program at Strang Cancer Prevention Center, truly provided the inspiration and motivation that has resulted in the writing of this book. These wonderful and diverse people were almost unanimously of the frame of mind to say "please don't tell me what to do—tell and show me how to do it." In the process of answering their similar nutrition questions and referring them to various nutrition newsletters, books, and cookbooks, I realized a single and cohesive resource to address all or most of their needs did not exist.

Many of us know that numerous scientific organizations recommend five to nine fruit and vegetable servings per day to lower risk of cancer and other diseases. Unfortunately, this information is of limited use unless we know what a *serving* of fruit or vegetable is and how to include more of them into our diets when cooking, snacking, or dining out. Furthermore, although there are no "bad" fruits or vegetables, some stand out above others due to their high levels of protective vitamins, minerals, and phytochemicals (naturally occurring cancer fighters found in plant foods). In this book we have compiled the most comprehensive up-to-date food/phytochemical lists (see chapter 3) to familiarize you with which plant foods may be the most beneficial.

Encouraging studies looking at substances in soybeans and their potential to ward off or retard cancer has put this legume in the center of much media attention. I have worked with many people who want to take advantage of some of the health benefits they have heard about, but bad tofu experiences caused them to throw in the towel. The availability and use of soybeans and soy products is now extensive. The comprehensive section on soy (see pages 40–47) outlines the numerous soy products available, their many uses, and where to find them. I have created many recipes that include soy, and in the recipes provided by chefs, notations indicate when a soy product can be substituted or added.

The recipes included in this book are not just "good enough" for health food—you will find them tasty, attractive, and appealing for any occasion. Unlike many healthy recipes, they do not require that you adjust your palate to a lower standard. Nutritional comments and analyses serve to provide "light" lessons in the nutrient and phytochemical composition of the ingredients and of the prepared dishes. For example, when the amounts of a protective nutrient such as vitamin A or C or fiber are substantial, the value is indicated as a percentage of the Daily Value (similar to "Nutrition Facts" food labels). Finally, remarks provided for many of the recipes indicate the possibilities for variation, additions, substitutions, and pairing with other foods—an important factor in keeping you excited about healthy eating and in the kitchen.

In the last decade the increase in dialogue between M.D.'s (medical doctors), R.D.'s (registered dietitians), and chefs has advanced our relationship to one of collaboration and camaraderie. In *The Strang Cookbook for Cancer Prevention* we have further expanded this bridge of communication and sharing of disciplines to include laboratory, clinical, and epidemiologic scientists. Dr. Michael Osborne, president of Strang Cancer Prevention Center, had the vision that this book could also be an easy-to-understand resource for the layperson and health professional alike by including the scientific background for *why* we should make these dietary changes. Dr. Susan Oliveria, Director of Epidemiology at Strang Cancer Prevention Center, has performed the daunting task of summarizing the extensive and complex literature on cancer prevention and diet, in a clear and accessible manner. Dr. Oliveria has provided the why-to for this how-to guide.

There is a terrific amount of valuable information in this book, but don't let the details overwhelm you. Improving your diet is an evolving process of learning, implementing, and enjoying. These changes can be introduced gradually without going to extremes. The personal and social pleasure of dining need not be forsaken in your quest for better health. Buon Appetito!!!

LAURA PENSIERO, R.D.

# CHAPTER 1

# The Science Behind Diet and Cancer

**C**ancer is a devastating disease, responsible for shortening lives and throwing families into crisis. Many people think it can't happen to them, but most of us know at least one family member or friend who has cancer. It is a very real disease that can afflict each and every one of us, although there are some people who are more susceptible than others because of lifestyle or heredity.

On the positive side, however, we can do something about reducing our risk for developing cancer even though there is no "magic bullet" to prevent or cure the disease. Believe it or not, the power to decrease our chances of getting cancer is at our fingertips—knowledge is this power. Information is readily available so that we can all learn what to do on a day-to-day basis to help prevent cancer. And we know diet is key to helping fight cancer; in fact, about 30 percent of all cancer deaths can be attributed to a poor diet. This might not sound new to many of us who have seen on television or read in the newspaper that certain aspects of our diet can protect us against cancer. The media conveys this information to us daily in the form of "headlines" and "sound bites." But we are also bombarded by conflicting studies and misinformation.

What should we believe and more importantly what should we eat? What does a study really mean to you and when should you make a change in your diet based on scientific findings? We begin by showing you how to understand the results you hear about each day and make the most of them to reduce your risk of developing cancer. Understanding the role of diet in cancer prevention is the first step to make a change! We will then show you how to make those changes while enjoying a diet that is healthy, fun, and tasty with the help of professional chefs who have created a vast array of exciting and delicious recipes that are simple enough for almost anyone to prepare.

# What Is Cancer?

Cancer is a proliferation of cells that grow uncontrolled and may eventually metastasize and spread, invading other major organs in the body. This multistaged process called carcinogenesis begins with the "initiation" of cancer cells. Initiation is then followed by "promotion," during which initiated cells are stimulated to grow by causal factors. The entire process (initiation, promotion, and, finally, detection of cancer) takes from at least ten to thirty years.

Initiation of a cancer cell may occur through exposure to carcinogenic (cancer-causing) substances in our environment or may occur spontaneously. These substances have the potential to damage the cell's makeup and cause a genetic malfunction. If the process stops at this point, there is probably little danger of cancer developing. However, if these initiated cells are exposed to cancer "promoters," stimulation will occur leading to uncontrolled growth and ultimately cancer. It is important to remember that it usually takes continued exposure to both initiators and promoters over a relatively long time in order for cancer to occur. Some carcinogenic substances have the ability to act as both initiators and promoters.

Since cancers take time to develop, aging (midlife and older) is probably the strongest factor increasing a person's cancer risk. This is particularly important for the U.S. population, where the average life expectancy has risen consistently over time. As the population ages, we might expect to see an increase in the total number of cancers simply due to longevity.

Cancer causes a significant amount of disease and mortality. It is the second leading cause of death after cardiovascular disease in the United States. More than *2 million new cases of cancer will be diagnosed and approximately 560,000 people will die of cancer in 1997.* It is important to identify risk factors that can be modified to help prevent cancer.

## Carcinogenic Process

Exposure to carcinogens ➜ Initiation of tumor ➜ Tumor promotion ➜ Progression ➜ Precancerous cells ➜ Malignant tumor ➜ Metastasis

Here are some examples of carcinogens and promoters:

| **Carcinogens** | **Promoters** |
| --- | --- |
| air pollution | alcohol |

chemicals                              cigarette smoke
cigarette smoke                        dietary fat
radiation                              excess caloric intake
ultraviolet radiation (sunlight)       hormones
viruses                                pollutants (like asbestos)

# Why Study Diet?

Although scientists have been able to identify both genetic and environmental factors as causes of cancer, much is still to be learned. Genetic factors are those traits that are determined by your genes or heredity. Environmental factors are all the things we are exposed to on a daily basis including the air we breathe, the water we drink, the food we eat, and the lifestyles we choose. Many people believe that heredity plays a major role in causing most cancers. However, a major scientific report by the Office of Technology and Assessment of the U.S. Congress published in 1981 suggested that cancer is an avoidable disease and up to 80 percent of cancers can be attributed to environmental factors. These scientists estimated that 10 to 70 percent of all cancer was caused by diet. Since then these estimates have been refined and we now believe that *diet contributes to 20 to 40 percent of all cancer*. Because some forms of cancer can be attributed to both genes and environment, diet may be especially important in individuals who have a family member with cancer.

The role of diet in cancer prevention has been the focus of intense interest with hundreds of studies showing a link between diet and cancer. Initially diet was implicated as a cause of cancer based on observations that cancer rates varied among countries and people in these countries also had different diets. Studies of migrants showed that people who moved to another country actually acquired the cancer rates of their new host country. For instance, a more than fivefold variation exists in breast cancer rates around the world. It has been shown that women who migrate from countries with a low incidence of breast cancer, such as Japan, to countries with a high incidence of breast cancer, such as the United States, acquire the "higher" rates of their new country. These observations implicated diet and other environmental factors as possible causes of breast cancer and implied that genetic factors were of lesser importance. (If inherited factors were solely responsible for breast cancer we would not expect the rates to change so dramatically once women moved to a new country.) These studies also gave investigators hints as to the amount of time it takes for cancer to develop.

Studies on diet and cancer have been conducted in both animals and humans. Animal experiments are done in controlled situations where the investigator controls the animal's intake of the dietary factor of interest. Studies such as these often serve as the basis for studies in humans. Because animals are physiologically different from humans and because they are usually fed extremely high amounts of the dietary factor of interest, the relevance of these findings to people can be questionable. *Results of animal experiments do not necessarily apply to humans.*

Epidemiologic studies are conducted in large groups of people and seek to describe how much cancer exists as well as the causes or risk factors for specific cancers. *The goal of an epidemiologic study is to try to show a common factor in those people who have cancer and relate this to the biological understanding of how this factor might cause cancer.* The results of these studies can be directly applied to humans.

Epidemiologists calculate the risk of disease in those who are exposed to a certain factor as compared to those who are not exposed. These "risks" are often referred to as the "odds" of developing disease. They are a measure of the strength of the relationship between the factor and disease, and how important the factor is in causing or preventing disease. Examples of epidemiologic studies that had important public health impact on cancer prevention were those that showed a link between cigarette smoking and lung cancer. The risk or odds of lung cancer is about tenfold in smokers as compared to nonsmokers. This means smokers are ten times more likely to develop lung cancer compared to nonsmokers.

Whether or not the study results are "statistically significant" may also be reported. Statistical significance estimates how likely the results are due to chance, that is, a fluke finding. If the results are statistically significant, then chance is an unlikely explanation. Statistical significance is controversial and often can be misinterpreted. It is important to know that even if a study's findings are not statistically significant they still may be meaningful.

We often hear in the news that a certain factor "causes" cancer. In actuality, causation is difficult to prove in epidemiology and the results cannot be used to predict if a person will develop cancer. It is generally accepted that smoking causes lung cancer, but we all have heard of the person who smokes and lives to be a hundred years old! From a scientific standpoint it is difficult to say in every situation that if a person smokes he or she will get cancer. It is even more complicated when looking at nutritional factors because the relationship is not as strong or clear-cut. Thus, epidemiologists will refer to a factor as increasing or decreasing risk and usually avoid the term "cause."

Diet has been the focus of numerous research studies because it is believed that it accounts for a large amount of the cancer we see in our society. Studying the relationship between dietary intake and cancer is difficult because it is hard to measure diet: we all eat differently and our diets vary greatly on a day-to-day basis. The ability of a person to remember what he or she eats is limited and it is difficult to pinpoint what time period during a person's life is important in influencing cancer development. For instance, are we interested in the diet consumed as a child, adolescent, or adult? Even if the time period of interest is during the adult years, is it the food we ate yesterday or five years ago that is important? We can speculate that it is most likely the diet many years prior to the diagnosis of cancer or the food we ate over many years that is most significant. Various dietary factors may act during different time periods to increase or decrease cancer risk.

To further complicate studying the link between diet and cancer, it has been shown that the total calories consumed and the amount of energy expended in physical activity can affect the results. Other lifestyle factors may be related to nutrition and the development of cancer. As an example, smokers often have a poor diet and both of these factors, smoking and diet, are related to specific cancers. It is hard to know what caused the cancer: the smoking or the poor diet. Recent developments in statistical methods and computing techniques have made it possible to adjust for these potential "confounding factors."

When should a person make a lifestyle or behavior change based on research findings? We usually hear about the results of studies through the media: television, newspapers, magazines, or radio. When you see or hear these reports be sure to understand who is being interviewed. Is it the author of the study? Try to balance the information by taking into consideration comments about the study reported by scientists or experts other than the authors. The reason the media publicizes a study is because the findings are newsworthy and unusual. Avoid the news "headlines" and read or listen to the details, which will generally give a more fair description of the study results.

Most media reports are based on studies that have been published in major medical journals which have undergone peer review. This is a process whereby a scientist's research is scrutinized by other professionals in the relevant field of study and then a decision is made to publish or not based on the merits of the work. In most instances, these news reports should be interpreted cautiously because the results are preliminary. *No definitive conclusion should be made based on a single study; instead, the "totality" of the evidence is most important: What is the general consensus or conclusion based on the results from all the studies published about a particular topic?* Be careful of reports about anecdotal findings where one person or a few people report their personal experiences. You should wait until medical experts reach a consensus.

Obtaining medical information, particularly with respect to diet, can be confusing and contradictory. Look at the big picture. For instance, many cancers can be directly attributed to poor diet, smoking, and obesity, while pesticides, medical X rays, and food additives account for an extremely small amount of cancer. Some reliable sources of health information include the National Cancer Institute, American Cancer Society, Centers for Disease Control, and National Institutes of Health. These agencies serve the public interest. There are also health newsletters and books published by medical institutions that can be valuable resources for medical information. For a listing of medical, health, and nutrition information resources see the appendix.

# Overview of Diet and Cancer

Scientists have attempted to assess the connection between cancer and many different aspects of diet, including foods such as fruits and vegetables, nutrients in foods such as fat, and other substances such as phytochemicals. It has been estimated that diet is responsible for 20 to 40 percent of all cancers, maybe as high as 70 percent. Fruit and vegetable consumption has consistently been shown to have a beneficial effect on cancer. High red meat consumption has been shown to increase the risk of developing colon cancer, while saturated fat from animal sources has been linked to prostate cancer. High intake of salty foods and cured foods probably causes stomach cancer, although in the United States this does not account for much cancer because stomach cancer is rare. It is also thought that excess calories early in life increases the risk of breast cancer, although the evidence is not conclusive.

Lifestyle factors related to nutrition, such as alcohol consumption, obesity, and physical activity, are also linked to cancer. Physical activity appears to protect against colon cancer and may be helpful for decreasing risk of breast and prostate cancer. Obesity has been linked to many cancers including endometrial, breast, colon, and ovarian. Alcohol consumption has been strongly linked to cancers of the digestive tract (oral cavity and esophagus) and liver. Also, tobacco consumption is most notably linked with cancers of the lung and oral cavity.

The process of carcinogenesis takes at least ten to thirty years, beginning with initiation of cancer cells followed by promotion of these existing cells. Diet probably is important during the initiation phase whereby certain foods or nutrients may serve to increase detoxifying enzymes that help stop the initial stimulation and growth of the cancer cells. At the same time, certain nutrients and foods such as fat may serve as promoters for already initiated cancer cells.

## Fruits and Vegetables

*Fruits and vegetables protect against cancer!*
More than two hundred studies have shown that people who consume a diet high in fruits and vegetables reduce their risk for cancer, specifically, cancer of the esophagus, stomach, mouth, lung, bladder, colon, rectum, larynx, and cervix. The evidence is strong and there is a consensus in the scientific and medical community that fruits and vegetables protect against these cancers. Fruits and vegetables have also been shown to be beneficial for breast, pancreatic, endometrial, and kidney cancer and may have an effect on prostate and ovarian cancer, although the evidence is not as conclusive. *There is about a twofold increased risk of cancer for those people who have the lowest intake (bottom*

*twenty-fifth percentile) of fruits and vegetables as compared to those who have the highest intake (top twenty-fifth percentile).*

Fruits and vegetables contain nutrients and minerals, such as vitamins A, C, and E, folic acid, and fiber. They also contain phytochemicals, naturally occurring substances found in plants thought to protect against cancer, including allium compounds, indoles, plant polyphenols, and carotenoids as well as many others. It has been suggested that the vitamins, minerals, fiber, and phytochemicals found in fruits and vegetables have anticarcinogenic properties and help to ward off cancer (acting as antioxidants, detoxifiers, and blocking agents). Other anticancer functions include repairing damaged cells, inhibiting tumor formation, decreasing cell proliferation, and increasing immune activity.

Scientists are only beginning to explore the role of these phytochemicals. It is not possible at this time to measure the amount of most phytochemicals that people eat because we cannot isolate and quantify these substances in foods. Thus, it is difficult to study the link between a particular phytochemical and cancer. We must rely on results from studies assessing the relationship between fruit and vegetable consumption and cancer risk. Furthermore, there are many substances in fruits and vegetables and it is probably not one nutrient or chemical that protects against cancer, but a combination of these.

The beneficial effect of fruit and vegetable consumption on overall health is not limited to cancer. A favorable effect has been observed for other chronic diseases including heart disease, cataracts, diabetes, diverticulosis, and stroke. Fruits and vegetables are also naturally low in calories and may be important in maintaining ideal body weight and controlling obesity.

Studies have shown that Seventh-Day Adventists, who practice vegetarianism, overall have about half the cancer mortality of the general U.S. population. Vegetarians have a lower risk of lung and colon cancer, as well as a decreased risk of bladder and prostate cancer. These individuals usually have other associated healthy behaviors (generally they do not smoke or drink) that contribute to this reduced risk of cancer. Their diets usually consist of adequate fruits, vegetables, fiber, and calcium, and are generally low in total and saturated fat. Obesity is a risk factor for many cancers and vegetarians tend to have weights that are within recommended weight guidelines; this may also explain their decreased risk of cancer. Some studies suggest that vegetarian women may be at decreased risk of breast cancer, although this remains to be confirmed.

Despite the healthful properties of fruits and vegetables, some consumers worry that they may contain "chemicals," such as nitrates and pesticides. *Nitrates* are chemicals that are naturally occurring in fruits and vegetables as compared to *nitrites*, which are added to preserved meats and pickled vegetables to inhibit growth of microorganisms. Nitrates can be changed to nitrites with the help of bacteria present in the mouth or stomach. These nitrites can then undergo a process called nitrosation to form N-nitroso compounds. These N-nitroso compounds are carcinogenic in animals and presumably have adverse effects in humans.

**nitrates → nitrites → N-nitroso compounds (nitrosamines)**

It would seem reasonable to conclude that fruits and vegetables containing nitrates might promote cancer because of the potential for conversion to N-nitroso compounds. *However, the evidence does not support the assumption that nitrates found in fruits and vegetables are a cause of cancer. In fact, there is a strong, consistent, beneficial effect of fruits and vegetables on the risk of stomach, esophageal, and oral cancer.* This protective result is probably related to the presence of high levels of vitamins C and E that help reduce the formation of N-nitroso compounds.

Pesticide levels in fruits and vegetables have been the concern of many advocacy groups seeking to limit our environmental exposure. Most pesticides are naturally occurring, produced by plants themselves as a defense mechanism and present little danger to our food supply. Synthetic (man-made) pesticides used in coloring or preservation have not been shown to cause cancer. However, a conservative approach would include limiting our exposure to man-made pesticides. This can be done by thoroughly washing produce or buying organically grown products. It should be noted that there is no proven beneficial effect of these organic products on cancer risk.

There is overwhelming evidence to support a recommendation for increased consumption of fruits and vegetables. Americans do not meet the recommended two servings of fruit plus three servings of vegetables daily. In a 1995 survey, the average daily intake of fruits and vegetables was 3.3 servings for men and 3.7 servings for women. Only 20 percent of Americans consumed five or more servings of fruits and vegetables daily. From a public health standpoint implementing this change would make a huge impact on decreasing cancer.

## Protein

Foods high in animal protein include meat, poultry, eggs, and dairy. The effects of animal protein (especially that obtained from red meat) on risk of cancer have been studied extensively. Results from studies consistently show that people who eat a diet high in animal protein derived from red meat have an increased risk of colon and prostate cancer. There is some evidence to suggest that prostate, pancreatic, and endometrial cancer may also be associated with an increased consumption of animal protein and that kidney cancer may be higher in people who consume fried or sautéed meats.

A possible explanation for the link between protein and cancer is that diets high in animal protein are also high in saturated fat (which is associated with increased risk for some cancers) and/or that carcinogens (heterocyclic amines) may be created during the cooking process. However, other factors associated with a high meat-fat diet may also be implicated, such as low fiber and antioxidant intake and high intake of cholesterol. It is difficult to separate these effects when studying the association between meat consumption and cancer risk.

Protein from plant sources, particularly soy products, has been associated with decreased risk for some cancers. Also fish, an excellent source of protein, has omega-3 fatty acids shown to be important in cancer prevention.

## Fat

A diet high in fat has been associated with the development of many cancers as well as heart disease. Studies have shown that people who eat a high amount of fat, particularly saturated fat derived from animal products, have a greater likelihood of developing certain cancers, especially prostate and colon. The relationship between colon cancer and fat may be related to red meat intake. Endometrial, ovarian, and lung cancer are possibly linked to a high fat intake. Fat might induce certain cancers by affecting hormone levels and synthesis, increasing the body's exposure to bile acids or promoting tumor growth. The breakdown of fat may produce free radicals, which are highly unstable molecules with the potential to cause cell damage. Also, high fat intake may be a marker for low fiber, fruit and vegetable consumption that could be more important in influencing cancer risk than fat per se.

It has been suggested that increased total fat intake is a cause of breast cancer, but this remains controversial. Initially, both animal and human studies supported an adverse effect of fat intake on breast cancer. Since then studies generally have been less supportive, and overall it appears that diets high in animal fat during midlife are not associated with breast cancer risk. The studies did not measure diet during puberty or adolescence, which may be the critical time period (because of the growth and development of breast tissue). Furthermore, these studies did not look at women with very low intakes of fat (less than 15 percent of daily calories), which may provide some benefit. It remains to be seen if there is a beneficial effect of very-low-fat diets on breast cancer risk. But since a high intake of fat can increase the risk for other cancers as well as heart disease, it is prudent to limit our consumption.

A few epidemiologic studies suggest that olive oil, one type of fat, is beneficial in reducing breast cancer risk. This is a promising area of research and work is ongoing. Omega-3 fatty acids (sometimes called marine or fish oils) have also been of interest because of the observation that cancer rates are lower in populations where the diet is composed of a high proportion of these fatty acids, such as the Eskimos in Alaska and Greenland and the Japanese. Diets that contain a high proportion of these omega-3 fatty acids as compared to fatty acids from vegetable oils have been shown to slow or prevent the growth of tumors, particularly mammary and colon tumors in animals, possibly by inactivating hormones that promote certain cancers.

### Fiber

Fiber has been identified as a potential preventive for breast, colon, and pancreatic cancer. Some studies have also shown a beneficial effect for rectum, oral cavity, and stomach cancer. The role of fiber intake in the prevention of breast cancer is not conclusive, but it has been suggested that fiber can bind with and reduce circulating levels of estrogen. Cumulative exposure to estrogen has been strongly associated with an increased risk of breast cancer and fiber may be beneficial by reducing a woman's exposure to estrogen.

Fiber may protect against colon cancer by increasing fecal bulk and normalizing the bowel function. Hypothetically, this would mean that potential cancer-causing agents have less contact with the lining of the intestines. Fiber may also decrease or dilute the bile acids in the fecal matter that are thought to increase cell proliferation. Also, fiber may be a "marker" for fruit and vegetable consumption (because fruits and vegetables are high in fiber) and the evidence is much stronger for a protective effect of fruits and vegetables on cancer risk as compared to fiber.

## Vitamins and Minerals

Vitamins and minerals are nutrients that are present in food but can also be obtained from vitamin supplements (pill form). Since a beneficial effect of fruits and vegetables on cancer risk has been consistently observed in studies, it is reasonable to think that the *vitamins and minerals* contained in fruits and vegetables might protect against cancer. The role of particular vitamins and minerals in the prevention of cancer has been investigated in studies. Although vitamins and minerals do not definitively prevent cancer, anticancer properties have been observed for certain cancers.

### → VITAMINS, MINERALS, AND CANCER ←

**Antioxidants: Vitamins A, C, E, and Selenium**

*Carotenoids.* Overall, a high intake of carotenoids (those which are vitamin A precursors and include beta-carotene) has been linked to a decreased risk of many cancers, including endometrial, stomach, ovarian, breast, colon, pancreatic, prostate, bladder, cervical, lung, oral cavity, esophageal, and laryngeal.

*Beta-carotene (precursor vitamin A).* The relationship between beta-carotene and lung cancer is the most consistent relationship observed for vitamins and cancer. An increased intake of beta-carotene appears to decrease a person's risk for developing lung cancer; however, this has not been observed in large studies with beta-carotene *supplements*, which suggests that the active agent is probably not beta-carotene but likely something else contained in beta-carotene–rich foods.

*Vitamin A (preformed retinol).* Vitamin A has been shown to be beneficial for breast cancer, although not definitively.

*Vitamin C.* Vitamin C appears to protect against esophageal, oral, stomach, laryngeal, cervical, and pancreatic cancer in people who have a high intake of this antioxidant vitamin. There have been studies that suggest lung, breast, and colorectal cancer may also be reduced, although the results are not as strong or consistent.

*Vitamin E.* Some forms of oral cancer and possibly lung cancer may be decreased if a diet high in vitamin E–rich foods is consumed. In some studies there has been a suggestion of a beneficial effect on stomach, cervical, laryngeal, kidney, and skin cancer. With respect to breast cancer, there are conflicting results, although some studies suggest a beneficial effect of vitamin E.

*Selenium.* The studies assessing the relationship between selenium intake and cancer have been conflicting, although some have suggested a beneficial effect on stomach, esophagus, breast, prostate, colon, rectal, and lung cancer.

**Other Vitamins and Minerals**

*Calcium and vitamin D.* A link between increased intake of calcium and vitamin D and reduced risk of colon cancer has been proposed, although the evidence is not convincing at this time.

*Folic acid (folate).* Folic acid is beneficial in reducing the risk of both cervical and colon cancer and maybe lung.

*Magnesium.* It has been suggested that magnesium deficiency may impair immunity or promote the cancer process. Further research is necessary, but initial studies have suggested a link between low intake of magnesium and kidney cancer.

*Iron.* Recently there has been speculation that too much iron may be linked to cancer, especially in people who have iron absorption defects (called iron overload or hemochromatosis). Individuals with this condition may absorb up to two times more iron from food and supplements than those without this defect and store it in major organs like the liver, pancreas, heart, and brain. However, based on animal experiment studies and human studies there is inconclusive evidence to support a link between iron and cancer.

## Antioxidants, Free Radicals, and Cancer

Antioxidants act as scavengers of "free radicals," by-products of normal metabolism, before they can cause harm to the body. Free radicals are missing an electron (a negatively charged particle) from their chemical structure and are thus highly unstable. Because of their unstable nature, they can undergo a process called oxidation, the process whereby free radicals take electrons and transfer them, leaving a new free radical. This is damaging to the body's cells and will continue as a chain reaction unless an enzyme or free radical scavenger (antioxidant) stops the process.

If left unchecked, free radicals can cause oxidative damage: genetic damage, uncontrolled cell growth and cancer, heart disease and other degenerative diseases, and aging. Exposures to certain environmental factors, including radiation, ultraviolet light, alcohol, cigarette and marijuana smoke, air pollutants, smog, pesticides, herbicides, drugs, fried foods, inflammation, and very strenuous physical activity (such as marathon run-

---

✦ **PROPOSED ANTICANCER FUNCTIONS OF**

**Carotenoids (Including Beta-Carotene)**
*Proposed anticancer functions:* antioxidants; metabolized to vitamin A, which helps cell differentiation (cancer cells are characterized by lack of differentiation); may inhibit cell proliferation
*Other functions:* improves immune response; lowers cholesterol levels; may reduce heart disease, stroke, anti-inflammatory disorders, and cataracts

**Vitamin A (Preformed Retinol)**
*Proposed anticancer functions:* plays a role in regulating cell differentiation; may prevent malignant transformation of cells; may enhance immune function

**Vitamin C**
*Proposed anticancer functions:* antioxidant; inhibits the formation of N-nitroso compounds (carcinogens implicated in stomach cancer); enhances immune system; plays a role in the synthesis of connective tissue proteins; may be important in inhibiting tumor growth and promoting cell differentiation
*Other functions:* protects against atherosclerosis by interfering with oxidation of LDL cholesterol; may protect against cataracts

**Vitamin E**
*Proposed anticancer functions:* antioxidant; inhibits formation of N-nitroso compounds (carcinogens implicated in stomach cancer); modulates immune function to work against tumors; protects cells from malignant transformation
*Other functions:* may protect against heart disease (atherosclerosis) and cataracts

ning), can promote the production of these free radicals. However, normal metabolism is responsible for most free radical production.

• The body has built-in defense mechanisms against this oxidation process, including enzymes and antioxidants that search for these unstable free radicals. It is thought that foods rich in vitamins A, C, and E, carotenoids, and phytochemicals work together as antioxidant free radical scavengers.

Although many studies suggest that vitamins protect against certain forms of cancer, the evidence is not compelling enough to "prove" vitamins protect against cancer. Nevertheless, we do know that diets high in vitamin- and mineral-rich fruits and vegetables definitely protect against many forms of cancer. Even if the studies on vitamins and minerals do not provide conclusive evidence of a beneficial effect, it is prudent for all people to follow the recommendations of eating five to nine servings of fruits and vegetables each day.

---

## SELECTED VITAMINS AND MINERALS ✦

### Selenium
*Proposed anticancer functions:* enhances antioxidant activity of vitamin E; increases immune response; produces enzymes that protect against oxidative damage; suppresses cell proliferation; may alter metabolism of carcinogens so they produce less toxic substances

### Calcium
*Proposed anticancer functions:* regulates cell function (reduces proliferation and enhances differentiation of cells); may bind with bile acids and fatty acids to decrease the exposure of the colon to carcinogens and reduce risk of colon cancer; may increase immune response
*Other functions:* reduces risk of osteoporosis

### Vitamin D
*Proposed anticancer functions:* may retard formation or progression of tumors
*Other functions:* reduces risk of osteoporosis

### Folic acid (Folate)
*Proposed anticancer functions:* essential for DNA synthesis (low levels may cause errors in DNA synthesis and genetic defects); may enhance immunity
*Other functions:* protects against heart disease and birth defects

### Magnesium
*Proposed anticancer functions:* enhances immunity; competes with cancer-causing agents; a deficiency may trigger and/or promote the cancer process

## Vitamin and Mineral Supplements

Studies that have specifically looked at vitamin and mineral supplements (as opposed to vitamins from food sources) have shown a decreased risk of some cancers: individuals who take vitamin E supplements are at a reduced risk of oral, prostate, and colon cancer and are protected against heart disease; vitamin A supplementation has been shown to protect against colon and breast cancer; and vitamin C supplementation decreases the risk of breast, colon, and bladder cancer. Selenium supplementation reduces the risk of lung, prostate, and colorectal cancer. However, research conducted to date does not support a *strong* effect of vitamin and mineral *supplements* per se on cancer risk. Before vitamin supplementation is recommended for preventing cancer, its role in cancer prevention needs more research; however, there may be a positive effect of vitamin supplementation for people from countries that have high rates of stomach and esophageal cancer. Studies of vitamin supplementation (vitamin A, zinc, riboflavin, beta-carotene, vitamin E, and selenium) have been conducted in China, where the rate of both esophageal and stomach cancer is high. The results show that vitamin A, zinc, and riboflavin taken together reduces the risk of esophageal cancer, whereas beta-carotene, vitamin E, and selenium may be beneficial for stomach cancer.

The idea of taking a vitamin supplement to compensate for deficiencies in their diet appeals to many people. Although the chemical structure of a particular vitamin supplement is the same as that of the vitamin found in food sources, absorption and utilization by the body may be different. It is known that diets rich in foods containing certain vitamins and minerals help to prevent cancer; however, these foods may contain other substances, such as phytochemicals, that work in conjunction with vitamins and minerals to confer benefit.

# Other Dietary Factors

There has been much speculation about the role of alcohol, caffeine, salt, and "charcoal grilling" in causing cancer. What part do they play in our diet, and how do they increase or decrease our risk of cancer?

## Alcohol

Studies have consistently shown that alcohol is the cause of many cancers, including breast, esophageal, oral cavity, laryngeal, and liver. There have also been studies linking alcohol consumption to colon, rectal, and pancreatic cancer. It appears that the risk of cancer is dependent on the amount of alcohol consumed; that is, as alcohol intake rises so does risk of cancer. With respect to breast cancer, as little as one drink per day increases the risk 20 to 30 percent. Women who are heavy drinkers increase their risk to 60 to 70 percent.

It is speculated that alcohol acts as a tumor promoter. The ethanol contained in alcoholic beverages appears to be the promoting agent and may alter the liver's ability to metabolize carcinogens. Alcohol consumption is also associated with inadequate nourishment in moderate and heavy drinkers, which may indicate a deficient supply of the antioxidant vitamins C, E, and beta-carotene. Stores of folic acid and vitamins A, C, and E (which have cancer-fighting properties), may be depleted by alcohol consumption. Also, alcohol may interact with dietary fats to enhance the cancer-promoting effects.

It has been shown that alcohol interacts with smoking to increase cancers of the oral cavity, larynx, and esophagus. In one large study of oral cavity cancer, a 36-fold increased risk was observed in people who were both heavy drinkers and smokers.

Alcohol is responsible for an estimated 3 percent of cancer deaths. Reduction or elimination of alcohol clearly reduces the risk of developing many cancers. Moderate drinking is defined as about two drinks a day for men and one drink a day for women. A beneficial effect of moderate alcohol consumption on coronary heart disease has been observed, but this needs to be balanced with the associated increased risk of cancer.

## Caffeine

Is caffeine really bad for you? Caffeine is a natural ingredient contained in coffee, tea, soft drinks, cocoa, and some medications. Considered a drug with biochemical and physiological effects, it can cause heart palpitations and raise blood pressure and cholesterol levels (usually at high levels of consumption) in some people. In the past caffeine (in coffee) has been implicated as a cause of cancer, heart attacks, infertility, miscarriages, osteoporosis, and glaucoma. Because of its widespread consumption, the relationship between caffeine and disease has been studied extensively.

There is little evidence that caffeine or coffee in moderation causes heart attacks. The relationship between coffee consumption (with or without caffeine) and breast, ovarian, bladder, pancreatic, rectal, and colon cancer has been investigated. *The World Health Organization and the American Cancer Society both support the evidence that indicates no association between caffeine (or coffee) and cancer.* (Coffee does not cause these cancers!) Two cups of coffee a day is generally acceptable and presents little health hazard for most people, although four to five cups a day may be a problem.

Furthermore, the totality of research studies do not show that caffeine is a risk factor for decreased fertility, birth defects, or glaucoma. Some studies have shown that caffeine intake may be a risk factor for osteoporosis, because it promotes excretion of calcium from the body, although the studies are conflicting. It appears that adequate calcium intake may balance any negative effect of caffeine consumption on osteoporosis.

## Salt

It has been suggested that food additives contribute to cancer. In fact, no food additive other than salt has been shown conclusively to cause cancer. Salted, smoked, and cured foods can increase the risk of developing some forms of cancer. A high intake of salted foods, including smoked and cured products, can account for much of the stomach cancer observed throughout the world, especially in Asian countries. In the United States, stomach cancer is rare, probably because these foods are not a mainstay of our diet. Salted foods often contain nitrites that can undergo nitrosation during the cooking process and produce N-nitroso compounds. These compounds are potent toxins and animal carcinogens. Also, salted Chinese-style fish, which is rarely consumed by Americans, has been linked to nasopharyngeal cancer in children. It is estimated that salt contributes to 1 percent of total cancer mortality.

## Cooking Process

The ordinary process of cooking can promote the formation of chemical compounds such as heterocyclic amines (from heating amino acids or proteins), polycyclic hydrocarbons (from charring meat), and nitrosamines (from gas cooking or barbecuing). The formation of these compounds is dependent on the type of food, cooking method (frying, broiling, or barbecuing), time, and temperature (above 100 degrees centigrade or 212 degrees Fahrenheit). Studies thus far have not measured directly the intake of these chemical compounds and are not conclusive, but it is reasonable to limit our intake because it is known that these compounds are cancer-causing. However, levels of intake shown to be carcinogenic in animals are many times higher than those consumed by people: the effects of moderate intakes are unclear; research is ongoing.

In this chapter, we have outlined what you need to know to understand how diet plays a crucial role in preventing cancer. With this information, you can begin to make those changes that will ultimately lead to reducing your cancer risk. Now that you have the knowledge, you need to acquire the right tools to be successful. The next chapter tells you how to do just that!

# CHAPTER 2

# Lowering Your Risk of Cancer through Diet

It is important to view your eating habits as a lifetime commitment to good health, rather than a temporary inconvenience to endure until a short-term goal is reached. The word *diet* has too many negative, unpleasant connotations, and is usually associated with bland meals, deprivation, hunger, and guilt. You don't have to starve to eat right, nor do you need to deprive yourself of many of your favorite foods. An occasional splurge will not ruin you as long as the exception does not become the rule. Extremes, either very high or very low in certain nutrients such as calories, fat, protein, or carbohydrates, are not the answer for a lifetime of good health, appropriate weight, and overall well-being. The key is moderation! After wading through all the gimmicks and "quick fixes," we will demonstrate that the real "secret" to healthy eating is to plan long-term goals based on variety, balance, and moderation—goals that you can both meet and maintain. It is essential to develop a nutrition plan that is right for you and your lifestyle.

## Strang Cancer Prevention Center Guidelines for Reducing Your Risk of Cancer

These suggestions are adapted from the American Cancer Society Dietary Guidelines:

**1.** *Choose most foods from plant sources.* Eat five or more servings of fruits and vegetables each day. This will ensure that your diet is rich in vitamins A and C, as well as minerals and phytochemicals that may reduce the risk of cancer. Eat several servings from other plant sources, such as minimally processed whole grains, breads, cereals, and legumes (beans, peas, and lentils). *If you follow these suggestions, your fiber intake will likely be within the recommended range of 25 to 35 grams per day.*

**2.** *Limit intake of high-fat foods, particularly from animal sources.* Limit meats, especially high-fat meats, such as some cuts of beef and pork. Eat moderate portions of other lean animal protein sources, such as chicken, fish, and low-fat dairy products.

**3.** *Reduce intake of potentially carcinogenic (cancer-causing) substances.* Limit or eliminate the following from your diet:

- smoked foods, which absorb some of the tars that arise from the smoking process and contain numerous carcinogens
- nitrite-preserved foods, such as hot dogs, ham, and other processed meats. Nitrites can combine with proteins in your stomach to form cancer-promoting chemicals. Vitamin C–rich foods may help prevent this from occurring, so if you occasionally eat foods preserved with nitrites, be sure to consume a fruit or vegetable rich in vitamin C.
- grilled foods (avoid charring)
- salt-cured foods, such as bacon and many types of ham
- alcoholic beverages. Regular alcohol consumption may promote certain cancers; heavy drinking is strongly linked to liver cancer. If you drink, it should be infrequently and in moderation.

**4.** *Be physically active; achieve and maintain a healthy weight.* Be moderately active for thirty minutes or more on most days.

**5.** *Eat a variety of foods each day.* Variety assures the intake of a spectrum of protective nutrients and phytochemicals.

**6.** *Moderate sugar intake.* Although there is no evidence to support a link between sugar intake and cancer, limiting intake of sugar and other "empty calories" (calories without nutrients) leaves more room for foods rich in fiber, vitamins, minerals, and phytochemicals. High consumption of sugar-laden foods often results in excessive intake of calories and fat, making it difficult to maintain a healthy weight.

The first place to start making changes is with macronutrients, or energy (calorie)-yielding nutrients. Macronutrients include fat, carbohydrates, protein, and alcohol. The balance among them is an important factor in maintaining an appropriate weight and in preventing disease.

## General Caloric Requirements

The table below gives the U.S. Department of Agriculture method of estimating your daily caloric needs: multiply your body weight (in pounds) by your corresponding level of activity.

|  | Sedentary | Moderately Active | Active |
|---|---|---|---|
| Males | 16 | 20 | 30 |
| Females | 15 | 18 | 25 |

For example, if you are a 125-pound female who gets infrequent exercise (sedentary), you require approximately 1,875 calories daily (125 pounds × 15), which allows for a maximum fat intake of about 40 grams (based on a target of 20 percent of calories from fat; see the table of fat gram allowances on page 23).

It should be noted that the actual number of calories needed to maintain a stable weight might vary among individuals by as much as 30 percent due to factors that influence metabolic rate, such as frame size, muscle mass, fitness level, decreased requirements with age, and genetic variations. If you weigh more than 30 percent of your "ideal" body weight (see page 20), use your ideal body weight as the basis for the caloric formula above.

Keeping tabs on your fat intake, until it becomes second nature to you, is an easier way to make healthy changes in your diet than making more complex calculations of caloric and nutrient contents. Initially, however, it is a good idea to get an approximation of your caloric intake (over the course of a few days) until you are confident that the fat allowance is indeed no more than 20 to 25 percent of your total calories. You can do this fairly simply by using recipes from this book, which give caloric values, checking labels, or consulting any handy counter guide or nutrition software program. Consultation with a registered dietitian will provide the most accurate estimate of your calorie requirements.

Here is a quick rule-of-thumb estimate to give you a good idea whether your weight is "ideal" or within a healthful range. You can also refer to the graph on page 20. (The weight status and caloric and fat requirements for children and pregnant or lactating women follow different guidelines.)

Women:   Allow 100 pounds for the first 5 feet of height
         Add 5 pounds for each additional inch of height
Men:     Allow 106 pounds for the first 5 feet of height
         Add 6 pounds for each additional inch of height
Example: If you are a 5'8" male your ideal weight = 106 + 48 (6 × 8) = 154 pounds.

Individual variations by up to 10% (more or less) than this derived value still may fall between a normal weight range due to differences in body frame size and muscle mass.

If your actual weight exceeds this estimate by 20 to 30 percent, consult a nutrition professional to help you begin an effective weight-loss program. Once again, since fat is the most concentrated source of calories in your diet, you will discover that limiting your fat intake can help considerably in your efforts to maintain a healthy weight.

---

**Are You Overweight?**

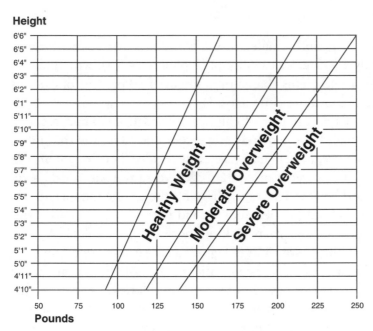

To use this graph, find your height in feet and inches (without shoes) along the left side of the graph. Trace the line corresponding to your height across the figure until it intersects with the vertical line corresponding to your weight in pounds (without clothes). The point of intersection lies within a band that indicates whether your weight is healthy or is moderately or severely overweight. The higher weights apply mainly to men, who have more muscle and bone.

Source: USDA Center for Nutrition Policy and Promotion

# BMI

Body Mass Index (BMI) is a method of determining fat or mass. BMI is calculated by dividing weight in kilograms by height in meters squared. It derives a single value that can be compared to standards established by scientists. Health researchers and practitioners are increasingly leaning towards BMI as a more reliable indicator of "ideal" body weight as compared with height/weight tables. Keep in mind, BMI, like other methods, can be influenced by muscle mass (a person with a high muscle density will yield higher BMI, although their body fat may be quite low).

How do you determine your BMI?

1. Convert your weight to kilograms: multiply your weight in pounds by 0.45.
2. Determine your height in centimeters: multiply inches by 2.5. This will provide your height in centimeters.
3. Divide your height in centimeters by 100 to determine your height in meters.
4. Multiply this number by itself for meters squared.
5. Divide your weight in kilograms by height squared. This is your BMI.
6. Compare this value to the standards below.

Standards for BMI:

|  | Females | Males |
|---|---|---|
| Underweight | <19 | <20 |
| Desirable BMI | 19–24 | 20–25 |
| Overweight | 25–30 | 26–30 |
| Obese | >30 | >30 |

Example: 160 pounds, 5'10" (70 inches), male:

1. 160 pounds x 0.45=72 kilograms.
2. 70 inches x 2.5= 175 centimeters.
3. 175 centimeters ÷ 100 = 1.75 meters.
4. 1.75 meters x 1.75 meters = 3.06 meters squared.
5. 72 kilograms ÷ 3.06 meters squared = 23.5 (BMI).
6. Desirable BMI.

You can also forgo the math and refer to chart below. Find your height and weight and then plot your BMI. Compare your BMI to the standards above.

| BMI | 19 | 20 | 21 | 22 | 23 | 24 | 25 | 26 | 27 | 28 | 29 | 30 | 35 | 40 |
|---|---|---|---|---|---|---|---|---|---|---|---|---|---|---|
| 4'10" | 91 | 96 | 100 | 105 | 110 | 115 | 119 | 124 | 129 | 134 | 138 | 143 | 167 | 191 |
| 4'11" | 94 | 99 | 104 | 109 | 114 | 119 | 124 | 128 | 133 | 138 | 143 | 148 | 173 | 198 |
| 5' | 97 | 102 | 107 | 112 | 118 | 123 | 128 | 133 | 138 | 143 | 148 | 153 | 179 | 204 |
| 5'1" | 100 | 106 | 111 | 116 | 122 | 127 | 132 | 137 | 143 | 148 | 153 | 158 | 185 | 211 |
| 5'2" | 104 | 109 | 115 | 120 | 126 | 131 | 136 | 142 | 147 | 153 | 158 | 164 | 191 | 218 |
| 5'3" | 107 | 113 | 118 | 124 | 130 | 135 | 141 | 146 | 152 | 158 | 163 | 169 | 197 | 225 |
| 5'4" | 110 | 116 | 122 | 128 | 134 | 140 | 145 | 151 | 157 | 163 | 169 | 174 | 204 | 232 |
| 5'5" | 114 | 120 | 126 | 132 | 138 | 144 | 150 | 156 | 162 | 168 | 174 | 180 | 210 | 240 |
| 5'6" | 118 | 124 | 130 | 136 | 142 | 148 | 155 | 161 | 167 | 173 | 179 | 186 | 216 | 247 |
| 5'7" | 121 | 127 | 134 | 140 | 146 | 153 | 159 | 166 | 172 | 178 | 185 | 191 | 223 | 255 |
| 5'8" | 125 | 131 | 138 | 144 | 151 | 158 | 164 | 171 | 177 | 184 | 190 | 197 | 230 | 262 |
| 5'9" | 128 | 135 | 142 | 149 | 155 | 162 | 169 | 176 | 182 | 189 | 196 | 203 | 236 | 270 |

Height (in feet and inches)

| Height (in feet and inches) | | | | | | | | | | | | | | |
|---|---|---|---|---|---|---|---|---|---|---|---|---|---|---|
| 5'10" | 132 | 139 | 146 | 153 | 160 | 167 | 174 | 181 | 188 | 195 | 202 | 207 | 243 | 278 |
| 5'11" | 136 | 143 | 150 | 157 | 165 | 172 | 179 | 186 | 193 | 200 | 208 | 215 | 250 | 286 |
| 6' | 140 | 147 | 154 | 162 | 169 | 177 | 184 | 191 | 199 | 206 | 213 | 221 | 258 | 294 |
| 6'1" | 144 | 151 | 159 | 166 | 174 | 182 | 189 | 197 | 204 | 212 | 219 | 227 | 265 | 302 |
| 6'2" | 148 | 155 | 163 | 171 | 179 | 186 | 194 | 202 | 210 | 218 | 225 | 233 | 272 | 311 |
| 6'3" | 152 | 160 | 168 | 176 | 184 | 192 | 200 | 208 | 216 | 224 | 232 | 240 | 279 | 319 |
| 6'4" | 156 | 164 | 172 | 180 | 189 | 197 | 205 | 213 | 221 | 230 | 238 | 246 | 287 | 328 |

Weight (in pounds)

# The Fat Facts

Whether or not they want to admit it, Americans are having a love affair with fat. An oily substance that is one of the principal components of living cells, fat is essential in the diet; however, too much fat puts people at risk for significant health complications. Many elements of American cuisine include fat: T-bone steaks, dairy products, salad dressings, condiments (sour cream, cream cheese, butter), and processed foods (commercial chips, cookies, and crackers). Other cultures offer diets richer in fruits, vegetables, and whole grains. Because Americans consume more fat, their incidence of heart disease and cancer is significantly higher than that of people who eat a traditionally low-fat diet.

To lower your risk of both heart disease and cancer, it is recommended that you limit your fat intake to 20 to 25 percent of your total calories (in some instances underlying medical conditions warrant lower or higher fat intakes). Because individuals require different amounts of calories, fat intake is expressed as a percentage of caloric intake. The guideline of 20 to 25 percent should not be used for individual foods, but for your whole day or even week. If your average fat intake in a meal is 40 percent of calories, you can offset it by limiting two or more subsequent meals to 15 to 20 percent. In addition, you may have a day where your fat intake is at 40 percent of calories; you can come out even if you balance total fat intake for the next two days at 15 to 20 percent of calories. This amount allows for moderate portions of animal protein and limited amounts of added fat in cooking and seasoning of food and even an occasional rich dessert.

The best way to stay close to this guideline is to assess your daily target for maximum amount of fat in grams. Once you know the number of grams of fat you can consume each day, reading labels and making decisions becomes much easier. To assess your daily fat intake:

**1.** Determine your daily calorie requirements (see page 19).
**2.** Multiply your total calories by 0.20 (20 percent of total calories).
**3.** Since each gram of fat has 9 calories, divide the number you get in step 2 by 9.

Example: If you require 1,800 calories a day: 0.20 × 1,800 = 360 (fat calories).

360 ÷ 9 calories/gram = 40 grams of fat per day. If you don't want to do the math, refer to the table below after assessing your caloric requirements.

| | | Fat Gram Allowances | | |
|---|---|---|---|---|
| Daily Calorie Intake | Max. Fat Grams at 20% Calories Fat | Max. Daily Calories from Fat (at 20%) | Max. Fat Grams at 25% Calories Fat | Max. Daily Calories from Fat (at 25%) |
| 1100 | 24 | 220 | 31 | 275 |
| 1200 | 27 | 240 | 33 | 300 |
| 1300 | 29 | 260 | 36 | 325 |
| 1400 | 31 | 280 | 39 | 350 |
| 1500 | 33 | 300 | 42 | 375 |
| 1600 | 36 | 320 | 44 | 400 |
| 1700 | 38 | 340 | 47 | 425 |
| 1800 | 40 | 360 | 50 | 450 |
| 1900 | 42 | 380 | 53 | 475 |
| 2000 | 44 | 400 | 56 | 500 |
| 2100 | 47 | 420 | 58 | 525 |
| 2200 | 49 | 440 | 61 | 550 |
| 2300 | 51 | 460 | 64 | 575 |
| 2400 | 53 | 480 | 67 | 600 |
| 2500 | 56 | 500 | 69 | 625 |
| 2600 | 58 | 520 | 72 | 650 |
| 2700 | 60 | 540 | 75 | 675 |
| 2800 | 62 | 560 | 78 | 700 |

To figure out the percentage of calories from fat in a meal, recipe, or food product:

**1.** Determine the number of grams of fat.

**2.** Multiply the grams of fat by 9 (every gram of fat has 9 calories)—this will provide the total calories from fat.

**3.** Divide this number by the total number of calories from the meal or food.

**4.** Multiply by 100 and you will have the percentage of calories from fat.

Example: If a recipe contains 300 calories and 10 grams of fat: 10 grams fat × 9 calories per gram = 90 calories from fat. 90 fat calories ÷ 300 total calories = 0.30 × 100 = 30 percent calories from fat.

Beware: fat grams add up quickly. A tablespoon of olive oil in a homemade salad dressing will cost you 15 grams; a small serving (4 ounces) of meat, fish, or poultry can be 10 to 15 grams; each teaspoon of butter, regular margarine, and other oils is another 5 grams. That's why it's important to moderate your intake of lean protein sources and added fats.

The "Nutrition Facts" labels of commercial food products contain information on the fat content of particular foods in the "Total Fat" section that you can use to choose products that fit into your total fat allotment for the day. Be sure to adjust for the portion size you actually consume. See "Lowering Fat in Your Diet" on page 29 for more information on keeping your fat intake on target without lots of gram counting.

Not all fat is created equal. Dietary fat is composed of two major types of fatty acids: saturated and unsaturated. Unsaturated fatty acids are further classified as either polyunsaturated or monounsaturated. Foods that contain fat usually have a combination of all three fatty acids, although they are generally classified by the predominant fatty acid.

## Saturated Fats

Saturated fats are "saturated," or loaded, with the hydrogen atoms they carry. You should make the greatest effort to avoid these fats. A diet high in saturated fat can lead to high blood cholesterol levels, and may be associated with increased risk of certain types of cancer. Saturated fats are usually solid at room temperature, and are the visible fats that you can see in foods such as bacon. Although saturated fat comes in the highest ratios in foods of animal origin (beef, lamb, pork, veal, poultry, and full-fat dairy products), some vegetable-based products, such as coconut and palm oils (used in commercial baked goods) and solid vegetable shortenings, contain saturated fat. Coconut and palm oils, in fact, derive approximately 86 percent of their calories from saturated fat. The vegetable oils in many commercial food products also undergo a solidifying process called hydrogenation, that further increases their levels of saturation. Hydrogenation is the process used to make vegetable shortenings and margarine.

## Cholesterol

Cholesterol is a waxy fatlike substance. Your body needs some cholesterol to help form cell walls, hormones, and vitamins. But too much cholesterol in your bloodstream can cause fatty deposits to build up on artery walls. This can lead to heart attacks and strokes.

Blood cholesterol comes from two sources. Your liver makes all the cholesterol your body needs. Blood cholesterol levels are also related to the foods that you eat, particularly foods high in saturated fat. Surprisingly, the cholesterol found in food has less influence on blood cholesterol levels than does saturated fat. This type of cholesterol is called dietary cholesterol and it is found *only* in foods of animal origin, such as butter, dairy products, and meats. So it's not such a big deal when a food label says *cholesterol free* for a product such as peanut butter or vegetable oil, because these foods have *always* been cholesterol free. Don't be confused: *cholesterol free* does not mean *fat free!* Some plant foods that are high in saturated fat, such as coconut and palm oils, do not contain cholesterol.

Even though the relationship between dietary cholesterol and cancer is not strong, you should limit your intake of foods that contain substantial amounts of cholesterol because they generally contain high levels of saturated fat, which has been associated with cancer.

## Unsaturated Fats

Olive oil is a type of unsaturated fat called monounsaturated. Olive oil is the predominant dietary fat source in Mediterranean countries like Greece, Italy, and Spain. The rate of breast cancer in these countries is lower than that of the United States (even though the overall total fat intake is about the same). A few epidemiologic studies suggest that olive oil is beneficial in reducing breast cancer risk, but research in this area is continuing. It has been shown that monounsaturated fat (in place of saturated fat) has a positive effect on blood lipid (fat) levels. Monounsaturated fat reduces "bad" low-density lipoprotein (LDL) cholesterol and elevates the levels of "good" high-density lipoprotein (HDL) cholesterol, reducing the risk of heart disease.

Another type of unsaturated fat, polyunsaturated, is made up of *omega-6's*, found in vegetables, and *omega-3's*, which are most often present in fatty fish. Some plants have the potential to provide omega-3 fatty acids. The body can convert linolenic acid, a type of fat found in canola oil, flaxseeds, soybeans, walnuts, and some leafy green vegetables, into omega-3 fatty acids (see page 28). Moderate dietary intake of omega-3 fatty acids, found in substantial amounts in salmon, bluefish, swordfish, trout, tuna, and striped bass, may have a protective effect against heart disease and certain types of cancer.

Interest in the omega-3 fatty acids has been based on the observation that cancer rates are lower in populations where the diet is composed of a high proportion of these fatty acids. When compared to diets that contain omega-6 fatty acids from vegetable oils like corn and safflower, diets that contain a high proportion of omega-3 fatty acids have been shown to slow or prevent the growth of tumors, particularly mammary and colon tumors in animals, possibly by inactivating hormones that promote certain cancers. Other beneficial effects of omega-3 fatty acids include reduction of cholesterol and triglyceride levels and lowering of blood pressure. They may also improve symptoms of inflammatory diseases like rheumatoid arthritis and ulcerative colitis, as well as immune function.

The omega-6's and their effect on cancer risk has also been a focus of interest. It appears that certain polyunsaturated fats may actually *increase* the risk for some cancers; however, this has been shown mainly in animal studies with little support from human data.

The relationship between omega-3 fatty acids and omega-6 fatty acids is competitive and interrelated. When dietary intake of one is out of proportion, the other can control important biochemical reactions in the body. Researchers believe that a 1:1 ratio of omega-3 to omega-6 may be important in the prevention of heart disease. The American diet contains about ten omega-6's to one omega-3. This disproportion may lead to the overproduction of hormones, which in turn can cause formation of blood clots, promote the buildup of plaque on artery walls, and disturb immune function. A healthy immune system is vital to warding off certain types of cancer. Here are some ways to increase your omega-3 intake.

- Include an omega-3–rich fish source in your diet two to three times per week.
- Sprinkle whole flaxseed on rolls, muffins, or breads before baking or add it to waffles, pancakes, muffins, or quick breads. For more information about flaxseed and its uses, contact the Flax Council of Canada (800) 817-9894, or visit their web site at http://www.flaxcouncil.ca.
- Substitute ground flax flour for up to 10 percent of the flour in baked goods. Because of its high fat content (omega-3's), cut the fat in the recipe by up to one-third by replacing the moisture with water, juice, or fruit puree.
- Use all oils sparingly, and use olive, canola, flaxseed, soybean, and walnut oils more frequently than other vegetable oils.
- Limit omega-6–rich foods, such as salad dressings, margarine, and mayonnaise.
- Avoid fish oil capsules unless prescribed by your physician. The most concentrated source of omega-3's, these supplements can cause overdose, which may lead to excessive bleeding, increased risk of hemorrhagic stroke, adverse drug interactions, and, in some instances, high cholesterol.

---

**→ PROPOSED ANTICANCER FUNCTIONS OF OMEGA-3 FATTY ACIDS ←**

*Proposed anticancer functions:* slows or prevents cancerous tumor growth; stimulates the immune system; inhibits cancer-promoting hormones

*Other functions:* lowers blood pressure; reduces serum triglycerides and low-density lipoprotein cholesterol; increases clotting times; alleviates symptoms of psoriasis, rheumatoid arthritis, and ulcerative colitis

---

## Olestra

In January 1996, the Food and Drug Administration (FDA) approved a new type of fat called Olestra for use as an ingredient in potato chips and other savory snacks. Though Olestra is made from real fatty acids, giving it similar taste, "mouth feel," and frying capacity, its chemical structure is such that it cannot be absorbed in the intestinal tract. Because it is not absorbed, it contributes no calories or fat grams to one's daily diet.

Sounds good, right? The problem is that as Olestra travels through the gut unabsorbed, it carries with it the fat-soluble vitamins A, D, E, and K. It has also been shown to lower levels of circulating carotenoids, those colorful compounds in fruits and vegetables that may help prevent cancer. Procter & Gamble, the maker of this product, fortifies Olestra-containing foods with vitamins A, D, E, and K, but beta-carotene and other carotenoids are not, and cannot be, completely replaced. There is no doubt that diets high in fruits and vegetables help prevent cancer and heart disease, and it is likely that carotenoids contained in these foods play a significant role. There are other drawbacks of Olestra-containing foods: at varying levels of intake consumers have reported mild to severe gastrointestinal discomfort, such as cramping, flatulence, and diarrhea. Procter & Gamble is now seeking approval for use of Olestra as an ingredient in ice cream, oil, salad dressing, and cheese. Little scientific data are available on the health effects of Olestra. Some experts believe the safety of this "drug" has not been proved and Procter & Gamble is required to conduct long-term studies of its health effects. Avoid fake foods containing fat that seem too good to be true, and eat smaller portions of the real thing.

## Fatty Acid Food Sources

### High in Monounsaturated Fatty Acids

**Best Sources**

| | |
|---|---|
| canola oil* | olives/olive oil |

**Good Sources**

| | |
|---|---|
| almonds/almond oil | lard[†] |
| avocados | margarine[†] |
| beef fat[†] | palm oil[†] |
| hazelnuts | peanuts/peanut oil |

### High in Polyunsaturated Fatty Acids

#### OMEGA-6'S (linoleic acid)

| | |
|---|---|
| corn oil | soybeans/soybean oil* |
| cottonseed oil | sunflower seeds/sunflower oil |
| safflower oil | walnuts/walnut oil* |
| sesame oil | |

*Also contains significant amounts of linolenic acid (omega-3).

[†]Fatty acid ratio is greater than 40 percent monounsaturated, but also contains greater than 40 percent saturated fatty acids.

## OMEGA-3'S

### Best Sources

| | |
|---|---|
| anchovies | sablefish |
| Atlantic bluefish | salmon‡ |
| catfish‡ | sardines |
| herring | whitefish |
| mackerel | |

### Good Sources

| | |
|---|---|
| pompano | striped bass‡ |
| shark | swordfish |
| smelt | trout‡ |
| squid | tuna |

### Moderate Sources

| | |
|---|---|
| carp | ocean perch |
| cod | pollack |
| flounder | sea bass |
| grouper | shellfish: clams, oysters, mussels, lobster, shrimp, scallops |
| haddock | |
| mahimahi | snapper |

## PLANT SOURCES OF OMEGA-3'S (linolenic acid):

canola oil
flaxseed/most flaxseed products (flour, bread)/flaxseed oil
leafy green vegetables (kale, spinach, Swiss chard)
soybeans/some soy products/soybean oil
walnuts/walnut oil

It is acknowledged that some fats are better than others with respect to prevention of heart disease and cancer, but your total fat intake should be moderate. This will help keep you at an appropriate weight and will lower your risk for many chronic diseases, including heart disease and cancer. Does this mean the less fat you eat the healthier you will be? Not necessarily; it is possible to eat too little fat. Fat serves several vital functions in the body. Fats carry vitamins A, D, E, and K across the intestinal wall into the

‡Wild or sea-caught versions of these fish have significant levels of omega-3 fatty acids. Keep in mind that farm-raised fish are fed grains (rather than feeding on marine plants) and therefore may contain omega-6 rather than the protective omega-3 fatty acids.

bloodstream. In fact, vitamin E is found predominantly in fatty foods of plant origin. Essential fatty acids, such as linolenic and linoleic, which are provided only through the diet, are needed to make hormones and maintain healthy cells. Over a long period of time, diets with less than 10 percent of calories from fat can put you at risk for vitamin and essential fatty acid deficiencies. Diets high in saturated and hydrogenated fat (the kind found in commercial snack foods and baked goods) can also lead to essential fatty acid deficiency if they are low in monounsaturated and polyunsaturated fats. The bottom line is to go easy on the fat-free and other processed foods. Moderation and variety are the keys to balancing your fat intake.

## Lowering Fat in Your Diet

Decreasing the amount of fat you eat can be achieved with a little planning and good decision making when shopping, cooking, and dining out. By using good quality cooking equipment, some of today's hottest chefs have refined the art and techniques of healthy cooking. A sampling of their methods include high temperature oven roasting (for meat, fish, poultry, fruits, and vegetables), searing food in nonstick pans to achieve flavor and browning, and using fruit and vegetable purees to replace some or all of the fat in soups, sauces, and baked goods. By applying some of their basic techniques and making healthy substitutions for high-fat ingredients, you can substantially cut the amount of fat in your diet and never miss it.

### COOKING AND BAKING

- Trim the fat off meat and limit portion sizes.
- Bake, broil, roast, boil, braise, sear, sauté (with minimal oil or stock in a nonstick skillet), steam, or grill rather than fry.
- Roast firm-fleshed fish, such as snapper, halibut, or cod, "en papillotte" (in paper). Inside the fold of parchment paper, sprinkle the fish with fresh herbs and a splash of white wine (or broth). Seal at the edges with egg whites, folding over repeatedly. Well-sealed foil wrap can also be used. This method of cooking really concentrates the flavors of the herbs and fish, allowing you to forget all about fat.
- Use a rack in the pan when cooking meats to allow fat to drip down.
- Use nonstick pans and bakeware to limit the amount of fat in cooking and baking. Use a limited amount of fat (about $1/2$ teaspoon per serving) to sauté or sear food in a nonstick pan. Heating oil until it is very hot—almost smoking—and then turning down the heat to medium-high before adding the food will help to achieve good browning and flavor with a minimum of fat.

- Sauté foods in broth, water, or wine instead of butter or oil.
- Steam or oven-roast vegetables.
- Prepare soups and stocks at least a day in advance so that fat can be skimmed off the top more easily. Add starches such as beans (cooked), peas, potatoes, or rice when preparing soup. Cook until tender, then puree all or half of the soup. The starch will give it a creamy consistency and will thicken the soup.
- Limit the use of butter, margarine, oils, cream, regular salad dressing, lard, commercial baked goods (containing hydrogenated fats or tropical oils such as palm and coconut), and shortening.
- Try nonfat powdered milk in baking. Low-fat baked goods typically do not brown well. Adding one or two tablespoons of dry milk will help you to achieve a golden brown color.
- Halve the amount of fat called for in savory recipes, such as soups, stews, sauces, and casseroles.
- When baking, use fruit purees made from apples, bananas, prunes, soy, or flaxseed flour to replace part of the fat. Replace unsweetened chocolate with unsweetened cocoa powder: for every ounce of chocolate, substitute 3 tablespoons of cocoa. Because fat adds flavor to baked goods, enhance flavor by increasing or adding ingredients such as citrus zests, various extracts, and sugar when you cut fat from a recipe.

SUBSTITUTE . . .

- fish, poultry without skin, and lean meats for higher fat meats
- nonfat or 1 percent milk for whole milk
- low-fat or fat-free sour cream for the full-fat versions; 1 or 2 percent milk or half the amount of fat-free sour cream for cream in "cream" soups and sauces
- 1 cup of milk mixed with 1 tablespoon of cornstarch or 3/4 cup of evaporated skim milk mixed with 1 tablespoon of all-purpose flour for cream in cooking. Whisk the mixture into a soup or sauce and bring to a boil. Reduce the heat and maintain a low boil until creamy and slightly thickened, about two minutes (the cornstarch or flour will prevent the milk from breaking when heated).
- 1 whole egg plus 2 egg whites for 2 whole eggs in cooking and baking
- reduced-fat cheeses, such as cottage, part-skim mozzarella and ricotta, farmer, soy, for high-fat cheeses; and lower-fat versions of Swiss, Cheddar, goat's milk, and cream cheeses
- soy sausages for regular sausages to add flavor (and protein) to a soup or stew; smoked turkey or lean smoked ham in bean soups that call for hocks

- fruit or vegetable salsas, chutneys, or flavorful mustards for mayonnaise on sandwiches
- pureed 1 percent or nonfat cottage cheese or "yogurt cheese" for mayonnaise as a sandwich spread or as a base for dressings adding fresh herbs or seasonings, such as tarragon, thyme, parsley, cilantro, saffron, curry, cayenne, tomato paste or pureed sun-dried tomatoes, and a pinch of olive or anchovy paste (see tip on page 32)
- pureed 1 percent or nonfat cottage cheese for ricotta cheese in cooking and baking
- acidic dairy products, such as yogurt or buttermilk, for part of the liquid ingredients in baking to help prevent gluten (a protein found in flour) from developing and tenderize the baked goods.

---

### ✦ MAKE YOUR OWN VINAIGRETTES ✦

Traditional vinaigrettes are made with a ratio of three parts oil to one part vinegar. To spare fat, combine equal parts of oil (preferably extra virgin olive oil), a good-quality vinegar (balsamic, sherry, fruit-flavored, herb-infused, and rice wine vinegars work well), and water. For more flavor, substitute stock or fresh juice for water. A pinch of fresh herbs or mustard can also add flavor. Vegetable purees, such as red pepper, watercress, spinach, or roasted garlic, can contribute nutrients, color, a creamier texture, and flavor (see Roasted Red Pepper Vinaigrette, page 172).

---

- turkey or chicken breast (skin removed) or tuna salad (prepared with a small amount of olive oil, reduced-fat mayonnaise, or mustard) for high-fat luncheon meats, such as bologna, ham, or salami
- fresh fruit, pretzels, baked tortilla chips with salsa, raw vegetables, air-popped popcorn, low-fat cheese, whole-grain low-fat crackers, flavored rice cakes, cereal, or sorbet for high-fat snacks, such as potato chips, cold cuts, high-fat cheese, cookies, chocolate, nuts, or ice cream
- small portions of low-fat or fat-free sweets for the regular versions. (Remember, they still have calories!)
- broth-based or vegetable puree soups for cream-based soups
- high-fiber, low-fat breakfast cereals or a bagel with a light layer of reduced-fat cream cheese (or any other type of low-fat cheese) for high-fat muffins or scones; include a piece of fruit with your breakfast to add nutrients and replace fat
- thin-crust pizza topped with vegetables for pizza with sausage or pepperoni; blot any surface fat with a napkin

> To make yogurt cheese, drain nonfat plain or vanilla yogurt through a funnel lined with cheesecloth or mesh overnight in the refrigerator. This will remove the "whey," the distinctive, tart flavor specific to yogurt. The "cheese" that remains is creamy and bland and can be seasoned with condiments or herbs or sweetened for cooking, baking, or spreading.

# Protein

Getting enough protein is rarely a health concern for most Americans. The average American under sixty-five years of age consumes 50 percent more protein than the Recommended Dietary Allowance (RDA) (46 to 63 grams per day for adults, depending on age and sex). Two-thirds of the protein intake is from meat, fish, poultry, or dairy; the remaining one-third is from plant sources, such as legumes, grains, cereals, and vegetables. Animal protein sources provide high-quality protein and vitamins $B_6$, $B_{12}$, and zinc (nutrients that are hard to get from a strict vegetarian diet), and contain a form of iron that is easily absorbed by the body. However, they also contain significant amounts of total fat, saturated fat, and cholesterol. Researchers have linked diets high in animal protein to increased risk of heart disease and certain types of cancer. People whose intake of protein is moderate and more predominantly from plant sources also consume less fat and more fiber, vitamins, minerals, and other substances such as phytochemicals. They are healthier in general and are less prone to these diseases.

Why are high protein diets so popular? Every decade or so high protein diets are repackaged as a "new" concept for weight loss. The most recent wave of these books blames the increase in obesity on excessive carbohydrate intake, which supposedly causes insulin resistance and thus weight gain in many people. In fact, the relationship between insulin resistance and obesity is just the opposite: insulin resistance is often the *result* of obesity, not the cause of it. Furthermore, these diets "work" by limiting food choices and food groups and, in the final analysis, total calories. Most nutrition experts agree that weight control is a matter of "calories in = calories out." Whenever calorie intake exceeds calories burned, whatever the source of the calories—carbohydrate, protein, or fat—the excess will be stored as fat. The exceptions to this rule are rare medical conditions that cause irregular metabolism or interfere with the body's ability to digest and absorb nutrients. As for the safety of high-protein diets, there is no evidence that protein intake up to 50 percent greater than the RDA poses detrimental health consequences, provided that intake of animal protein and fat are not excessive and the individual does not have any conditions or diseases that compromise kidney function. In the long run, however, these diets can be problematic if protein foods replace fruits, vegetables, and high fiber grains and cereals.

## How Much Protein Do You Need?

The protein RDA for adults is 0.8 grams per kilogram of body weight or 0.36 grams per pound of body weight.

For a 125-pound (57-kg) female → 125 × 0.36 equals 45 grams protein/day
For a 170-pound (77-kg) male   → 170 × 0.36 equals 61 grams protein/day

When you consider that an 8-ounce steak (half the portion served in many restaurants) provides approximately 56 grams of protein, you realize how easy it is to get adequate protein and even more. By keeping animal protein at around 6 ounces per day (two 3-ounce servings), while increasing plant protein sources, you will meet key nutrient requirements (vitamin $B_{12}$, iron, and zinc) and at the same time be moderating your total fat, saturated fat, and cholesterol intake. With careful planning, a totally plant-based vegan diet can meet all of your body's nutrient requirements. According to the RDA guidelines approximately 8 to 10 percent of your daily calories should come from protein. With 20 to 25 percent of calories set aside for fat, the remaining calories in your diet are for nutrient-rich complex carbohydrates (about 65 to 72 percent). If these percentages become too confusing, simply assess your protein requirements using the formula above, then familiarize yourself with the protein content of the different food categories listed below or use food labels to count grams.

## Protein Sources

### Lean Protein Sources

MEAT/POULTRY/GAME/FISH AND SHELLFISH (**6 to 8 grams protein per ounce***)

#### Beef

All beef cuts are trimmed "choice" or "select" grades. Because these grades tend to be very lean, longer moist heat cooking methods such as stewing or braising help to tenderize them. Keep in mind, even lean beef contains significant amounts of saturated fat and cholesterol, so if you eat beef, choose from lean cuts on an occasional basis, not more than three to four times a month.

**Sources**

| | |
|---|---|
| arm, chuck | flank |
| bottom round | tenderloin |
| calves liver[†] | top loin |
| eye round | top round |

### Pork

Fresh pork tenderloin is a terrific alternative protein source for those who are all "chickened out." It is almost as lean as skinless chicken breast, and is very tender. Pork tenderloin and loin chops cook quickly, so be careful not to overcook. Searing, grilling, roasting, or braising are other cooking techniques to consider for these cuts of pork. For marinating ideas see Marinated Pork Tenderloin with Smashed Orange-scented Sweet Potatoes on page 251. Another form of pork, extra-lean ham, can be as low in fat as 1.5 grams per ounce; however, you should still limit consumption because even "fresh" hams often contain nitrites.

#### Sources

| | |
|---|---|
| arm-shoulder, lean, trimmed | loin chop, lean, trimmed |
| center loin, lean, trimmed | tenderloin, lean, trimmed |
| ham, extra lean | |

### Poultry

Poultry, particularly chicken, is one of the most popular protein sources. Without its skin, breast meat from turkey or chicken can contain less then 1 gram of fat per ounce. Recommended cooking methods include roasting, stewing, sautéing (with a minimal amount of fat in a nonstick skillet), grilling, braising, or poaching.

#### Sources (skin removed)

| | |
|---|---|
| chicken breast | domestic turkey breast |
| chicken leg | domestic turkey, dark meat |
| chicken liver[†] | |

### Game

As consumer demand for game has increased in recent years, different varieties have become more available in some supermarkets, gourmet specialty shops, and from butchers. Many types of game can also be purchased through mail order sources. Wild game tends to have even less fat than ranch-raised varieties; however, the taste is typically more "gamey" and is not quite as tender. Because game meat tends to be so lean, it will dry out quickly, particularly when roasting. Be careful not to overcook it. For nonpoultry game such as buffalo, elk, or venison grill or sear quickly (medium rare to medium) in a hot nonstick pan with a little oil. This will preserve juices and tenderness. Other cooking methods for boar, rabbit, or venison include careful roasting or braising in flavorful liquids such as stocks, fruit juices, wines, or combinations. Flavorings and seasoning, which compliment game include: fresh herbs such as thyme, rosemary, sage (for stronger flavored game), and tarragon; frozen, fresh, or dried berries (great additions to a sauce, and fresh and dried berries are nice garnishes); juniper berries; peppercorns; currant preserves; and roasted garlic.

### Sources

| | |
|---|---|
| buffalo | rabbit, wild and domestic |
| duck breast | rhea |
| elk | squab |
| ostrich | venison |
| pheasant | wild boar |
| quail breast | wild turkey, breast and dark meat |

### Fish and Shellfish

Even some fattier fish, high in good omega-3 fatty acids, are low in total fat as compared with many other protein sources. For information about the protective type of fat found in wild and sea versions of fattier fish, see page 28. There are many varieties of fish with 3 or less grams of fat per serving. To keep the fat down in these already low-fat protein choices, avoid breading and frying and heavy butter and/or cream-laden sauces. Use simple cooking techniques such as grilling, roasting, pan searing, poaching, or steaming to keep the fat low and allow the full flavors of the fish to come through.

### Sources

| | |
|---|---|
| bluefish, Atlantic | salmon, king or chinook, coho, chum, sockeye, Atlantic |
| catfish | |
| cod, Atlantic‡ | scallops‡ |
| crab‡ | sea bass |
| flounder‡ | shrimp‡ |
| grouper‡ | snapper |
| haddock‡ | sole‡ |
| lobster, northern, spiny‡ | striped bass |
| ocean perch | swordfish |
| oysters‡ | trout, seatrout, wild rainbow trout |
| pike‡ | tuna, bluefin, yellowfin, albacore (water packed) |
| pollack‡ | |
| rockfish | |

### LOW-FAT DAIRY

Skim or low-fat dairy products are convenient and are high-quality protein sources. Check the Nutrition Facts label. "Reduced-fat" cheeses typically have 25 percent or less fat than the regular versions. This amount can still be high. For example, a reduced-fat Cheddar may still have 7 grams of fat per ounce. "Low-fat" means no more than 3 grams of fat per one-ounce serving.

### Milk and Yogurt (portion sizes as indicated)
skim or 1 percent milk (all types): 8 grams protein per cup
evaporated skim milk: 8 grams protein per 4 fluid ounces
non-fat or fat-free yogurt: 13 grams protein per cup

### Cheeses (labeled "low-fat"—7 to 10 grams protein per ounce; portion size is 1 ounce)

| | |
|---|---|
| American | mozzarella |
| Cheddar | Muenster |
| cottage ($^1/_2$ cup) | ricotta |
| Monterey Jack | Swiss |

### Eggs and Egg Substitutes
whole eggs: 6 grams protein, 5 grams fat each
egg whites: 7 grams protein, 0 grams fat (for 2 egg whites)
egg substitute: 7 grams protein, 0 grams fat per $^1/_4$ cup

## Plant Protein Sources

After computing your daily protein requirement, note how easy it is to achieve it with plant sources alone. Plants that are good protein sources also tend to be rich in fiber, vitamins, minerals, and protective phytochemicals. The macronutrient profile of most plant foods is a mixture of carbohydrate and protein. Fat levels will vary from none to quite high.

**Myth:** People who exercise frequently require substantially more protein than the Recommended Dietary Allowance (RDA).

**Fact:** High protein powders, drinks, capsules, and bars are unnecessary for frequent exercisers. The RDA furnishes sufficient protein to build and repair muscle. Considering that most people, including vegetarians, exceed the RDA for protein, there is no need to supplement protein in the form of food or amino acids. Professional athletes and weight trainers may require slightly more protein than the RDA, but they also require higher calorie levels, which in itself often leads to higher protein intake. An extra 8 grams of protein a day can be added with one glass of milk (1 percent or nonfat, regular, or soy). A cup of nonfat or low-fat yogurt provides 13 grams of protein, so why buy expensive supplements?

*Sources*

dried (cooked) or canned beans: 7 to 8 grams protein, 0 to 1 gram fat per 1/2 cup

other starches (rice, pasta, breads, and cereals): 3 grams protein per serving (serving sizes vary)

nuts and seeds[§]: 4 to 8 grams protein, 5 to 10 grams fat per 1/4 cup

soybeans: 14 grams protein, 7 grams fat per 1/4 cup boiled

vegetables: 2 grams protein, 0 grams fat per serving (1/2 cup cooked, 1 cup raw = 1 serving)

## Vegetarianism

People who consume a vegetarian diet have a decreased risk of developing cancer. Almost 7 percent of the U.S. population consider themselves vegetarian, more than a 250 percent increase in the last two decades. Some people define themselves as vegetarians because they omit poultry, fish and seafood, and red meat from their diet. Less than 1 percent of Americans are vegetarians by the following criteria, but their numbers are growing:

*Lacto-ovo vegetarians* consume dairy foods and eggs, but no meat, fish, or poultry.
*Lacto vegetarians* eat dairy foods, but no eggs or any other animal products.
*Vegans* do not eat animal foods of any type.

Even within these classifications a great deal of variation may exist with respect to which animal products are avoided; therefore, a diet's adequacy should be evaluated on individual intake rather than classification. If a wide variety of foods is eaten each day, a vegetarian diet can be easy and healthy. The more food groups that are eliminated, however, the more attention is required to assure that nutrients are replaced by other foods.

---

*The sources listed contain 3 grams or less of fat per cooked ounce (dry heat cooking). Values do not reflect any fat added during cooking or from sauces.

[†]Though high in cholesterol (you get a day's worth in a 3-ounce serving), liver still has only 3 grams or less of fat per ounce and is an economical protein source rich in vitamins A, $B_{12}$ and other B vitamins, zinc, copper, iron, and phosphorous. However, liver is the animal tissue most likely to contain pesticides as well as antibiotic or drug residues. Even though the USDA randomly checks liver and other meats for toxic levels of these substances, liver should be only an occasional source of protein. Some natural food stores, supermarkets, and butchers sell meat from animals not treated with hormones or antibiotics and these may provide a healthier source of liver.

[‡]very low in fat: contains 0.5 grams or less of fat per cooked ounce.

[§]high in fat; limit portion sizes

Here are the American Dietetic Association's recommendations for people who follow vegetarian diets:

- Consult a registered dietitian or other qualified nutrition professional, especially during periods of growth, pregnancy, breast-feeding, or recovery from illness.
- Minimize intake of less nutritious foods, such as sweets and fatty foods.
- Limit egg intake to 3 to 4 yolks per week.
- Choose whole or unrefined grain products instead of refined products.
- Choose a variety of nuts, seeds, legumes, fruits, and vegetables, including good sources of vitamin C to improve iron absorption.
- Choose low-fat or nonfat varieties of dairy products, if they are included in the diet.
- For infants, children, and teenagers, ensure adequate intake of calories, vitamin D, calcium, iron, and zinc. (Intakes of vitamin D, calcium, iron, and zinc are usually adequate when a variety of foods and sufficient calories are consumed.)
- If exclusively breast-feeding premature infants or babies beyond four to six months of age, take vitamin D and iron supplements beginning from birth or at least by four to six months, as your doctor recommends.
- Take iron and folate (folic acid) supplements during pregnancy.
- Vegans should use properly fortified food sources of vitamin $B_{12}$, such as fortified soy beverages or commercial breakfast cereals, or take a cyanocobalamin supplement. If sunlight is inadequate, vegans should take a vitamin D supplement during pregnancy or while breast-feeding. You may not be getting enough sunlight if you do not spend a lot of time outdoors, or do spend a fair amount of time in the sun, but wear sunscreen to block out ultraviolet rays. Also, if you are a northern resident, you may need to consider vitamin D supplementation during winter months when the sun's ultraviolet rays are not strong, preventing the body from synthesizing vitamin D.

It is not necessary to completely give up animal products to reap the health benefits of a vegetarian-style diet. These four small changes are the starting point in making the transition to a more vegetarian diet:

**1.** *Moderate portion sizes of meat, fish, and poultry.* Keep portion sizes to 3 to 4 cooked ounces, about the size and thickness of the palm of your hand. Be flexible; if you have eaten a meat-free breakfast and lunch, enjoy that 6-ounce fish portion served to you in a restaurant. In general, however, meat should not take up more than one quarter of the space on your dinner plate, with the remaining area left for grains, legumes, and vegetables.

**2.** *Use meat as a side dish or condiment.* When meats are used in soups, stews, casseroles, or stir-fries, you can use a lot less (2 to 3 ounces per serving) with the remaining bulk of ingredients being grains, legumes, and vegetables.

**3.** *Eat more meatless meals.* Try eliminating meat from one meal per day and then move on to a couple of days per week. Replace meat with plant protein sources, especially soybeans and soy products. Cooking ideas include using ratatouille or beans with pasta; vegetable curries or chili with tofu; burritos with vegetables, rice, and beans; salads with grains, vegetables, and beans.

**4.** Adapt a vegetarian plan that suits your lifestyle and preferences (lacto, lacto-ovo, vegan). If you adopt a vegan plan, choose foods fortified with nutrients found in animal foods.

---

Vegetarian diets can still be high in fat. Limit or avoid dishes that contain moderate to high amounts of avocado, oil, nuts, olives, cheese, mayonnaise, or salad dressings.

---

### Good Sources of Nutrients in a Vegetarian Diet

| Vitamin B$_{12}$ | Vitamin D | Calcium | Iron* | Zinc | Protein |
|---|---|---|---|---|---|
| fortified soy beverages | fortified soy beverages | tofu curded with calcium | green leafy vegetables | legumes | grains |
| fortified cereals | some fortified cereals | broccoli | collard greens | nuts | legumes |
| some brands of nutritional yeast | sunlight | bok choy | kale | tofu | nuts |
| | | collard greens | spinach | whole grains | seeds |
| | | kale | Swiss chard | whole wheat bread | soybeans and soy products |
| | | legumes (peas and beans) | turnip greens | | vegetables |
| | | orange juice enriched with calcium | dried fruit | | |
| | | fortified soy beverages | iron-fortified breads and cereals, especially whole wheat | | |
| | | soybeans | legumes | | |
| | | turnip greens | tofu | | |

*Eat these iron-rich plant foods with fruits, vegetables, or juices high in vitamin C to improve iron absorption.

**Myth:** Vegetarian diets require that different plant foods, such as whole grains, legumes, vegetables, seeds, and nuts, be combined at the same meal to assure all protein requirements are met.

**Fact:** It was previously thought that plant foods need to be combined in such a manner that all essential and nonessential amino acids are available with each meal (protein complementing). We now know that this is unnecessary as long as a variety of foods is consumed throughout the day. Additionally, soy protein is nutritionally equivalent to the protein value of foods from animal origin and thus can serve as a sole source of protein.

**Myth:** Spirulina, seaweed, and fermented soy products such as tempeh can be reliable sources of vitamin $B_{12}$ for vegetarians who do not eat any animal products.

**Fact:** Spirulina, also called blue-green algae or plant plankton, is a hot seller in health food stores where it is often touted as a superfood that can prevent and cure many modern ills. The truth about spirulina is that it is rich in carotenoids, particularly beta-carotene. It is also a good plant source of protein and sometimes contains vitamin $B_{12}$. The problem is that 80 to 94 percent of the vitamin $B_{12}$ in spirulina, seaweed, and fermented soy products may be inactive analogs, types not useful to the human body. The form of $B_{12}$ that is physiologically active for human beings is cyanocobalamin. It is available in fortified breakfast cereals and beverages, nonfermented soy products, some brands of nutritional yeast, and in multivitamin formulas.

**Myth:** Macrobiotic diets can both prevent and cure many types of cancer.

**Fact:** There is no evidence that macrobiotic diets can stop cancer once the diagnosis has been made. In fact, they can lead to or advance malnutrition in some cancer patients who are unable to meet their calorie and protein requirements on such regimes. Inadequate nutrition can harm the immune system, which may further impair the body's ability to fight cancer. From a prevention standpoint, however, the stages of macrobiotic diets that do not advance to the restrictive Zen stage (consisting of only brown rice and water) are consistent with dietary recommendations for cancer prevention. They include foods such as whole grains, fruits, and vegetables and moderate amounts of tofu and fish.

## Soy

The soya plant, the most widely eaten plant in the world, provides a quality source of protein to billions of people daily. The "fruits" of the soya plant are used mostly in Asian diets, but they are becoming a popular source of protein elsewhere as scientists begin to understand the vital role they may play in disease prevention.

Soy has been in the headlines since studies linked the intake of this bean to lower risk of heart disease and cancer. Phytochemicals in soybeans are thought to contribute beneficial effects. One group of compounds, called isoflavones, is a phytoestrogen, a plant form of estrogen. Isoflavones are much less potent than human estrogen but can still interfere with the action of human estrogen by mimicking its role in the body and causing less to be produced. Isoflavones are of great interest to investigators studying the link between diet and breast and prostate cancer.

Soybeans also contain plant sterols, which may block estrogen and hinder cell division, possibly preventing cancer cells from multiplying. Protease inhibitors found in soybeans and other legumes may slow the rate of division in cancer cells, allowing time for genetic repair and interruption of the carcinogenic process.

Most people are bewildered about how to incorporate more soy into their daily diet. No longer is soy just about tofu. There are many convenience products available that are not only healthy, but also very tasty. Soy products include soybeans, soy milk, soy-based yogurt, tofu (firm and silken), tempeh, miso, soy flour, isolated soy protein, textured soy protein, soy "meat products," soybean oil, soy cheese, and soy sauce.

**Soybeans** range in size from as small as a pea to as large as a grape. The beans can be any combination of yellow, black, red, green, or brown. Though their flavor is bland, their nutritive value is rich—they are high in protein, low in carbohydrates, and high in a desirable oil that is often extracted and sold as soybean oil.

A harvest bean, soybeans are generally available at Asian markets, some supermarkets, health or natural food stores, and from local producers during late summer to late fall. They are available dried all year long.

## USES

- After presoaking, use in soups, stews, and casseroles.
- Buy "sprouted" (or sprout your own) and use in salads and stir-fries.
- Steam or boil for 10 to 15 minutes and eat plain or seasoned.

**Soy milk** is a creamy beverage made from dried soybeans that have been soaked in water and then crushed and boiled. The remaining liquid, soy milk, is lactose free and can be used by those who are lactose intolerant or allergic to cow's milk. It is available plain and in a variety of flavors, such as vanilla, chocolate, almond, and mocha, and like regular cow's milk, its content ranges from fat free to full fat (unlike that of cow's milk, the type of fat in soy milk is predominantly unsaturated). Unfortified soy milk is high in protein, B vitamins, and some minerals; however, it does not contain significant amounts of calcium or vitamin D and $B_{12}$, as does fortified cow's milk. More recently, however, soy milk producers are fortifying their products with these important nutrients.

Soy milk is available at health and natural food stores and most supermarkets.

USES

- Drink as a hot or cold beverage.
- Pour over hot or cold breakfast cereals.
- Use in cooking or baking as a substitute for milk or cream.
- Use soy milk for a milk shake (see page 299).

**Soy yogurt** is made by adding bacterial culture to soy milk. The fat content and flavors vary like those of dairy yogurt.

Soy yogurt is available at health and natural food stores.

USES

- Use as a part of breakfast or lunch.
- Try as a snack.
- Use in fruit smoothies or protein shakes.

**Tofu** is the curd remaining when soy milk is coagulated and the whey is discarded. Different coagulants are used in its production, including nigari, a natural compound of sea water or calcium sulfate (tofu curded with calcium sulfate provides a substantial source of calcium). Recently, low-fat or "lite" tofus have reached the market and contain the beneficial properties of the soybean without all the fat.

High in nutrients and cholesterol-free, tofu is available at health and natural food stores and some supermarkets. Commercially sealed packages of tofu have less bacteria than the kind sold floating in water. Cooking tofu until it reaches an internal temperature of 160° F kills all bacteria.

*Firm tofu* is a dense form of tofu that holds its shape nicely in cooking.

USES

- Add to soups or stews to increase protein. Since tofu is bland in taste, it works better with well-seasoned foods like Indian, Southwestern, and Asian dishes, rather than subtle flavors.
- Marinate and grill, sear, or bake and then use as an animal protein replacement in a meal or inside a sandwich.
- Substitute for ground beef in spaghetti sauce, tacos, and burritos.
- Crumble and add bread crumbs and seasonings to make tofu burgers.
- Scramble with vegetables and seasonings.

*Silken tofu* is a soft variety that contains more water than firm tofu and becomes creamy when pureed or blended.

### USES

- Blend with fresh fruit and soy milk to make a protein-rich fruit "smoothie."
- Puree and combine with seasonings to make a low-fat sandwich spread to replace mayonnaise. Seasoning suggestions include curry, saffron, tomato paste or pureed sun-dried tomatoes, olive paste, anchovies, cilantro, basil, or rosemary. Use to blend tuna or chicken salad.
- Use as a replacement for sour cream in cooking or in place of cream cheese in baking.
- Use as a base for a creamy salad dressing.

**Tempeh** is a fermented soy patty made in combination with another grain, such as rice or barley. It has a nutty, "mushroomy," meatlike flavor and its texture makes it perfect for marinating, grilling, searing, or baking.

Tempeh is sold in blocks of various sizes (sometimes already marinated), often frozen, at health and natural food stores and some supermarkets.

### USES

- Grill or oven-roast with barbecue sauce and make a sandwich.
- Grate and use in veggie burgers with other grains and seasonings; use grated tempeh in soups, stews, chilies, and casseroles to add protein and a meaty texture.
- Use as a replacement for tuna or chicken in a salad.

**Miso** is a paste formed when water, salt, soybeans, rice, or barley and a fermenting agent are mixed. There are a variety of types of miso, which are distinguished by their colors and tastes. Miso is high in protein and low in fat, but high in sodium. It should be used sparingly and people who are salt sensitive or hypertensive should avoid miso as a soy protein source. Fortunately, after being aged in cedar vats for up to three years, the flavor is intense and small amounts go a long way.

You'll find small and large plastic tubs of miso in the refrigerated section of health and natural food stores and some supermarkets.

## USES

- Use yellow miso (or light miso), which is less intense and less salty, to make a salad dressing.
- Enrich soups, sauces, or vegetable stocks with red miso (made with a barley); it adds both color and flavor.
- Use dark miso, which has the most intense flavor, as a soup base.

**Soy flour** is made from roasted soybeans that are rolled into flakes and then ground. Soy flour is loaded with soy protein (approximately 50 percent by weight), is an excellent source of isoflavones, and adds color, texture, and moistness to baked goods. Since it contains no gluten, soy flour needs to be mixed with all-purpose or bread flour (20 percent:80 percent, respectively) when making yeast-raised products. In preparing quick breads, muffins, and cookies, up to 30 percent soy flour can be used. Full-fat soy flour can be very high in fat, so look for defatted, "low-fat" soy flour, which is also a more concentrated source of protein.

Soy flour is available at health and natural food stores.

## USES

- Substitute for one-quarter to one-half of the wheat flour in baking. Unless you are using defatted soy flour, it contains more fat (in part, linolenic fatty acids—the good kind) than wheat flour so cut the fat in the recipe by up to one-quarter.
- Replace 1 egg in baked goods with 1 tablespoon of soy flour and 1 tablespoon of water.
- Use in frying and sautéing. Because of its composition, soy flour absorbs less fat in cooking than does its wheat counterpart.
- Toasting the flour on a baking sheet in the oven or in a dry skillet (while stirring) on the stove until lightly browned produces a nutty aroma and flavor, and helps with browning of baked goods.

---

- Baked foods brown more quickly when using soy flour, so decrease the baking time or lower the cooking temperature.
- Because even defatted soy flour contains some oils, it is best to store it in the refrigerator or freezer to prevent spoilage.
- Soy flour is fine and gets compressed or packed easily, so sift it before using it in recipes.

**Isolated soy protein** is made from defatted soy flour. Isolated soy protein is at least 90 percent protein: most of the carbohydrate and fat have been extracted. It is a good source of isoflavones and has a variety of uses. Because it is a fat-free source of high-quality protein, isolated soy protein is often found in weight-loss beverages, infant formulas, meal-replacement or "energy boosting" bars, and "muscle-building" protein powders. It can be purchased generically or under a variety of labels. If you cannot locate a generic source of soy protein isolate, look for a protein powder in which soy protein isolate is listed as a first or second ingredient.

Isolate soy protein is available at health and natural food stores.

## USES

- Blend with fruit and/or yogurt shakes.
- Add in baking (muffins, quick breads, or cookies) or cooking (puddings, soups, and casseroles) to increase protein content.

**Textured soy protein** is also made from defatted soy flour. The flour is compressed until the protein changes texture to a granular or chunky form. Textured soy protein is high in protein, isoflavones, calcium, and iron, and is generally low in fat and calories. It is sold dry and can be rehydrated with stock or water before being used in recipes.

Textured soy protein is available at health and natural food stores.

## USES

- Once rehydrated, use as an extender (or a medium to add both protein and bulk), replacing some or all of the ground beef, turkey, or chicken (and fat) in chili, meat loaf, hamburgers, tacos, sloppy joes, or casseroles.

**Soy "meat products"** are made to look, smell, and taste like the real thing. Products include soy-based vegetarian sausages, hot dogs, hamburgers, bacon, and cold cuts. One needs to read labels carefully when shopping for these products because, in some cases, they are very high in fat and sodium and have been chemically preserved. Unless they have been vitamin and mineral fortified, they are not an equivalent replacement for protein derived from animal products.

Soy "meat products" are available at health and natural food stores.

USES

- Use as an occasional replacement for animal protein products.

**Soybean oil** is pressed from soy flakes and is a common ingredient in commercial baked goods. The flavor is subtle and is therefore good for cooking foods whose flavor you do not want influenced by the cooking oil. Due to its high smoking point, it is also good for sautéing or cooking in a wok, which require high heat. Although soybean oil does not contain isoflavones, it does have other beneficial compounds. Unlike most other vegetable oils, it contains a significant amount of linolenic fatty acids, essential fatty acids that are not produced in the body. Linolenic fatty acids can be converted to omega-3 fatty acids in the body. As with all oils and fats, however, it should be used sparingly.

Soybean oil is available at health and natural food stores and most supermarkets.

USES

- Use for sautéing or cooking in a wok.
- Use in baking.
- Try in salad dressings (in this case you may wish to use a rich-flavored vinegar and/or chopped herbs).

**Soy cheese**, made from the "milk" of soybeans, is a terrific alternative to dairy cheese. Varieties include mozzarella, Cheddar, Muenster, Monterey Jack (with or without jalapeño), and American. Most soy cheeses are not fat free, but they have about half the fat of the dairy equivalents and are very low in saturated fat. The fact that they do contain some fat makes them suitable for cooking, as they melt well. In a cooked dish such as lasagne it's difficult to tell the difference from dairy cheese.

Soy cheese is available at health and natural food stores and most supermarkets.

USES

- Grate and use in casseroles, lasagne, tacos, burritos, omelets, or any other recipe that calls for cheese (see Mexican Lasagne, page 204).
- Use soy ricotta to replace dairy ricotta in baking and cooking.
- Try soy American cheese on a grilled cheese and tomato sandwich.
- Use in macaroni and cheese.

**Soy sauce**, *shoyu*, or tamari is made by adding mold to roasted soybeans and wheat. After a few days they are mixed with sea water and brewed in fermentation tanks for up to one year, after which the liquid is pasteurized. Soy sauce does not contain isoflavones; however, it is a great flavoring agent in cooking. Similar to miso, it is very high in sodium (even the low-sodium varieties), so it should be avoided by those with salt sensitivity or those who have high blood pressure.

Soy sauce is available at health and natural food stores and supermarkets.

### USES

- *Chinese soy sauce* is stronger in flavor and very salty, while Japanese soy sauce, tamari, is sweeter and less salty. Both can be used in stir-fries, sauces, marinades, and salad dressings.

Many soy products are also available through mail-order sources. For resource and reference information about soy and soy products, call 1-800-TALK-SOY (1-800-825-5769), between 8 A.M. and 4 P.M. (CST) weekdays. This line is sponsored by the United Soybean Board.

# Carbohydrates

Carbohydrates are the major energy source in the human diet. They are the least expensive energy source and the majority of the world's population relies on carbohydrates to meet most of its energy requirements. Foods rich in complex carbohydrates (starches or fiber) are generally rich in vitamins, minerals, and phytochemicals. The calories derived from fruit are almost exclusively from carbohydrates. Grains, cereals, legumes, and vegetables contain protein and, in some cases, fat, but they are composed of significantly more carbohydrate by weight.

Carbohydrates are chemical ring compounds made solely of carbon, oxygen, and hydrogen. The number and structure of the rings determine the type of carbohydrate. Carbohydrates are distinguished as *simple carbohydrates*, containing one or two rings, or *complex carbohydrates*, containing many rings. Complex carbohydrates are further differentiated as starches, which are digestible, and fiber, which is not digestible.

Simple carbohydrates include monosaccharides (fructose, glucose, and galactose) and disaccharides (sucrose, maltose, and lactose) that are split when digested. Common simple sugars include sucrose (fructose and glucose joined together), what we call table sugar; fructose, the main sugar in fruit (also used to make the high fructose corn syrup used in many commercial products); and lactose (glucose and galactose) found in milk. Many other words that appear in ingredients lists indicate that the product contains sugar. If you are trying to moderate your intake of empty calories from sugar, look for the following ingredients (the higher they appear in ingredients lists, the greater the amount present):

| | |
|---|---|
| beet sugar | honey |
| brown sugar | invert sugar |
| cane sugar | maltodextrin or dextrin |
| confectioners' sugar (powdered) | maple syrup |
| crystallized cane sugar | molasses |
| dextrose | raw sugar |
| fructose | sucrose |
| high fructose corn syrup | turbinado sugar |

Starches from complex carbohydrates are chains of hundreds of glucose molecules. Starting with the digestive enzymes in the mouth all the way to the small intestine, starches are broken down to form individual glucose molecules that are then absorbed for energy or storage in muscle or fat. The rate at which complex carbohydrates are digested and absorbed is significantly slower than that of simple carbohydrates. Complex carbohydrates are found predominantly in grains, cereals, legumes, fruits, and vegetables. They have much more nutritional value and typically less fat than foods high in simple carbohydrates.

**Myth:** Simple carbohydrates, particularly refined white sugar, can cause cancer as well as other diseases.

**Fact:** Although sugar should not be a major component of your diet, especially if you are watching calories, researchers have not found a direct link between sugar and ill health. There are medical conditions, such as diabetes and elevated trigylcerides (a type of fat found in the bloodstream), that do warrant restrictions on sugar and other simple carbohydrates, but for most people, sugar intake does not impose health dangers. Furthermore, all types of sugars (and complex carbohydrates) are broken down to the body's primary energy source, glucose. Whether refined or unrefined, sugar is not a source of any major nutrient except calories. For this reason, you should limit your sugar intake to leave room for nutrient-packed complex carbohydrates.

# Fiber

It may appear odd that something undigestible could be touted as good for you. But such is the case with fiber, which is less an essential nutrient than an important element of internal maintenance. Fiber is a nonabsorbable complex carbohydrate that comes from the cell walls of plants. Most of the foods that are good sources of fiber have endured little or no "processing," such as whole-grain breads, bran, oats, brown rice, vegetables, and legumes.

There are two different types of fiber, and each serves different dietary functions: those that are soluble in water and those that are not. *Insoluble fiber,* such as cellulose, hemicelluloses, and lignan, is found in wheat and rye bran, seeds, nuts, and vegetables. It passes intact through the intestinal tract, helping potential carcinogens exit rapidly. This laxative action is thought to be an effective preventive measure against colon cancer, as well as a means to forestall other problems such as hemorrhoids or diverticulosis.

*Soluble fiber,* such as pectins, gums, and mucilages, is found in many fruits, some vegetables, oatmeal, oat bran, barley, and legumes. It is also used in commercial food products to provide fatlike consistency and texture without the fat. Soluble fiber absorbs water and nutrients in the stomach. This action slows food absorption, and the fiber's bulky texture creates a feeling of fullness that tends to reduce overall food intake (a nice benefit for people who are watching their weight). Soluble fiber is also associated with prevention of heart disease and colon cancer. It binds with bile acids, which help to absorb cholesterol and other lipids (fats), and increases their excretion. The water-holding capacity of soluble fiber may also have a dilutional effect on the potential damaging effects of bile acids while positively modifying the bacterial flora (or the resident bacterial growth) in the colon.

The amount of dietary fiber consumed daily by the average North American is 10 to 20 grams. The U.S. National Cancer Institute recommends 25 to 35 grams of dietary fiber per day. However, you should watch your dietary fiber intake, because too much of it can cause bloating and gas and give you loose stools. To meet these guidelines with minimal undesirable side effects, increase your fiber intake gradually.

There is no need to count the number of grams of fiber in every food you consume. There are some basic concepts which will help you work your way up to the recommended 25- to 35-gram range daily:

- Fruits and vegetables contain, on average, 2 grams of fiber per serving. Although some do contain higher or lower amounts, by eating a variety of fruits and vegetables, your intake should average out to this level. Reaching the minimum of your fruit and vegetable goal (5 servings per day) will satisfy about 40 percent of your dietary fiber goal.

    *Fiber = 10 grams*

- Eat a small bowl of hot or cold cereal. If you prefer a cereal that does not have much dietary fiber, increase the fiber by sprinkling a couple of teaspoons of unprocessed bran on top or add some 100 percent bran cereal.

    *Fiber = 3 grams*

- Eat two slices of whole wheat or pumpernickel bread (approximately $1^1/2$ to $2^1/2$ grams per slice).

  *Fiber = 4 grams*

- Eat $1^1/2$ cups pasta *or* 1 cup brown, wild, or basmati rice *or* $3/4$ cup of barley, polenta, or bulgur (cooked).

  *Fiber = 3 grams*

- When you're able to tolerate the above additions to your diet, add $1/2$ cup of any kind of beans or lentils (for example, black beans, chickpeas, pinto beans, white beans), which will provide about 5 to 8 grams of fiber.

  *Fiber = 5 grams*

  **Grand total = 25 grams**

When you consistently tolerate approximately 25 grams of dietary fiber per day, you can slowly bump it up by adding high-fiber cereal and fiber-containing soy products. You can also increase portion sizes and varieties of grains and beans, and increase fruit and vegetable servings (aim for nine servings per day).

**Myth:** Fiber supplements are an alternative to eating foods high in fiber.

**Fact:** Fiber supplements do not make up for dietary fiber. Fiber is a complex substance. Within the two major categories of fiber, soluble and insoluble, there are many subcategories that may provide some of the beneficial effects associated with high-fiber diets. Fiber supplements usually contain only one type of fiber, such as psyllium or cellulose, and none of the nutrients found in high-fiber foods, although some can help with regulating laxation and lowering cholesterol. High-fiber foods like fruits and vegetables also contain other beneficial phytochemicals.

## Good Sources of Fiber

### *Grains*

|  | Grams of Fiber per Serving |
|---|---|
| Kellogg's All Bran ($1/2$ cup) | 10 |
| Nabisco 100% Bran ($1/2$ cup) | 12 |
| General Mills Fiber One ($1/2$ cup) | 13 |
| oatmeal, cooked (1 cup) | 4 |
| Wheatena, cooked ($3/4$ cup) | 5 |

| | |
|---|---|
| whole wheat bread (2 slices) | 3.5 |
| pumpernickel bread (2 slices) | 4 |
| whole wheat pita bread (1 each) | 5 |
| whole wheat tortilla | 3 |
| bran muffin (medium, 2¹/₂ ounces) | 4 |
| brown rice, cooked (1 cup) | 3.5 |
| basmati rice, cooked (1 cup) | 2.5 |
| wild rice, cooked (1 cup) | 3 |
| amaranth, cooked (¹/₂ cup) | 4 |
| barley, cooked (¹/₂ cup) | 3 |
| bulgur, cooked (¹/₂ cup) | 4 |
| couscous, cooked (1 cup) | 2.5 |
| hominy grits, yellow, regular, cooked (1 cup) | 8 |
| millet, cooked (1 cup) | 3 |
| pasta, cooked (1¹/₂ cups) | 3.5 |
| polenta, cooked (³/₄ cup) | 3 |

## Beans (¹/₂ cup, cooked)

| | |
|---|---|
| adzuki | 6 |
| black | 8 |
| chickpeas or garbanzo | 5 |
| fava | 5 |
| kidney, red | 7 |
| lentils | 7 |
| lima | 7 |
| mung | 8 |
| navy | 7 |
| pinto | 7 |
| soybeans | 5 |
| white (Great Northern and cannellini) | 6 |

## Fruits (1 medium item=serving, unless indicated)

| | |
|---|---|
| apple, with skin | 3 |
| banana | 2 |
| blueberries (1 cup) | 3 |
| cantaloupe, cubed (1 cup) | 1.5 |
| cherries, pitted (20) | 4 |

| | |
|---|---|
| figs (2) | 3 |
| grapefruit ($^1/_2$) | 1 |
| grapes (1$^1/_2$ cups) | 2 |
| kiwi | 2.5 |
| mango, pitted ($^1/_2$) | 2 |
| nectarine | 2 |
| orange | 2 |
| peach | 1.5 |
| pear | 4 |
| pineapple ($^3/_4$ cup) | 1.5 |
| plums (2) | 2 |
| prunes, uncooked (3) | 1.5 |
| raisins ($^1/_4$ cup) | 1.5 |
| raspberries (1 cup) | 6 |
| strawberries (1$^1/_4$ cups) | 3 |
| tomato, raw | 1.5 |

## Vegetables ($^1/_2$ cup cooked, unless indicated)

| | |
|---|---|
| asparagus | 2 |
| broccoli | 2 |
| Brussels sprouts | 3 |
| butternut squash | 3 |
| cabbage | 2 |
| carrots | 3 |
| carrots, raw, shredded (1 cup) | 3 |
| cauliflower | 1.5 |
| corn | 2 |
| eggplant | 1 |
| green beans | 1.5 |
| iceberg lettuce, raw (1 cup) | 0.5 |
| kale | 1.5 |
| peas | 3 |
| potato, with skin (1 medium) | 4 |
| pumpkin, mashed | 3 |
| rutabagas | 2 |
| spinach | 1.5 |
| sweet potato, without skin | 2 |
| Swiss chard | 2 |

| | |
|---|---|
| turnips | 1.5 |
| zucchini | 1 |

## Bean Basics

Beans are a nearly perfect food. As a source of carbohydrate, they are "complex," and are therefore more slowly digested and absorbed, making them an ideal carbohydrate. They are a great source of protein, providing 7 to 9 grams per $1/2$ cup, and most varieties contain only a trace amount of fat. Beans are loaded with fiber, ranging from 5 to 8 grams per $1/2$ cup, depending on the variety. The B vitamins, thiamin, niacin, $B_6$, and folate, and important minerals, such as iron, calcium, phosphorus, and potassium, are abundant in most types of beans. The iron in beans is more readily absorbed when beans are accompanied by vitamin C–rich foods, such as tomatoes, potatoes, peppers, broccoli, and citrus fruit or juices.

Beans contain insoluble fiber, the kind that promotes regularity and lowers risk of colon cancer, and soluble fiber, the type that is helpful for lowering blood cholesterol and controlling blood glucose. Many types of beans also contain the same cancer-protective phytochemicals (isoflavones, plant sterols, and protease inhibitors) that are found in soybeans.

Like most high-fiber foods, beans are useful for weight control. They are slowly absorbed and have the capacity to draw and hold water in the stomach and the gut, producing a feeling of fullness and delaying the return of hunger. Additionally, they add weight and volume to food without many added calories. By weight, an ounce of cheese provides approximately 100 calories, an ounce of beans, 40 calories.

Some people avoid beans for any or all of the following reasons: beans cause flatulence or gas, beans take too long to cook, and/or people do not know what to do with them. However, all of these problems have solutions.

**Preventing gas from beans.** The complex sugars in beans, oligosaccharides, cannot be digested by the human gut. In the lower intestine these molecules encounter the resident bacteria that eat the oligosaccharides and, as part of their own metabolic process, give off various gases. Flatulence is more often a problem with people who eat beans infrequently; it becomes less of a problem for those who eat beans regularly. If you do not tolerate beans well, start with small doses, such as the amount you might sprinkle on a salad, and slowly work your way up.

Some cooking methods may also decrease the likelihood of flatulence. Cook beans thoroughly; uncooked starch is much harder to digest and can result in gas and bloating. Cooked beans should mash easily when pressed between two fingers.

The U.S. Department of Agriculture (USDA) recommends the following solution to minimize flatulence from beans: use 9 cups of water for each cup of beans, and soak for four to five hours. Before beans are soaked, they should be rinsed and sorted to remove any grit, pebbles, or broken pieces. The process of soaking beans softens and rehydrates them and breaks down the oligosaccharides. Lentils, split peas, and black-eyed peas generally do not need soaking. Discard the soaking water and add 9 cups of fresh water, then cook for a half hour and drain; if the beans are not completely cooked (most types won't be), add fresh water, cook again, and drain once more. This technique works, but it can be tedious and can also wash away some of the water-soluble nutrients.

Changing the soaking water frequently (two to three times) is an alternative to the USDA method. Draining and adding fresh tap water after each soaking should degrade the oligosaccharides. Rinse the beans after they have been soaked and do not cook the beans with the soaking liquid. To minimize gas and reduce sodium when using canned beans, rinse after draining. Adding baking soda or salt to beans when they soak or cook toughens the beans and, in the case of baking soda, destroys some nutrients.

**Soaking and cooking beans.** On average, most beans need to soak for four hours (with two to three water changes). Exceptions are soybeans and fava, or broad beans, which should be soaked overnight. Although a few more nutrients are lost, there are ways to cut soaking times by two and a half to three hours. Simply place rinsed and picked-over beans in a large saucepan and cover with 3 inches of unsalted water. Bring to a boil and continue for ten minutes. Drain the beans and cover with 3 inches of cold water. Soak for thirty minutes. Drain and discard water, rinse, and proceed to cook beans in fresh water.

In general, beans double their volume in cooking. One cup of most dried beans will yield 2 to 2$^{1}/_{2}$ cups cooked (approximately four portions for a side dish). The exceptions are soybeans and chickpeas, which triple their volume.

### Cooking Times for Beans after Four Hours of Soaking

| Type | Cooking | Pressure Cooking |
| --- | --- | --- |
| adzuki | 1 hour | 15 minutes |
| black | 1$^{1}/_{2}$ hours | 15 minutes |
| black-eyed peas* | 45 minutes | 10 minutes |
| chickpeas (garbanzos) | 2–2$^{1}/_{2}$ hours | 25 minutes |
| fava beans† | 3 hours | 40 minutes |
| Great Northern | 1 hour | 20 minutes |
| kidney | 1 hour | 20 minutes |
| lentils, brown* | 35 minutes | not appropriate |
| lentils, green* | 40 minutes | not appropriate |
| lentils, red* | 30 minutes | not appropriate |
| lima | 1–1$^{1}/_{2}$ hours | 20 minutes |

| | | |
|---|---|---|
| mung | 1 hour | not appropriate |
| navy | 1½–2 hours | 25 minutes |
| peas, split* | 30 minutes | not appropriate |
| peas, whole | 45 minutes | 15 minutes |
| pink | 1 hour | 20 minutes |
| pinto | 1–1½ hours | 20 minutes |
| soybeans† | 3–3½ hours | 30 minutes |
| white (cannellini) | 1 hour | 20 minutes |

*Do not require soaking.
†Require twelve hours of soaking.

If soaking and cooking beans just does not fit into your schedule, do not skip the beans. Try a good-quality canned bean. Avoid brands that list preservatives, added salt, and/or sugar in the ingredients. Remember to drain and rinse before using.

## USES

- Sprinkle chickpeas, pinto beans, or black beans over a salad.
- Prepare bean puree soups using black beans or white beans. Other soups that include beans, but are not typically pureed, include minestrone, lentil, and pasta e fagioli.
- Use beans (canned are great too) to add texture, flavor, fiber, and protein to other soups, stews, chilis, and casseroles.
- Add beans to pasta or rice.
- Puree beans to replace other high-fat sauces.
- Top bruschetta or toasted bread with bean salsas.
- Prepare or purchase lightly dressed bean salads.
- Make vegetarian terrines or pâtés.
- Prepare bean spreads to replace butter or high-fat dips. Some ideas include white bean spread, bean dips made with pinto beans, jalapeños, and spices, or hummus (see Healthy Hummus, page 115).

## Fluids

It is important that you remember to drink enough fluid with your fiber-rich diet. Unless you have a medical condition that limits fluid intake, a minimum of eight 8-ounce glasses daily is recommended. This should help move the fiber through your intestinal tract and prevent constipation, gas, and discomfort. Do not count caffeinated or alcoholic beverages toward your fluid goals. They are diuretics and will actually set you back. Limit high-calorie, nutrient-empty beverages, such as soda and "fruit drinks" that contain little or no fruit, and moderate your intake of caffeine-free diet sodas, sugar-free iced teas, lemonades, and fruit drinks that contain artificial sweeteners. Save room for more nutritious beverages. Some beverage ideas include:

- Water (spring, mineral, or seltzer)
- Milk (nonfat or 1 percent regular or soy milk)
- All natural juices (if you do not squeeze your own juice or use a juicer, read labels to make sure that you are actually buying 100 percent juice, not a "fruit drink" that may contain only 10 percent real juice). If you are watching your weight, go easy on fruit juices and instead try vegetables juices, which have fewer calories. Another option is to "spritz" or add fruit juice to a glass of seltzer or carbonated mineral water. Limit the amount of juices that you count as fruit and/or vegetable servings. Although they are nutritious, they contain slightly less vitamins, minerals, and phytochemicals, and do not have nearly the amount of fiber as whole fruit and vegetables.
- Decaffeinated coffees and teas

Green teas, and to a lesser extent black teas, also contain flavonoids, catechins, and theaflavins, which may play a role in cancer prevention. Green tea is consumed mostly in Asian countries; Americans generally consume black tea. Lower rates of certain types of cancer in Asian populations are thought to be partially a result of green tea consumption. Green tea is made by steaming or drying tea leaves at high temperature with little processing. This heating stops the process that would inactivate polyphenols. Phytochemicals are potent antioxidants and may promote enzymes that rid the body of carcinogens. Black tea leaves are exposed to the air and allowed to ferment or oxidize for several hours (but still contain polyphenols). When brewing tea, be sure to let it steep for at least 3 1/2 minutes to get the full concentration. When shopping for tea, be sure the ingredients on the label list "tea" first. Iced, powdered, or bottled tea is okay, but these can be laden with sugar.

Coffee consumption is not linked to an increased risk of cancer. In fact, coffee contains caffeic and ferulic acids (other types of plant polyphenols) that may have a role in cancer prevention. Still, moderate your coffee drinking, because excessive caffeine intake can lead to loss of calcium in urine.

# The Importance of Fruits and Vegetables

Numerous studies have found a lower incidence of cancer among people who eat large amounts of fruits and vegetables. While it is not yet clear what nutrients or substances or what mechanisms may be responsible for this health-promoting effect there are several theories being studied. Nutrients such as vitamin C, vitamin A and related substances, or vitamin E may offer protection through their antioxidant properties. Other components like fiber or plant substances (phytochemicals) may have a beneficial effect. An important extra benefit of vitamin-rich foods is that they provide minerals, calcium, zinc, and iron, which may be associated with a decreased risk of cancer. These minerals are also vital for good health because they play a known role in the prevention of diseases such as anemia and osteoporosis.

It is likely that increasing fruits and vegetables will decrease the intake of fat-containing foods and thus have a favorable effect on obesity and coronary heart disease. A great deal of research is going on to determine how fruits and vegetables confer their health benefits. One thing is certain: a wide variety of fruits and vegetables (a total of five or more servings per day) will be beneficial to your health.

Most vegetables are excellent sources of vitamins A and C, yet dark-green leafy vegetables like spinach, romaine, and kale—and yellow, orange, and red vegetables—are among the most valuable. Citrus fruits and juices and virtually all summer fruits are good sources of these vitamins.

Vegetables from the cabbage patch (cruciferous vegetables) also may reduce cancer risk. They are good sources of fiber as well as important vitamins and minerals. Several servings each week of this type of vegetable (Brussels sprouts, cabbage, broccoli, cauliflower, rutabagas, and turnips) are part of a healthy diet.

Five to nine fruit and vegetable servings may sound like a lot, but it really is not difficult to get within this range. To determine if you are close you must first know what a serving is.

## ONE VEGETABLE SERVING EQUALS

- 1 cup of raw leafy vegetables such as spinach, lettuce varieties (dark in color), escarole, Swiss chard, collard greens, cabbage, or other leafy greens. For these vegetables, cooked, a serving equals 1/2 cup.
- 1/2 cup of other vegetables, raw or cooked, including broccoli, carrots, cauliflower, peppers, green beans, or squash
- 3/4 cup vegetable juice (such as carrot or tomato)*
- 1 medium potato or sweet potato
- 5 to 6 asparagus spears
- 1 medium tomato

ONE FRUIT SERVING EQUALS

- 1 medium apple, orange, pear, or peach
- 1 small banana
- 2 medium plums, figs, or tangerines
- $1/3$ cantaloupe
- $1/8$ honeydew melon
- 15 small grapes or cherries
- $1/2$ cup cut-up raw, cooked, or canned fruit
- $3/4$ cup raspberries, blueberries
- 8 large strawberries or $1^1/4$ cups
- $1/4$ cup dried fruit
- $3/4$ cup (6 fluid ounces) fruit juice*

---

*Your fruit and vegetable intake should include:*
- One vitamin A–rich selection daily
- One vitamin C–rich selection daily
- At least one high-fiber (greater than 5 grams per serving) selection daily
- Several servings each week of cabbage family (cruciferous) vegetables

---

## 25 Tips to Help You Meet Your Daily Fruit and Vegetable Goal

**1.** Add more vegetables and less meat to recipes for soups, stews, casseroles, stir-fries, burritos, or pastas, such as lasagne.

**2.** Make vegetables the entrée and meat and starches the side dishes.

**3.** Add more vegetables to store-bought sauces or soups.

**4.** Use grilled, roasted, or raw vegetable slices on sandwiches.

**5.** Puree cooked vegetables and use them as sauces or add them to risotto to increase flavor and creaminess.

**6.** Try vegetable puree soups.

**7.** Add fruit to breakfast cereals.

**8.** Have fruit juice for breakfast and a fruit snack each day.

**9.** Make fruits and vegetables visible. Leave fresh fruit out in bowls on tabletops. Place cut and washed vegetables, such as carrots, pepper slices or rings, broccoli, or cauliflower florets in air-tight, see-through containers in the refrigerator (add a little water to the bottom if you plan to keep them more than one day).

*Limit the number of servings counted from juices because they have much less fiber compared with whole fruits or vegetables. For diabetics, fruit juice portion sizes are considered $1/2$ cup due to the high content of natural sugar.

10. Keep dried, frozen, and canned fruits and vegetables on hand for busy days.

11. If you eat convenience frozen foods, supplement the meal with a tossed green salad and a fruit dessert (choose dark green lettuce leaves when possible).

12. Expand your use of unfamiliar vegetables, such as broccoli rabe, collard greens, kale, and tropical fruits, such as mango, papaya, or kiwi.

13. If you do not like a particular vegetable, try a different cooking method. For example, if you don't like turnips, try oven-roasting turnips with other vegetables or mashing them with potatoes.

14. Add fruit to yogurt or "blenderize" them together to make fruit "smoothies."

15. Try ethnic cuisines, such as Mediterranean, Middle Eastern, or Asian, that use lots of fruits and vegetables.

16. Shred vegetable scraps you might ordinarily throw away. Use them in casseroles, stir-fries, soups, or slaws or make a vegetable stock with them.

17. Add dried or grated fruits and vegetables to baked goods, such as muffins or quick breads.

18. Serve entrées with fruit or vegetable chutneys, compotes, or relishes.

19. Use fruit and vegetable salsas or relishes on sandwiches.

20. Add fruits and vegetables to salads (see Healthy Tuna Salad, page 161).

21. Select or prepare desserts with fruit or fruit coulis (or sauces).

22. Top pizza with vegetable combinations and cut back on the cheese.

23. Top pancakes or French toast with fresh berries or fruit compote rather than butter and syrup.

24. Make omelets using 1 whole egg plus 2 egg whites per serving. Add fresh or leftover cooked vegetables, such as broccoli, spinach, asparagus, peppers, onions, and tomatoes.

25. Munch on fresh-cut vegetables while making dinner so that you are not tempted to reach for chips.

## Your plate should look like this . . .

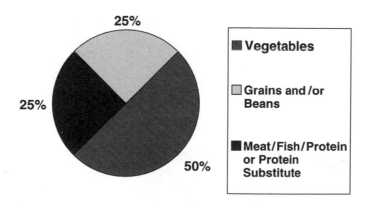

25%

25%

50%

- Vegetables
- Grains and/or Beans
- Meat/Fish/Protein or Protein Substitute

## Carotenoids in Fruits and Vegetables

Numerous foods contain carotenoids, including many plant species. A high intake of carotenoids is linked to a decreased risk of many types of cancer. Of the more than six hundred identified carotenoids, the amounts found in foods are known for only a select few, such as beta-carotene, alpha-carotene, beta-cryptoxanthin, lycopene, and lutein. The others exist in foods, lending pigment, and in some cases fragrance; however, their values have yet to be measured and there is no recommended dietary allowance for the various carotenoids. Fortunately, numerical values are not necessary for the individual trying to include more carotenoids in his or her diet. Selecting from a variety of colorful fruits and vegetables and eating the recommended five to nine servings per day is all you need to do. The list below is not exhaustive but does give numerous examples of fruits and vegetables containing significant amounts of carotenoids.

### Carotene Food Sources

apricots
arugula
basil, fresh
beets and beet greens
broccoli
broccoli rabe
cantaloupe
carrots
cherries
chicory greens
collard greens
coriander, fresh
corn
dandelion greens
dill, fresh
grapefruit, pink and red
guava
kale
lettuce, mâche
lettuce, red leaf
lettuce, romaine
mango

mint, fresh
mustard greens
nectarine
papaya
parsley, fresh
peaches
peas, green
peppers, all types
plums
rosemary, fresh
scallions
seaweed
spinach
squash, all winter varieties:
    acorn, butternut, delicata, golden
    nugget, hubbard, pumpkin,
    spaghetti, and more
squash, summer
squash, zucchini
sweet potatoes
Swiss chard, red and green
turnip greens

# Vitamins and Minerals

The Food and Nutrition Board of the National Research Council, an arm of the National Academy of Sciences, has developed nutrition recommendations since 1943. They are revised approximately every five years to reflect the latest nutrition research. The Food and Nutrition Board sets the Recommended Dietary Allowances (RDAs) for most vitamins and minerals based upon the nutritional requirements of the majority (97 to 98 percent) of the healthy population. There are no RDAs for carbohydrates or fat because needs are based on individual caloric requirements. There are also no RDAs for some vitamins and minerals that are essential to humans, because information about requirements is unavailable at this time. The RDAs have sometimes been criticized because they are primarily set at levels to prevent deficiency of vitamins and minerals and do not address the levels needed for prevention of disease. The Food and Nutrition Board has indicated that the prevention of chronic disease should be considered in the formulation of future RDAs. To date, the RDAs are the best standard for nutrition assessment of diet adequacy and are used as the basis for the Daily Values listed on the packaging labels of most foods and multivitamin supplements.

Most healthy people can meet the RDAs for their age and sex without supplementation. Vitamin and mineral supplementation *may* be required in some of these circumstances:

- Some vegetarians may not receive adequate calcium, iron, zinc, and/or $B_{12}$.
- People over sixty-five years old may require $B_{12}$ supplementation, because production of stomach acid (needed to extract and absorb $B_{12}$ from food) diminishes with age. Also, $B_{12}$ supplementation may be indicated in older people who have difficulty meeting their caloric requirements and have lower intakes of protein food sources containing $B_{12}$.
- People with low caloric intakes frequently consume diets that do not meet their nutritional needs for all nutrients. Intake of fewer than 1,200 calories per day should be medically supervised and generally requires a multivitamin and mineral supplement.
- Women who are pregnant or breast-feeding need more of certain nutrients, especially iron, folic acid, and calcium. At present, iron supplementation during pregnancy is practiced routinely in the United States. Two expert committees have called for more research to assess if iron supplementation should occur routinely during pregnancy or be evaluated on an individual basis.
- Certain disorders and diseases and some medications may interfere with nutrient intake, digestion, absorption, metabolism, or excretion and thus change requirements and/or make supplementation necessary. Check with your doctor.

- Newborns are given, under the direction of a physician, a single dose of vitamin K.
- Women with excessive menstrual bleeding may need to take iron supplements.
- People with limited milk intake and sunlight exposure may need vitamin D supplements.
- Calcium supplementation may be appropriate in some individuals, especially women.

Antioxidants such as vitamins C, E, and A, as well as many other substances in plants (phytochemicals), help to destroy or neutralize free radicals that have been implicated in cancer and heart disease, thereby protecting healthy cells. Although the evidence is not conclusive that vitamin and mineral supplements protect against cancer, the following supplements are considered safe for those people who occasionally do not have proper nutrition or who want a measure of added insurance.

## Vitamin C

Vitamin C seems to protect against some types of cancer, and supplementation up to 250 milligrams is considered safe for most people; however, a small segment of the population is at risk for kidney stones and iron overload with high intakes of vitamin C. Additionally, high doses of vitamin C can result in false negatives on fecal occult blood tests for colon cancer screening. Though the optimal level of vitamin C may exceed the current RDA (60 mg), research shows no benefit with vitamin C levels greater than 400 mg. Eating five fruit and vegetable servings per day will meet (and likely exceed by at least double) the RDA. For most people there is no danger and potentially some benefit to supplementing vitamin C. Keep dosages to under 400 mg per day.

### Vitamin C Sources in Fruits and Vegetables*

| *Best Sources* | milligrams (mg) |
|---|---|
| avocado, Florida, 1 medium | 24 |
| blackberries, raw, 1 cup | 30 |
| broccoli, boiled, 1/2 cup | 58 |
| Brussels sprouts, boiled, 1/2 cup | 48 |
| cabbage, red, cooked, 1/2 cup | 26 |

*Nutrient values obtained from Pennington, J. A. T., *Bowes & Church's Food Values of Portions Commonly Used* (16th ed.), J. B. Lippincott Company, 1994.

| | |
|---|---|
| cauliflower, boiled, 1/2 cup | 34 |
| chicory greens, raw, chopped, 1/2 cup | 22 |
| currants, European, black, 1/2 cup | 101 |
| elderberries, raw, 1 cup | 52 |
| grapefruit, pink and red, 1/2 medium | 47 |
| grapefruit juice, fresh, 8 fl. oz. | 60 |
| guava, raw, 1 medium | 165 |
| kale, boiled, 1/2 cup | 27 |
| kiwi, raw, 1 medium | 75 |
| lemon, raw, 1 medium | 31 |
| lime, raw, 1 medium | 20 |
| mango, 1 medium | 57 |
| orange, raw, navel, 1 medium | 80 |
| orange juice, fresh, 8 fl. oz. | 124 |
| papaya, raw, 1 medium | 188 |
| parsley, raw, chopped, 1/2 cup | 40 |
| peppers, bell, green, raw, 1/2 cup chopped | 45 |
| peppers, bell, red, raw, 1/2 cup chopped | 95 |
| peppers, bell, yellow, 1/2 large | 170 |
| peppers, hot chili, raw, 1 pepper | 109 |
| pineapple, raw, 1 cup pieces | 24 |
| potato, baked with skin, 1 potato | 26 |
| raspberries, raw, 1 cup | 31 |
| seaweed, laver (nori), raw, 3.5 oz. | 39 |
| snowpeas, frozen, 3 oz. | 24 |
| strawberries, raw, 1 cup | 85 |
| sweet potato, baked with skin, 1 | 28 |
| tomato, red, raw, 1 | 24 |
| tomato juice, 6 fl. oz. | 33 |
| turnip greens, boiled, 1/2 cup | 20 |

### Good Sources

| | |
|---|---|
| apricots, raw, 3 medium | 11 |
| artichoke, boiled, 1 medium | 12 |
| asparagus, 1/2 cup (6 spears) | 10 |
| banana, peeled | 10 |
| blueberries, raw, 1 cup | 19 |
| chard, Swiss, boiled, 1/2 cup | 16 |
| collard greens, boiled, 1 cup | 15 |

| | |
|---|---|
| cranberries, whole, 1 cup | 13 |
| fennel bulb, raw, 1 cup slices | 11 |
| mustard greens, boiled, 1/2 cup | 18 |
| okra, boiled, 1/2 cup slices | 13 |
| peas, green, boiled, 1/2 cup | 11 |
| persimmon, Japanese, raw, 1 medium | 13 |
| rutabagas, boiled, 1/2 cup cubes | 19 |
| soybeans, green, boiled, 1/2 cup | 15 |
| spinach, boiled, 1/2 cup | 9 |
| squash, butternut, boiled, 1/2 cup | 15 |

## Vitamin E

Vitamin E supplementation from 100 to 400 international units (IU), a level too difficult to get even with the most healthy diets, is generally considered safe and may decrease the risk of heart disease. Individuals who take vitamin E supplements are also at lower risk for certain types of cancer. For some people, the effect of vitamin E on blood clotting might interfere with a medication's intended benefit. Vitamin E supplementation should be kept between 100 and 400 IU. It is prudent to discuss vitamin E supplementation with your physician.

### Vitamin E Food Sources*

| *Best Sources* | milligrams (mg) *alpha-tocopherol* |
|---|---|
| almonds, dried, 1 oz. | 6.7 |
| almond oil, 1 tablespoon | 5.3 |
| breakfast cereals | † |
| cottonseed oil, 1 tablespoon | 4.8 |
| hazelnuts, 1 oz. | 4.4 |
| margarine, Mazola | 8.0 |
| mayonnaise, Best Foods/Hellmann's, 1 tablespoon | 11.0 |
| rice bran oil, 1 tablespoon | 4.4 |

*Nutrient values obtained from Pennington, J. A. T., *Bowes & Church's Food Values of Portions Commonly Used* (16th ed.), J. B. Lippincott Company, 1994.

†Levels of fortification vary.

*Green leafy vegetables, such as spinach, Swiss chard, kale, turnip greens, and seaweed kelp are fair sources of vitamin E, providing 0.5 to 1 mg of alpha-tocopherol per 1 cup (raw) serving.

| | |
|---|---|
| safflower oil, 1 tablespoon | 4.6 |
| sunflower seeds/kernels, dried, 1 oz. | 14.2 |
| sweet potato, raw, 1 medium | 5.9 |
| wheat germ, 1/4 cup | 4.0 |
| wheat germ oil, 1 tablespoon | 20.3 |

*Good Sources*

| | |
|---|---|
| asparagus, raw, 4 spears | 1.2 |
| avocado, raw, 1/2 medium | 2.3 |
| Brazil nuts, dried, 1 oz. | 2.1 |
| corn oil, 1 tablespoon | 1.9 |
| mango, 1 medium | 2.3 |
| olive oil, 1 tablespoon | 1.7 |
| peanut butter, 2 tablespoons | 3.0 |
| peanut oil, 1 tablespoon | 1.6 |
| peanuts, dried, 1 oz. | 2.6 |
| pistachios, dried, 1 oz. | 1.5 |
| rye flour, dark, 1 cup | 1.8 |
| soybean oil, 1 tablespoon | 1.5 |
| soy mayonnaise, 1 tablespoon | 2.9 |

## Vitamin A

Vitamin A has many forms. Most of our vitamin A comes from plant sources. Carotenes are a group of pigments ranging from yellow to orange found in fruits and vegetables like carrots, cantaloupe, and spinach (in many deep-green vegetables the chlorophyll masks the orange pigment). Beta-carotene is the most important relative to vitamin A activity, and is called a vitamin A precursor because it is converted to the vitamin in the body. Preformed vitamin A, or retinol, is the natural, active form found in animal products, such as eggs, liver, and other organ meats. Retinol equivalents (RE) is the preferred measure of vitamin A activity, because it takes into account the biological activity, the bioavailability or ability of the body to convert and use it, and the many forms of vitamin A. Vitamin A may be protective against certain types of cancer.

A man's RDA for vitamin A is 1,000 RE and a woman's is 800 RE. The beta-carotene and other carotenoids in one sweet potato provide 2490 RE. Vitamin A deficiency is rarely seen in countries where food is abundant or foods have been fortified.

Active vitamin A or retinol is fat soluble and can therefore be stored in the body. Two recent studies have demonstrated that vitamin A (retinol) toxicity can occur at levels lower than previously thought. In one study, levels of vitamin A at 25,000 IU over a period of time caused liver damage. Toxicity is particularly a concern for women of child-bearing years. In a large study, pregnant women who were taking more than 10,000 IU (the amount found in some multivitamin formulas) of preformed (active) vitamin A had a significantly higher risk of spontaneous abortions and birth defects in their infants.

Do not take single vitamin A supplements, particularly if you eat a lot of vitamin A–rich foods. If you take a multivitamin and mineral formula, be sure the vitamin A source is less than 5,000 IU or predominantly or completely in the form of precursor vitamin A (beta-carotene).

1 RE = 3.33 IU = 1 microgram retinol = 6 micrograms beta-carotene

## Vitamin A in Fruits and Vegetables*

| Best Sources | retinol equivalents (RE) |
|---|---|
| apricots, raw, 3 medium | 277 |
| broccoli, boiled, 1/2 cup | 108 |
| Brussels sprouts, boiled, 1/2 cup | 56 |
| cantaloupe, raw, 1 cup pieces | 516 |
| carrots, boiled, 1/2 cup | 1915 |
| chard, Swiss, boiled, 1/2 cup | 276 |
| chicory greens, raw, 1/2 cup chopped | 360 |
| collard greens, boiled, 1/2 cup | 349 |
| guava, raw, 1 medium | 71 |
| kale, boiled, 1/2 cup | 481 |
| mango, raw, 1 medium | 806 |
| papaya, raw, 1 medium | 612 |
| parsley, raw, 1/2 cup chopped | 156 |
| persimmon, Japanese, 1 medium | 364 |
| pumpkin, canned, 1/2 cup | 2691 |
| pumpkin, boiled, 1/2 cup mashed | 132 |
| seaweed, laver (nori), raw, 3.5 oz. | 520 |
| spinach, boiled, 1/2 cup | 737 |
| spinach, raw, 1 cup chopped | 376 |
| squash, acorn, baked, 1/2 cup cubes | 44 |
| squash, butternut, boiled, 1/2 cup | 714 |

*Nutrient values obtained from Pennington, J. A. T., *Bowes & Church's Food Values of Portions Commonly Used* (16th ed.), J. B. Lippincott Company, 1994.

| | |
|---|---|
| squash, hubbard, baked, $1/2$ cup cubes | 616 |
| sweet potato, baked with skin, 1 medium | 2488 |
| tomato, red, raw, 1 medium | 77 |
| turnip greens, boiled, $1/2$ cup | 396 |
| watermelon, raw, 1 cup | 58 |

*Good Sources*

| | |
|---|---|
| arugula, raw, 1 cup | 48 |
| asparagus, boiled, $1/2$ cup (6 spears) | 48 |
| cherries, raw, 20 each | 30 |
| corn, yellow, boiled, $1/2$ cup | 18 |
| grapefruit, pink and red, $1/2$ medium | 32 |
| okra, boiled, $1/2$ cup slices | 46 |
| peas, green, boiled, $1/2$ cup | 48 |
| plum, raw, 1 each | 21 |
| peppers, sweet, raw, $1/2$ cup chopped | 32 |
| peppers, bell, yellow, $1/2$ large | 44 |
| peppers, hot chili, raw, 1 pepper | 35 |

## Beta-Carotene

Beta-carotene is probably the most well known carotenoid. As mentioned previously, the body regulates the conversion of beta-carotene to vitamin A. Only 10 percent of the more than six hundred carotenoids have the ability to be converted to active vitamin A. Unlike vitamin A (retinol), beta-carotene is nontoxic even in large amounts. Studies strongly link diets high in beta-carotene and other carotenoid-containing foods to lower risk of certain types of cancer. The same may not be true for supplements. Numerous large and expensive studies have tried to link beta-carotene supplementation to lower risk of cancer. None has demonstrated such a relationship; in fact, an increased risk has been observed in smokers who take beta-carotene supplements. Considering these results, it is wise that smokers not take, or discontinue, beta-carotene supplements. For those who have not been able to quit smoking, the daily diet should contain an adequate amount of fruits and vegetables, because a diet high in fruits and vegetables has been linked to a decreased risk of lung cancer. (See "Vitamins and Minerals" in chapter 1 for more information on studies of beta-carotene and cancer risk.)

The amount of beta-carotene found in most multivitamins is generally less than amounts found to be potentially harmful and are considered to be acceptable. It is not prudent to megadose with a single carotenoid like beta-carotene, because it may undermine the importance of the many other carotenoids. Carotenoids are abundant in many fruits and vegetables and while only some of them can be converted to vitamin A, the remainder belong to an important group of food substances called phytochemicals that appear to have cancer-fighting properties. It is possible that beta-carotene and other precursor carotenoids provide cancer protection only in the presence of other phytochemical substances in fruits and vegetables that are not found in pills.

Evidence does not support a cancer-protective effect of beta-carotene supplements, but if you supplement beta-carotene individually or as part of an antioxidant formula, keep the dosage at around 6 to 9 mg (10,000 to 15,000 IU or 3,000 to 4,500 RE) daily. If you take a multivitamin and mineral formula, beta-carotene is the safest and preferred vitamin A source.

$$1 \text{ mg beta-carotene} = 1,000 \text{ mcg} = 1,666.7 \text{ IU vitamin A}$$

## Selenium

Selenium RDAs were established for the first time in 1989. Selenium is an antioxidant that can help prevent destruction of fat and cell membranes, and may block the action of some cancer-causing substances. Over the last thirty years studies in laboratory animals have demonstrated the ability of selenium to protect against many types of cancer, including cancers of the breast and esophagus. A recent ten-year study in which six hundred people took 200 micrograms (mcg) of selenium supplements daily, failed to demonstrate a protective effect against skin cancer, but researchers did observe a reduction in other cancer rates by about one-half. Selenium may also play a role in increasing "good" HDL cholesterol, which protects against heart disease. Although the research is encouraging, it is too premature to recommend selenium supplements at this time.

Toxicity is a real concern and has been seen with intakes as low as fifteen times the RDA. The Food and Nutrition Board of the National Academy of Sciences regards a total daily intake of 50 to 200 mcg as safe and adequate, and has established the RDA for selenium at 55 mcg daily for adult women and 70 mcg daily for adult men. The typical American diet provides this amount. Selenium is found most abundantly in animal protein foods, such as fish, meats, and poultry. Various plant foods, such as some minimally processed grains, nuts, legumes, and fruits and vegetables, contain significant amounts. Brazil nuts sold in their shells are an extraordinary source of selenium: two nuts can provide more than the RDA.

It is too early to make general recommendations for selenium supplementation, but don't worry about the 25 to 200 mcg that may be in a multivitamin supplement, and be sure to include selenium-rich foods in your diet. If you do supplement selenium, do not exceed 200 mcg daily; more is not better. The organic form of the supplement that contains selenium-enriched yeast is most similar to the kind found in food, and is the type used in recent research studies.

## Selenium Food Sources*

### Best Sources

| | |
|---|---|
| bass | molasses |
| beef | oysters |
| Brazil nuts | peanuts and peanut butter |
| cashews | red snapper |
| clams | salmon |
| cod | sunflower seeds |
| eggs | swordfish |
| haddock | tuna |
| lobster | turkey |
| mackerel | |

### Good Sources

| | |
|---|---|
| barley | navy beans |
| breakfast cereals (some) | oat bran |
| broccoli | ocean perch |
| brown rice | organ meats: liver, kidney, etc. |
| chicken | pasta |
| coconut | pinto beans |
| crab | pork |
| flounder/sole | rye flour |
| garlic | scallops |
| halibut | shrimp |
| lamb | soybeans |
| lentils | veal |
| mushrooms | |

*Selenium content of the growing soil is directly related to the amount found in plant foods. Levels of selenium in animal products depend on the quantity of these plants the animals consumed in their diet. The wide variation limits the information available in databases, so values are not provided for these foods.

## Folic Acid

Folic acid or folate (the form of folic acid found in foods) is a B vitamin that may be strongly linked to prevention of certain types of cancer (cervical and colon) and heart disease. Adequate folate intake during pregnancy can prevent birth defects related to the brain and spine. The relationship is so strong that the U.S. Public Health Service recommends that all women of child-bearing age consume 400 micrograms(mcg) of folic acid daily to reduce the incidence of spina bifida and other birth defects. The FDA has authorized use of health claims for food labels about the beneficial effects of folic acid and approved and guided the fortification of cereal and grain products with folate. It is preferable to meet folic acid requirements through diet rather than supplements because foods rich in folate also tend to be high in fiber and other cancer-protective nutrients, such as vitamins A and C. National surveys, however, indicate that the average intake of U.S. women is about 230 mcg. Folate intakes of 400 mcg daily can be met easily with diets rich in fruits, vegetables, grains, and especially some types of beans.

Because folic acid is a water-soluble vitamin that is not stored in the body, toxicity is not a major concern. For this reason, people who doubt the consistent adequacy of their dietary intake should make efforts to consume fortified food products, such as some breakfast cereals, or supplement with folic acid in the form of a multivitamin. Almost all multivitamins now contain 400 mcg of folic acid.

Folic acid can mask $B_{12}$ deficiencies, so be sure you consume $B_{12}$–rich foods (animal products, fortified cereals and beverages, and soy products). For animal products, a little goes a long way: $3^1/2$ ounces of cooked beef provides approximately 100 percent of the RDA for $B_{12}$.

## Folic Acid Food Sources*

| *Best Sources* | micrograms (mcg) |
| --- | --- |
| artichoke, boiled, 1 medium | 61 |
| asparagus, boiled, $1/2$ cup (6 spears) | 132 |
| avocado, Florida, 1 medium | 162 |
| beef liver, braised, 3.5 oz. | 217 |
| black beans, boiled, 1 cup | 256 |
| breakfast cereals (most), 1 cup[†] | 100 |
| Brewer's yeast, 1 tablespoon | 315 |
| chicken liver, simmered, 3.5 oz. | 770 |

*Nutrient values obtained from Pennington, J. A. T., *Bowes & Church's Food Values of Portions Commonly Used* (16th ed.), J. B. Lippincott Company, 1994.

| | |
|---|---|
| chickpeas, boiled, 1 cup | 282 |
| collard greens, frozen, boiled, 1/2 cup | 65 |
| cranberry beans, boiled, 1 cup | 366 |
| French beans, boiled, 1/2 cup | 132 |
| lentils, cooked, 1 cup | 358 |
| lima beans, boiled, 1 cup | 156 |
| pinto beans, boiled, 1 cup | 294 |
| red kidney beans, boiled, 1 cup | 229 |
| romaine lettuce, raw, 1 cup shredded | 76 |
| rye flour, dark, 1 cup | 77 |
| semolina flour, enriched, 1/2 cup | 61 |
| soybean flour, defatted, 1 cup | 305 |
| soybean flour, low-fat | 361 |
| soy nuts, dry roasted, 1/2 cup | 176 |
| spinach, boiled, 1/2 cup | 131 |
| split peas, cooked, 1 cup | 127 |
| sunflower seeds, oil roasted, 1 oz. | 67 |
| turnip greens, boiled, 1/2 cup | 85 |
| wheat germ, toasted, 1/4 cup | 100 |
| white beans, boiled, 1 cup | 145 |

### Good Sources

| | |
|---|---|
| beets, boiled, 1/2 cup slices | 45 |
| broccoli, boiled, 1/2 cup | 39 |
| Brussels sprouts, boiled, 1/2 cup | 47 |
| corn, yellow, boiled, 1/2 cup | 38 |
| endive, raw, 1/2 cup chopped | 36 |
| okra, boiled, 1/2 cup slices | 37 |
| orange, navel, 1 medium | 47 |
| orange juice† | |
| parsley, raw, 1/2 cup chopped | 46 |
| parsnips, boiled, 1/2 cup slices | 45 |
| peas, green, boiled, 1/2 cup | 51 |
| pepper, bell, yellow, 1/2 large | 48 |

†Levels of fortification vary depending on manufacturer.

## Calcium

Although calcium is most often associated with maintenance of the skeletal structure for bones and teeth, a number of other vital bodily functions depend on this important mineral, including blood clotting, muscle contraction and relaxation (particularly the heart), conduction of nerve impulses, and regulation of cell division. If your diet does not supply the proper amount of calcium, your body will automatically make up for the deficiency by drawing it from an emergency source—your bones. If dietary calcium remains inadequate for a prolonged period of years, bone deterioration may develop, which can lead to osteoporosis.

Osteoporosis, a reduction in bone mass or density, occurs more frequently in women than in men, and is particularly prevalent among postmenopausal women. As much as one-third of bone calcium may be lost before the condition is detectable through X-ray diagnosis. In fact, it usually goes undetected until bone fracture occurs, and by then it is usually too late to restore lost bone mass. Quite simply, it is much easier to prevent osteoporosis than it is to treat it, and a diet with the proper levels of calcium—coupled with a regular exercise schedule—is your best protection.

Adequate calcium intake may also protect against salt-sensitive and pregnancy-associated hypertension. High intakes of both dietary calcium and vitamin D (which aids in the absorption of calcium) are associated with reduced development of precancerous changes in the colon. Preliminary findings also suggest that vitamin D may have a protective effect against breast cancer.

Magnesium, another mineral that plays a role in bone building, may be diminished with high calcium intake. It is for this reason that many calcium supplements include magnesium. Magnesium-rich foods include whole grains, legumes, and green leafy vegetables. Preliminary findings support a possible link between adequate magnesium intake and prevention of kidney cancers.

## Calcium Requirements

In August 1997, The Food and Nutrition Board of the National Academy of Sciences released a report on Daily Reference Intakes (DRIs) which will expand and update the current RDAs. The goal of the RDAs is to prevent nutrient deficiency in the population. The DRIs are aimed at setting recommendations at levels to promote optimal health and prevent chronic diseases. Because of their definitive role in maintaining bone health, calcium and vitamin D were among the first nutrients in which recommendations were adjusted.

# New Dietary Reference Intakes for Calcium Issued by the National Research Council, August 1997

| Age | Adequate Intake (mg/day) |
| --- | --- |
| 0–6 months | 210 |
| 6–12 months | 270 |
| 1–3 years | 500 |
| 4–8 years | 800 |
| 9–13 years | 1,300 |
| 14–18 years | 1,300 |
| 19–30 years | 1,000 |
| 31–50 years | 1,000 |
| 51–70 | 1,200 |
| over 70 years | 1,200 |
| *Pregnancy and Lactation* | |
| under–19 years | 1,300 |
| 19–50 | 1,000 |

*Calcium Intake for women at menopause without estrogen replacement should increase towards 1500 mg/day.

All efforts should be made to meet your calcium requirements through dietary intake. Unfortunately, most people do not get enough calcium. On average, current intakes for women are about 600 mg per day. In some cases, it is difficult for people to reach their calcium requirements due to food preferences, intolerance to milk or milk products, and/or the high requirements of some age groups. After checking your calcium requirements, refer to page 74–75 to see the amounts in the foods you eat.

Consider supplementing calcium if you are:

- an adolescent or a young adult (fourteen to eighteen years old) and do not regularly consume four to five milk equivalents per day
- a male or female between the ages of nineteen and fifty or a female fifty to sixty-five who is taking estrogen *and* you do not regularly consume three milk equivalents per day
- a female at menopause who is not undergoing estrogen replacement
- more than fifty-one years old and do not regularly consume four milk equivalents per day
- pregnant or lactating

Certain health conditions preclude calcium supplementation. Check with your physician before supplementing. Though calcium supplementation is safe for the majority of people, there is no need for most people to consume more than 1,500 mg per day.

Drinking milk isn't the only way to get the recommended amount of calcium on a daily basis. A milk equivalent is a food source that may or may not contain milk and provides approximately the same amount of calcium as one milk serving (1 cup). Below are foods that are equivalent to one milk serving.

| | |
|---|---|
| Swiss cheese (1½ oz.) | custard (1 cup) |
| cottage cheese (2 cups) | tofu (8 oz.) |
| Cheddar cheese (1½ oz.) | cooked soybeans (2½ cups) |
| homemade macaroni and cheese (¾ cup) | greens: collards, kale, mustard, turnip (1 cup) |
| yogurt (1 cup) | sardines (6 to 7 medium) |
| ice cream (1½ cups) | salmon with bones (5 oz.) |

Calcium carbonate provides the most calcium per tablet (often 500 to 600 mg) and has the least lead of any calcium supplement (bone meal has the most). For some people, such as the elderly who produce less stomach acid, calcium carbonate is difficult to break down on an empty stomach and should be taken with meals. Calcium carbonate intake has been linked to constipation in some people. If increasing fiber and fluid intake does not help, try calcium citrate, which is as low in lead as calcium carbonate, but contains significantly less calcium per tablet (usually 200 to 300 mg), so you will need to take more to reach your target.

For best absorption, spread your calcium supplementation into at least two doses. If you regularly tend to forget the second dose, take one large dose. Getting in the habit of taking supplements with meals is a good way to remember. Calcium carbonate is best absorbed if taken immediately after eating: Calcium citrate is well absorbed whether taken between or with meals.

| Selected Calcium–rich Foods | | | |
|---|---|---|---|
| Food Item | Serving Size | Calcium Content (mg) | Calories |
| milk, skim lactose-reduced, calcium-fortified | 8 oz. | 302 | 85 |
| milk | 8 oz. | 500 | 90 |
| soy milk plus | 8 oz. | 300 | 150 |
| orange juice, calcium fortified | 8 oz. | 330 | 110 |
| yogurt | | | |
| fruit, low fat | 8 oz. | 343 | 230 |
| plain, low fat | 8 oz. | 415 | 145 |
| cheese | | | |
| mozzarella, part skim | 1 oz. | 207 | 80 |

| | | | |
|---|---|---|---|
| ricotta, part skim | 4 oz. | 335 | 190 |
| cottage, low fat (2%) | 4 oz. | 78 | 103 |
| iced milk, vanilla hard (4% fat) | 1 cup | 176 | 185 |
| soft serve (3% fat) | 1 cup | 274 | 225 |
| fish and shellfish oysters, raw (13–19 medium) | 1 cup | 226 | 160 |
| sardines, canned in oil, drained, including bones | 3 oz. | 372 | 175 |
| salmon, pink, canned, including bones | 3 oz. | 167 | 120 |
| shrimp, canned, drained | 3 oz. | 98 | 100 |
| vegetables bok choy, raw | 1 cup | 74 | 9 |
| broccoli (fresh, cooked, drained) | 1 cup | 136 | 40 |
| broccoli (frozen, cooked, drained) | 1 cup | 100 | 50 |
| soy beans (fresh, cooked, drained) | 1 cup | 131 | 235 |
| collards (fresh, cooked, drained) | 1 cup | 357 | 65 |
| turnips (fresh, cooked, drained) (leaves and stems) | 1 cup | 252 | 30 |
| tofu | 4 oz. | 108* | 85 |

*The calcium content of tofu may vary depending on processing methods. Tofu processed with calcium salts can have as much as 300 mg calcium per 4 ounces. Often, the manufacturer's label can provide more specific information.

**Myth:** Steaming milk for cafe latte or cappuccino destroys calcium or alters it so that it no longer can contribute to reaching your daily calcium goal.

**Fact:** Calcium levels of steamed milk are the same, cup for cup, as regular, cold milk. Steaming may cause a slight reduction in some vitamins, but it does not affect calcium. Coffee, a diuretic, may hasten loss of calcium excreted in the urine, but the amount is small, and in the case of cappuccino or cafe latte, this minor loss is more than made up for by the proportionally large amount of milk in these beverages. By selecting 1 percent or skim milk you can get 25 to 50 percent of your calcium requirement (depending on your needs) while keeping your fat intake low.

## Vitamin D

The National Academy of Sciences report raised the recommendations for vitamin D to 400 IU a day for people between fifty-one–seventy years and 600 IU for people seventy-one and older. Their guidelines for other adult age groups remain at 200 IU per day.

We need vitamin D to absorb calcium. There are 100 to 125 IU in a cup of milk. Other than fortified milk and cereals, there are not many food sources rich in vitamin D. Luckily, our body can make vitamin D. The skin contains a precursor of vitamin D and when exposed to the ultraviolet rays of the sun, the precursor turns into vitamin D. For older people the higher recommendations are difficult to achieve with diet alone, and they might consider a little bit of sunlight: a walk outside is good for older people because exercise will also help to maintain bone strength and muscle tone. Some people may also need to consider supplements to reach their recommended requirements (see below). Vitamin D is fat soluble (it can be stored in the body), so make sure you are not exceeding the Tolerable Upper Intake Level, established at 2000 IU/day for adults. Check the levels in milk, cereals, and all supplements (multivitamins, calcium, food and beverage supplements, etc.) and calculate your intake.

- adults under fifty years old who consume less than two milk servings per day
- men and women under fifty who have increased requirements and have less vitamin D precursor in their skin
- those who do not spend a lot of time outdoors, such as people who work at night and sleep during the day
- those who spend a fair amount of time in the sun, but wear sunscreen to block out ultraviolet rays
- those who live in northern climates where the sun is not strong enough to make vitamin D

## Buying Supplements

If you take supplements, multivitamin and mineral formulas are probably the best and easiest way to balance your vitamin and mineral intake and are generally considered safe. Taking individual supplements has its risks. As many vitamins and minerals compete for absorption or need to work together, supplementing excessive amounts of one can disturb levels or diminish or enhance the action of another. For instance, calcium competes with copper, iron, phosphorus, and zinc for absorption. Taking too much of any one of these nutrients can affect the balance between all of them. Although the supplemental iron in multivitamin formulas may benefit some people, adult men and post-menopausal women are unlikely to need or benefit from additional iron. Supplemental iron can cause more harm than good; a substantial portion of the population has a genetic predisposition to store iron (hemochromatosis). For these people, increased iron stores may result in an increased risk of cardiovascular disease or cancer.

The amount of preformed vitamin A (retinol) in multivitamins should be 5,000 IU or less. The new supplement labels include the percentage of vitamin A from (retinol or retinyl acetate) and the amount from beta-carotene. Other things to look for on multivitamin labels include:

- Daily Values. Under the Dietary Supplements Health and Education Act of 1994 (DSHEA), vitamin and mineral labels now must carry "Nutrition Facts" similar to the Nutrition Facts label on commercial foods. This will include percent Daily Values (%DV). Choose a supplement that provides 100 percent of the DVs rather than excessive or unbalanced quantities of nutrients.
- Expiration date. Vitamins and minerals do lose their potency over time, so be sure to purchase with adequate time to use before they expire.
- Storage instructions. Heat, humidity, and/or light destroys some nutrients.
- The vitamin should meet the U.S. Pharmacopeia (USP) standards for disintegration and dissolution of supplements. If vitamins and minerals are not dissolved by the time they reach the small intestine (thirty to forty-five minutes) absorption is unlikely. Look for a claim like "release assured" on the label.
- "Natural" vitamins are often combined with synthetic ones, and they are chemically the same. The exception is vitamin E. Natural vitamin E is absorbed more efficiently by the body, but many vitamins that call themselves natural may not have d-alpha tocopherol, the natural form of vitamin E. Look for this term as the source of vitamin E.
- Buy vitamins sold by reputable stores, but keep in mind that the highest priced supplement is not necessarily the best. Look at the sources of vitamins A and E and the overall completeness and balance of the formula. This is easier to assess with the new Nutrition Facts supplements labels.
- Source of dietary ingredient. Supplement labels now reveal from what source and of what quantity dietary supplements are derived: "Vitamin A (40 percent as beta-carotene)." Labeling of products containing herbal and botanical ingredients must also state the part of the plant from which the ingredient is derived.

The importance of reading labels cannot be overstated. Many foods are fortified with nutrients, and it is easy to unknowingly megadose simply by eating a breakfast cereal that provides nutrients at 100 percent of the Daily Values, taking a multivitamin and/or antioxidant formula, eating an energy bar at the gym (many are fortified with nutrients at the level of multivitamin supplements), and/or drinking a supplement beverage. If you take various supplements, add up the %DV of all sources to be sure that you are not taking too much.

# Nutrition Facts Labels

**Nutrition Facts**
Serving Size 1 Tablet

| Each Tablet Contains | %Daily Value |
|---|---|
| Vitamin A 5000 (40% as Beta Carotene) | 100% |
| Vitamin C 60 mg | 100% |
| Vitamin D 400 IU | 100% |
| Vitamin E 30 IU | 100% |
| Thiamin 1.5 mg | 100% |
| Riboflavin 1.7 mg | 100% |
| Niacinamide 20 mg | 100% |
| Vitamin B6 2 mg | 100% |
| Folic Acid 400 mcg | 100% |
| Vitamin B12 6 mcg | 100% |
| Biotin 30 mcg | 10% |
| Pantothenic Acid 10 mg | 100% |
| Calcium 162 mg | 16% |
| Iron 18 mg | 100% |
| Phosphorus 109 mg | 11% |
| Iodine 150 mcg | 100% |
| Magnesium 100 mg | 25% |
| Zinc 15 mg | 100% |
| Copper 2 mg | 100% |
| Potassium 80 mg | 2% |
| Vitamin K 25 mcg | * |
| Selenium 20 mcg | * |
| Manganese 3.5 mg | * |
| Chromium 65 mcg | * |
| Molybdenum 160 mcg | * |
| Chloride 72 mg | * |
| Nickel 5 mcg | * |
| Tin 10 mcg | * |
| Silicon 2 mg | * |
| Vanadium 10 mcg | * |
| Boron 150 mcg | * |

*Daily Value not established.

Nutrition Facts labels help consumers make good food choices. With the great variety of food products available, we have an excellent opportunity to exercise discretion when choosing the foods we eat. In addition, food manufacturers have responded to contemporary dietary concerns by providing many healthy choices. Making informed decisions in today's supermarket aisles has been made easier with the implementation of the Nutrition Labeling and Education Act (NLEA) in May 1994. These changes include a more comprehensive and understandable Nutrition Facts label to help consumers make knowledgeable food choices and understand how a particular food fits into the daily diet.

For good health and cancer prevention, the Strang Cancer Prevention Center recommends a maximum of 20 to 25 percent daily calories from fat. The new nutrition label includes "calories from fat." It is just one of the many items of diet-related information manufacturers are required to provide on their food products. There is also information on saturated fat, cholesterol, dietary fiber, and other nutrients that relate to today's health concerns.

Nutrition Facts labels include Daily Values (DV) based on current nutritional content. The Daily Value was developed to make labels more "user friendly." Daily Values reflect the amount of total fat, saturated fat, total carbohydrate, dietary fiber, and protein that is recommended based on a specified number of calories (most food labels provide Daily Values for 2,000- and 2,500-calorie diets). Daily Values for sodium, potassium, vitamins, and minerals stay the same no matter what the caloric level. You may require more or fewer calories and nutrients than those featured on the food label because factors such as height, weight, activity level, and gender influence your true caloric needs. In this situation the Daily Values would need to be adjusted. Use the formula on page 19 to estimate your calorie requirements.

The changes reflected on the Nutrition Facts label are extremely helpful, but there are still some pitfalls to watch for:

**1.** Don't confuse percent Daily Values with percentage of a total nutrient. A pizza may have a Daily Value for fat of 25 percent; do not confuse this with 25 percent calories as fat. Rather, this is one-quarter of the fat allowance for the entire day. If you eat fewer than 2,000 calories per day (not uncommon for women), this Daily Value percent would be more than 25 percent. The Daily Value requirements (except those for cholesterol, sodium, and fiber) must be adjusted downward for people who consume less than 2,000 calories daily. For most men, large women, and athletes, however, the Daily Values should be adjusted upward to compensate for their increased calorie needs. In general, a Daily Value of 20 percent should alert you that the food is high in that particular nutrient, and a Daily Value of 5 percent or less indicates that it is low.

2. A nutrient claim on a package like "90% fat-free" may sound good, but it does not mean that the product is low in fat, healthy, or that only 10 percent of calories come from fat. This percentage refers to the *total weight* of the product. In this case, if the product is 90 percent fat free by weight, then the rest is made up of fat. Because fat tends to weigh less than other ingredients, this could mean that 40, 50, or 60 percent of the total calories are from fat. It is always best to assess your fat gram allowance per day (or have it calculated by a registered dietitian) and then compare your daily fat gram "maximum" to the amount in the selected product.

3. What's in a serving? Although serving sizes on new labels are now standardized, they may not reflect how much you are eating. If you eat more or less than the standard amount, you'll need to adjust the Nutrition Facts accordingly.

4. Trans fatty acids may be hidden in foods. The new label does not tell you if trans fatty acids are present. Why is this important? Trans fats are formed when vegetable oils are hydrogenated to increase their shelf life and improve their texture for baking. Research suggests that they increase bad low-density lipoprotein (LDL) cholesterol just as saturated fats do. When reading ingredient lists, search for "partially hydrogenated oil" or "vegetable shortening." In the first case, this term indicates that trans fats are present; in the second, that they are likely to be present. Remember: foods that are "cholesterol-free," "low-cholesterol," "low in saturated fat," or "made with vegetable oil" are not necessarily trans fat–free. "Saturated fat–free" foods do not contain any trans fatty acids.

5. Restaurants using Nutrition Facts to support health or nutrition claims on their menus will base claims on comparisons to standardized recipes or portion sizes. For example, if a traditional slice of cheese cake has 32 grams of fat and a restaurant calls their version "lite," it must have at least 50 percent less (16 grams or less) per serving. Nutrition Facts from restaurants can be confusing because it may be unclear what the "standard" is based on.

## NEW GUIDELINES ENSURE THAT NUTRIENT CLAIMS MEAN THE SAME ON EVERY PRODUCT.

# Nutrition Facts

Serving Size 1 cup (228g)
Servings Per Container 2

**Amount Per Serving**

**Calories** 250   Calories from Fat 110

|  | **% Daily Value\*** |
|---|---|
| **Total Fat** 12g | **18%** |
| Saturated Fat 3g | **15%** |
| **Cholesterol** 30mg | **10%** |
| **Sodium** 470mg | **20%** |
| **Total Carbohydrate** 31g | **10%** |
| Dietary Fiber 0g | **0%** |
| Sugars 5g | |
| **Protein** 5g | |

| Vitamin A 4% | • | Vitamin C 2% |
|---|---|---|
| Calcium 20% | • | Iron 4% |

\*Percent Daily Values are based on a 2,000 calorie diet. Your daily values may be higher or lower depending on your calorie needs:

|  |  | Calories: | 2,000 | 2,500 |
|---|---|---|---|---|
| Total Fat | Less than | | 65g | 80g |
| Sat Fat | Less than | | 20g | 25g |
| Cholesterol | Less than | | 300mg | 300mg |
| Sodium | Less than | | 2,400mg | 2,400mg |
| Total Carbohydrate | | | 300g | 375g |
| Dietary Fiber | | | 25g | 30g |

Calories per gram:
Fat 9   •   Carbohydrate 4   •   Protein 4

**New heading** signals a new label.

**More consistent & realistic serving sizes,** in both household and metric measures.

**This new term** helps consumers meet dietary guidelines that recommend people get no more than 30 percent of their calories from fat each day. Remember, it's your total consumption over the whole day and not the percentage in one food or meal that's important.

**Use the % Daily Values** to easily compare products and to quickly tell if a serving of a food is high or low in nutrients.

**The list of nutrients** covers those most important to the health of today's consumers, most of whom need to worry about getting too much of certain nutrients (fat, for example) rather than too few vitamins or minerals, as in the past.

**The Daily Values** that have been set for certain nutrients are listed on larger packages for both a 2,000- and a 2,500-calorie diet. This information is based on current dietary guidance and can help you understand the basics of a good diet and plan healthy meals.

This shows the calorie content of the energy-producing nutrients.

### KEY

g = grams (about 28 grams = 1 ounce)
mg = milligrams (1,000 milligrams = 1 gram)

**Ingredients are still listed in descending order of weight.** The list is now required on almost all foods, even standardized ones such as mayonnaise and bread. The sources of some ingredients, such as certain flavorings, are stated by name to help people better identify ingredients that they avoid for health, religious, or other reasons.

INGREDIENTS: WATER, ENRICHED MACARONI (ENRICHED FLOUR [NIACIN, FERROUS SULFATE (IRON), THIAMINE MONONITRATE AND RIBOFLAVIN], EGG WHITE), FLOUR, CHEDDAR CHEESE (MILK, CHEESE CULTURE, SALT, ENZYME), SPICES, MARGARINE (PARTIALLY HYDROGENATED SOYBEAN OIL, WATER, SOY LECITHIN, MONO- AND DI-GLYCERIDES, BETA CAROTENE FOR COLOR, VITAMIN A PALMITATE), AND MALTODEXTRIN.

### PLEASE NOTE

Label terms used on meat-type products such as entrees, main dish products and dinners may have different criteria for nutrient levels. For more information on this type of product, call or write the food manufacturer.

## Nutrient Claims

Other changes in nutrition labeling include regulation of health and nutrient claims that food manufacturers can print on product labels. By law, the terms *low-fat, light,* and *cholesterol-free* now have standard definitions that mean the same thing for all foods. The new label terms can help you choose foods that are lower in calories, fat, cholesterol, and sodium, and higher in fiber, vitamins, and minerals.

You may find these common food label terms helpful in selecting the foods that contribute to good health.

**Free.** The product contains only a tiny or insignificant amount of fat, cholesterol, sodium, sugar, and/or calories. For example, a "fat-free" product will contain less than 0.5 gram of fat per serving.

**Low.** A food described as "low" in fat, saturated fat, cholesterol, sodium, and/or calories can be eaten fairly frequently without exceeding dietary guidelines. "Low in fat" means no more than 3 grams per serving. For restaurants, an item may be called "low-fat" if it contains less than 3 grams of fat in a serving greater than 30 grams (1 ounce). Main dishes or entire meals listed as "low-fat" must contain less than 3 grams of fat per 100 grams (3 1/2 ounces) and provide no more than 30 percent of calories from fat.

**Lean.** "Lean" and "Extra Lean" are USDA terms for use on meat and poultry products. "Lean" means the product contains less than 10 grams of fat, 4 grams of saturated fat, and 95 mg or less of cholesterol per serving. "Lean" is not as lean as "Low."

**Extra Lean.** "Extra Lean" means the product has less than 5 grams of fat, 2 grams of saturated fat, and 95 mg or less of cholesterol per serving. "Leaner than Lean" and "Extra Lean" are not as lean as "Low."

**Reduced, Less, Fewer.** These labels mean a diet product contains 25 percent less of a nutrient or calories. For example, hot dogs might be labeled "25% less fat than our regular hot dogs." Be wary and read the label; this product may still be very high in fat and saturated fat.

For restaurants, a menu item must have 25 percent less fat, cholesterol, sodium, sugar and/or/ calories than a standard recipe. For example, if the typical 3 1/2-ounce blueberry muffin has 300 calories per serving, then the "reduced-calorie" version must have no more than 225 calories.

**Light/Lite.** These labels mean a diet product has one-third fewer calories or one-half of the fat of the original. "Light in Sodium" means a product has half the usual sodium. Once again, this does not guarantee an acceptable level, so check the label. For restaurants, a menu item can be called "Light" or "Lite" only if it derives less than 50% of its calories from fat or contains one-third fewer calories or 50% less fat than a standard recipe.

**More.** One serving has at least 10 percent more of the Daily Value of a vitamin, mineral, or fiber than usual.

**Good Source of.** One serving contains 10 to 19 percent of the Daily Value for a stated vitamin, mineral, or fiber.

Health Claims

Relationships between specific nutrients or foods and the risk of disease or illness may now be claimed as long as they adhere to the specific requirements set forth for the approved claim. Furthermore, consumers must be able to identify the nutrient-disease relationship from the wording of the claim as well as the improtance of the nutrient's role in a daily diet.

The following are seven relationships between nutrients/foods and disease that may be described in authorized health claims.

- The role of calcium in preventing osteoporosis
- The relationship between fat and cancer
- How saturated fat and cholesterol contribute to coronary heart disease
- The beneficial effects of fiber-containing grain products, fruits and vegetables in preventing cancer
- Fruits, vegetables, and grain products that contain fiber and their role in fighting coronary heart disease
- The link between sodium and hypertension (high blood pressure)
- The beneficial role of fruits and vegetables in fighting cancer

# CHAPTER 3

# Phytochemicals: The New Functional Foods

**P**hytochemicals (*phyto* = plant) are sometimes referred to as functional foods (because they are thought to prevent disease). These compounds originate from plants and are responsible for the color, odor, and flavor of certain foods. They are not nutrients, having no calories or known nutritional value. A particular fruit or vegetable may contain hundreds of different phytochemicals. We do not have the ability to make phytochemicals in our body, but we can absorb them through the foods we eat.

Until recently, little was known about these functional foods and their potential to fight disease, especially cancer. Phytochemicals are now actively being studied and the National Cancer Institute (part of the National Institutes of Health) has focused research efforts on the anticancer constituents in these plant foods. Emphasis is on identifying and isolating new phytochemicals and studying their effects on cancer and other diseases.

We do not know exactly how phytochemicals work in the body, but it is thought that they may have antioxidant capabilities, as well as the potential to block and suppress carcinogens. Blocking agents increase enzymes that detoxify carcinogens and/or interfere with their activation. Suppressing agents oppose the carcinogenic changes in malignant cells by retarding or reversing the process, directly interfering with the promotion phase of carcinogenesis. In laboratory studies many phytochemicals have been shown to inhibit tumor development and growth in animals. There has been little research done on the long-term effects in people, but evidence is accumulating that phytochemicals may have the ability to decrease cancer and cardiovascular disease. Studies have shown that eating a diet high in plant-rich foods like fruits, vegetables, and grains decreases the risk of developing many cancers. These foods contain many phytochemicals, in addition to other nutrients and nonnutrients such as fiber, vitamins, minerals, and carbohydrates.

Phytochemicals are a complex group of food substances that includes many classes and subclasses. Although it is generally thought that phytochemicals might aid in preventing or treating cancer, each group appears to have unique and specific actions. Here is what we know about the different types of phytochemicals and how they may act to fight cancer.

## Major Classes of Phytochemicals

**Allium Compounds**
**Glucosinolates**
   dithiolthiones
   isothiocyanates
   sulforaphane
   indoles
**Plant Polyphenols**
   *Phenolic Acids*
      chlorogenic, caffeic, and ferulic acids
      curcumin
      ellagic acid
   *Flavonoids*
      catechins and theaflavins
      anthocyanins
      coumarin
      quercetin (rutin)
      kaempferol
      tangeretin and nobiletin
      phytoestrogens
      isoflavones (daidzein, genistein)
      coumestrans
      lignans
   *Capsaicin*

**Terpenes**
  *Monoterpenes*
    D-limonene
    myrcene
  *Diterpenes*
    carnosol
    rosmarinic acid
  *Triterpenes*
    glycyrrhizin
    6-gingerol
    zingiberene
  *Carotenoids*
    carotenes (tetraterpenes)
      vitamin A precursors
        alpha-carotene
        beta-carotene
        epsilon-carotene
      non–vitamin A precursors
        lutein
        lycopene
        gamma carotene
    xanthophylls (non–vitamin A)
      zeaxanthin
      cryptoxanthin
**Protease Inhibitors**
**Inositol (Phytic Acid)**
**Fatty Acids**
  linolenic acid (omega-3 fatty acid)
**Plant Sterols**
  sterols
  saponins

# Allium Compounds

Allium is found in plants of the genus *Allium*: chives, garlic, leeks, onions, and shallots. Studies have shown a decreased risk of stomach and possibly colon cancer in people who consume foods rich in allium. There is also some evidence from studies in laboratory animals that there is a beneficial effect on prostate, skin, and esophageal cancer. It is thought that the sulfur-containing compounds, called allicin and diallyl sulfide, may be the active ingredients that help to reduce cancer risk.

Garlic, a significant food source of allium, has received considerable attention. Manufacturers of garlic supplements have made many claims about its cancer-fighting ability. It is important to remember that although some studies support an anticancer effect of garlic, research is in the preliminary stages and no definitive conclusion can be made at this time. We do know that most of the research done to date has looked at garlic from fresh foods; supplements may not confer the same benefit. Because garlic is rich in vitamins and minerals, it is prudent to incorporate it into one's diet even though ongoing scientific studies have not "proved" that garlic protects against cancer.

---

#### ✦ ALLIUM COMPOUNDS ✦

*Proposed anticancer functions:* as a blocking agent, stimulates production of detoxification enzymes, which helps excrete carcinogens; decreases proliferation of tumor cells; antibacterial activity inhibits formation of N-nitroso compounds, which are associated with stomach cancer; may stimulate tumor-fighting immune cells

*Other functions:* lowers low-density lipoprotein blood cholesterol and blood pressure; inhibits blood clotting that can lead to stroke

---

### *Significant Sources of Allium Compounds*

| | |
|---|---|
| chives | onions, all types |
| garlic | shallots |
| leeks | |

# Glucosinolates and Indoles

Many studies have been conducted looking at the effect of vegetables containing high amounts of glucosinolates (cruciferous vegetables, such as cabbage, kale, broccoli, cauliflower) on risk of cancer. These phytochemicals have shown a consistent beneficial effect on cancer. People who consume large amounts of vegetables from this family are at decreased risk of developing cancers of the lung, stomach, colon, and rectum. Also, there appears to be a positive effect for prostate, endometrial, and ovarian cancer, but the findings are not as strong. Indoles are a breakdown product of glucosinolates and also seem to protect against cancers, especially those that are dependent on estrogen like breast and endometrial. A high intake of indoles has been shown to reduce recurrent laryngeal tumors.

> ↠ GLUCOSINOLATES ↞
>
> **Dithiolthiones, Isothiocyanates, Sulforaphane**
>     *Proposed anticancer functions:* antioxidant; promotes production of protective de-toxifying enzymes that block carcinogens; decreases activity of enzymes that promote carcinogenesis; may inhibit tumor growth
>
> **Indoles**
>     *Proposed anticancer functions:* promote production of enzymes that inactivate cancer-promoting estrogens and androgens; boost ability to detoxify carcinogens; increase immune activity

## *Significant Sources of Glucosinolates*

### Dithiolthiones, Isothiocyanates, and Sulforaphane

| | |
|---|---|
| broccoli | kale |
| Brussels sprouts | mustard greens |
| cabbage | radishes |
| cauliflower | turnips |
| horseradish | |

### Indoles

| | |
|---|---|
| bok choy | kale |
| broccoli | kohlrabi |
| Brussels sprouts | mustard greens |
| cabbage | rutabaga |
| cauliflower | turnips |
| collards | |

# Plant Polyphenols

The plant polyphenols are a large class of phytochemicals that are potent anti-oxidants. It is thought that they induce detoxification enzymes, prevent cancer at the initiation stage, and inhibit activity of enzymes involved in cancer progression. Results from animal studies have shown that polyphenols have anticarcinogenic effects. This class of polyphenols may have a beneficial effect on cholesterol, triglyceride fat, blood pressure levels, and cardiovascular disease. Antibacterial, antiviral, and anti-inflammatory properties have also been proposed.

## Phenolic Acids

The phenolic acids, a subgroup of the plant polyphenols, are found in various foods, including fruits and vegetables as well as some spices. The phenolic acids include chlorogenic, caffeic, and ferulic acids; curcumin; ellagic acid. It is believed that these substances act as cancer protectors by neutralizing or blocking carcinogens.

---

### ✦ PHENOLIC ACIDS ✦

**Chlorogenic, Caffeic, and Ferulic Acids; Curcumin; Ellagic Acid**
*Proposed anticancer functions:* antioxidant; blocking agent; tumor suppressor; neutralizes and reduces genetic damage caused by carcinogens like tobacco; anti-inflammatory

---

## Flavonoids

The flavonoids, another subclass of the plant polyphenols, are found in fruits, vegetables, and soy products. Flavonoids may reduce cancer by acting as antioxidants. Subclasses of the flavonoids include the catechins and theaflavins, quercetin, and coumarin. Another subclass of flavonoids, called phytoestrogens, may inhibit hormones thought to be involved in cancer promotion and development.

**Catechins and theaflavins.** Tea contains catechins (in green tea) and theaflavins (in black tea), which are part of the plant polyphenol family. Laboratory experiments have shown both green and black teas to be anticarcinogenic. Green tea has received most of the attention, and preliminary studies suggest it may decrease the risk for certain cancers and protect against heart disease. Specifically, decreased tumors of the skin, lung, esophagus, stomach, colon, liver, pancreas, and breast have been observed. It is thought that polyphenols contained in both green and black teas are responsible for this anticancer activity. Green tea has higher levels of polyphenols than black tea. Decaffeinated teas also appear to have some of these benefits. (Herbal teas are made using a different process than black or green tea and do not contain polyphenols.)

Relatively few studies have been conducted examining the link between tea and cancer. High tea consumption may explain why the lung cancer rates in Japan are only half those in the United States, even though the rate of cigarette smoking is nearly twice that of the United States. Not all studies have shown a beneficial effect; in fact, some have shown an *increased* risk of esophageal cancer in tea drinkers. This has been specifically attributed to drinking tea at burning temperatures, which causes injury to the esophagus.

At this time we cannot definitively "prove" that tea drinking decreases the risk for all cancers. This is a promising area of research. It is reasonable to conclude that tea is probably beneficial for esophageal and stomach cancers.

---

### → FLAVONOIDS ←

**Catechins and Theaflavins**
*Proposed anticancer functions:* powerful antioxidant; promotes production of detoxifying enzymes; inhibits tumor growth; may aid immune system and help rid body of potential carcinogens; anti-inflammatory
*Other functions:* may protect against atherosclerosis; cholesterol-lowering effect

**Anthocyanins, Coumarin, Quercetin, Kaempferol, Tangeretin, Nobiletin**
*Proposed anticancer functions:* antioxidant; blocking agent; promotes production of detoxifying enzymes; tumor suppressor

---

**Phytoestrogens.** Phytoestrogens are a subclass of flavonoids that have anticancer properties. They function as antioxidants, blocking enzymes that inactivate carcinogens, and suppressors of cell growth and division. Isoflavone-containing plants have a structure similar to human estrogen and contain hormones called phytoestrogens. More than three hundred plants have been identified with this estrogen activity, but the best sources are soy beans, soy products, and other legumes.

It is thought that these phytoestrogens act like human estrogens or sex hormones to help regulate female reproductive cycles. (Their action is that of weak estrogens, having much less potency than naturally occurring estrogens in the body. They help to reduce the level of the "stronger" estrogens by competing with and promoting excretion from the body.) These phytoestrogens compete with estrogen to block its promoting effects. These promoting effects can convert normal cells to cancer cells. Cancers of the breast, ovary, and uterus (endometrium) are dependent on hormones for growth and proliferation. Tamoxifen, a synthetic drug used to treat cancer, has a similar structure to the phytoestrogens'.

Studies have shown a five to eight times lower incidence of breast cancer in Asian women as compared to American women. Asian women from countries such as Japan, China, and Korea traditionally eat a diet high in soy foods and have lower circulating levels of estrogen compared to women who eat a Western diet. Some scientists believe the differences in soy intake may explain this variation in breast cancer rates; however, we cannot definitely say that consumption of soy products reduces the risk of breast cancer. Other factors related to lifestyle differences between Asian and American women may also be affecting the risk of breast cancer.

Soy may increase the length of the menstrual cycle, which would decrease the total exposure of a woman's body to estrogens. It has been observed that Asian women have a menstrual cycle that is two to three days longer than that of American women, and most of them do not experience menopausal symptoms. Phytoestrogens may function as hormone replacement for women during menopause, affecting hot flashes and mood swings. Because traditional hormone replacement therapy has been associated with an increased risk for some cancers, the potential of these substances to provide estrogen without raising cancer risk is being investigated as an alternative to estrogen replacement therapy for menopausal women.

Phytoestrogens may also have an effect on prostate cancer (a hormone-dependent cancer that occurs only in men) by blocking or reducing testosterone, which can foster growth of cancer. This theory is supported by the fact that estrogen has been shown to slow the growth of prostate cancer by affecting testosterone. Epidemiologic and laboratory experiments suggest that phytoestrogens lower the risk of prostate cancer. There is up to a thirtyfold variation in prostate cancer rates between Asian and American men. Men from Asian countries traditionally eat diets high in phytoestrogen-containing foods. These men do get prostate cancer, but their tumors seem to progress at a much slower rate, and mortality from this cancer is low.

---

### ⤳ PHYTOESTROGENS ⤆

**Isoflavones (Daidzein and Genistein)**
*Proposed anticancer functions:* may block growth of new vessels essential for some tumors to grow and spread by inactivating cancer enzymes; antiestrogen effects; stimulates differentiation of malignant cells
*Other functions:* lowers serum cholesterol and may prevent heart disease and osteoporosis

**Coumestrans and Lignans**
*Proposed anticancer functions:* antioxidant; may block or suppress carcinogenic changes

---

**Capsaicin.** Another subclass of the plant polyphenols, capsaicin is contained in hot chile peppers and produces the pungent characteristic burning sensation. Capsaicin appears to block carcinogenesis by neutralizing stomach carcinogens, but in large quantities may actually *increase* the risk of stomach cancer. Little is known about the effects of capsaicin and at this time results are preliminary.

---

→ **CAPSAICIN** ←

*Proposed anticancer functions:* blocks carcinogenesis; neutralizes carcinogens, but consumption of large quantities may be linked to stomach cancer
*Other functions:* anticoagulant; may help to prevent heart attack or stroke

---

## Significant Sources of Plant Polyphenols

### PHENOLIC ACIDS

#### Chlorogenic, Caffeic, Ferulic Acids

| | |
|---|---|
| apples | peaches |
| citrus fruits: grapefruits, | pears |
|    lemons, limes, oranges, tangerines | pineapples |
| coffee | potatoes |
| green peppers | strawberries |
| lettuce | tomatoes |

#### Curcumin

| | |
|---|---|
| curry | turmeric |
| mustard | |

#### Ellagic Acid

| | |
|---|---|
| cranberries | raspberries |
| grapes | strawberries |
| loganberries | walnuts |

### FLAVONOIDS

#### Catechins and Theaflavins

| | |
|---|---|
| berries, all types | green and black teas |

#### Anthocyanins

| | |
|---|---|
| apples | grapes |
| artichokes | licorice |
| berries | wine, varying amounts |

### Coumarin

| | |
|---|---|
| broccoli | fenugreek, component of some herbal teas |
| cabbage | squash |
| carrots | yams |
| citrus fruits: grapefruits, lemons, limes, oranges | |

### Kaempferol

| | |
|---|---|
| horseradish | radishes |

### Quercetin and Its Glycosides (e.g., Rutin)

| | |
|---|---|
| bell peppers | onions (with red skin) |
| berries | pea pods |
| broad beans or fava beans | potatoes |
| citrus fruits and juices | rosemary |
| eggplant | shallots |
| flaxseed | tomatoes |
| green and black teas | |

### Tangeretin and Nobiletin

tangerines

## PHYTOESTROGENS

### Isoflavones (Genistein and Daidzein)

| | |
|---|---|
| soybeans | soy products |

### Coumestrans

| | |
|---|---|
| bean sprouts | sunflower seeds |
| red clover | |

### Lignans*

| | |
|---|---|
| flaxseed | soybeans |
| rye | soy products |
| sesame seeds | wheat |

*Lignans are a type of fiber; for grains, the less processing, the more lignans.

# Terpenes

Terpenes are one of the largest classes of phytochemicals, and their subclasses number in the thousands. They exist in different forms, including monoterpenes, diterpenes, triterpenes, and carotenoids (tetraterpenes), and are found in most fruits and vegetables. The terpenes function predominantly as antioxidants; however, some terpenes, particularly those found in citrus fruits, stimulate enzymes to block carcinogens. They may also inhibit cholesterol production and enhance immune function. Taxol is a member of the terpene family and is used to treat breast and ovarian cancers. Taxol is not found in food but was first derived from the Pacific yew tree and is now made semisynthetically.

---

### ✧ TERPENES ✧

**Monoterpenes (D-limonene and Myrcene)**
  *Proposed anticancer functions:* antioxidant; blocking agent that increases protective enzymes that may interfere with carcinogens; may help differentiation of cells to non-malignant state
  *Other functions:* inhibits cholesterol production

**Diterpenes (Carnosol, Rosmarinic acid)**
  *Proposed anticancer functions:* potent antioxidant; increases detoxification enzymes; anti-inflammatory
  *Other functions:* may have antiviral properties

**Triterpenes (Glycyrrhizin,\* 6-Gingerol, Zingiberene)**
  *Proposed anticancer function:* may slow rate of growth of cancer cells; suppresses enzymes and hormones related to cancer; enhances immune function

---

## Significant Sources of Terpenes

### MONOTERPENES (INCLUDING D-LIMONENE)

| | |
|---|---|
| basil | caraway seeds |
| broccoli | cardamom |
| cabbage | carrots |

---

\*Glycyrrhizin is one subclass of triterpenes and is contained in true licorice root (found in health food stores and certain herbal teas). In excessive amounts glycyrrhizin can be toxic, so moderate consumption of both licorice root and licorice-containing products.

celery seed

citrus fruits: grapefruits, lemons,
   limes, oranges (especially their peels)

cucumbers

eggplant

fennel seeds and bulb

mint

nutmeg

parsley

peppers

spearmint

squash

star anise

thyme

tomatoes

yams

**Myrcene**

lemongrass

### DITERPENES

oregano (rosmarinic acid)

rosemary (carnosol)

### TRITERPENES

citrus fruits

licorice

soybeans and soy products

**6-Gingerol, Glycyrrhizin, and Zingiberene**

ginger

## Carotenoids

The carotenoids are a major subclass of the broad terpene group. Carotenoids are what give fruits and vegetables their yellow, orange, and red colors (dark-green vegetables and herbs also contain carotenoids; however, their colors are masked by the green pigment chlorophyll). The six hundred or more different carotenoids can be divided into two distinct subgroups: carotenes and xanthophylls. Although carotenes are known to be precursors of vitamin A, only 10 percent of all carotenes can be converted to vitamin A. Carotenes include beta-carotene, lycopene, and lutein. All are known for their anticancer properties. Carotenes have varying degrees of antioxidant properties, and some enhance immune response and protect skin cells against ultraviolet radiation. The second group of carotenoids, xanthophylls, function as antioxidants and include zeaxanthin and cryptoxanthin.

See page 60 for food sources.

---

### ✦ CAROTENOIDS ✦

*Proposed anticancer functions:* antioxidants; metabolized to vitamin A, which helps cell differentiation (lack of differentiation is a characteristic of cancer cells); may inhibit cell proliferation

*Other functions:* may reduce heart disease, stroke, and anti-inflammatory disorders; improves immune response; lowers cholesterol levels; may reduce cataracts

---

# Protease Inhibitors

Protease inhibitors are another major subclass of phytochemicals that act to limit the action of enzymes that break down protein. They are found predominantly in beans, seeds, and soy products. It has been suggested that these inhibitors act to slow the rate of cell division in cancer cells, allowing time for genetic repair. To date, there is little research on the effects of protease inhibitors in human cancer, but studies have shown a reduction of tumors in animals.

---

### ✦ PROTEASE INHIBITORS ✦

*Proposed anticancer functions:* prevents normal cells from being transformed to cancer cells; inhibits tumor promotion and cell proliferation; increases genetic repair of enzymes

---

### *Significant Sources of Protease Inhibitors\**

| | |
|---|---|
| grains: barley, oats, wheat, rye | soy |
| legumes | soy products |
| seeds | |

# Inositol (Phytic Acid)

Inositol is of plant origin and is found in legumes, cereals, and soybeans. An anticancer effect has been observed in laboratory experiments. In studies, diets high in fiber,

\*Levels are more significant if food is not extensively cooked.

which are also high in this phytochemical, have been linked to decreased cancers of the breast, colon, and pancreas.

---

### ✛ INOSITOL (PHYTIC ACID) ✚

*Proposed anticancer functions:* reduces cell proliferation; increases differentiation of cells; may bind with dietary minerals to decrease production of free radicals

---

## Significant Sources of Inositol (Phytic Acid)

all types of bran (rice, rye, wheat,
    oat, corn, soy)*
lima beans
nuts

sesame seeds
soybeans
soy products

# Fatty Acids

Linolenic acid is a fatty acid found in plant sources (linseed oils, walnuts, green leafy vegetables) that can be converted to omega-3 fatty acid.

---

### ✛ FATTY ACIDS ✚

**Linolenic Acids (Omega-3 Fatty Acid)**
*Proposed anticancer functions:* regulates prostaglandin production that reduces inflammation and may stimulate the immune system

---

See page 27 for food sources.

# Plant Sterols

Plant sterols are a type of fat that is similar to cholesterol. Vegetables contain significant amounts of plant sterols. There has not been any research done in humans so far, but a decreased rate of colon tumors in animals fed plant sterols has been shown. Saponins are a subclass of the sterol group.

*The less processed the bran, the more inositol.

---

### ⤳ PLANT STEROLS ⤶

**Sterols**
   *Proposed anticancer functions:* block estrogen promotion of breast cancer activity and act as differentiation agents of cancer cells during replication; suppress cancer growth
   *Other functions:* cholesterol-lowering properties

**Saponins**
   *Proposed anticancer functions:* influence genetic material in cancer cells not to multiply; reduce proliferation and decrease growth of various tumor cells
   *Other functions:* cholesterol-lowering properties

---

## *Significant Sources of Plant Sterols**

BEST SOURCES

|  | milligrams (mg) |
|---|---|
| almonds, dried, 1 oz. | 41 |
| amaranth, 1 cup | 47 |
| cashews, dried, 1 oz. | 45 |
| corn oil, 1 tablespoon | 132 |
| mayonnaise, 1 tablespoon | 40 |
| peanuts, unroasted, 1 oz. | 62 |
| pine nuts, pignolia, 1 oz. | 40 |
| rice bran oil, 1 tablespoon | 162 |
| sesame oil, 1 tablespoon | 118 |
| sesame seeds, whole dried, 1 tablespoon | 64 |
| soybeans, green, boiled, 1/2 cup | 45 |
| sunflower seeds/kernels, dried, 1 oz. | 152 |
| wheat germ oil, 1 tablespoon | 75 |

GOOD SOURCES

| | |
|---|---|
| apple, raw, with skin, 1 medium | 17 |
| apricots, raw, 3 medium | 19 |
| asparagus, boiled, 1/2 cup | 22 |
| bamboo shoots, raw, 1/2 cup | 14 |

*Nutrient values obtained from Pennington, J. A. T., *Bowes & Church's Food Values of Portions Commonly Used* (16th ed.), J. B. Lippincott Company, 1994.

| | |
|---|---|
| banana, raw, 1 medium | 18 |
| beets, raw, $1/2$ cup | 17 |
| Brussels sprouts, raw, $1/2$ cup | 11 |
| cantaloupe, raw, 1 cup | 8 |
| cherries, sweet, raw, 10 each | 8 |
| cucumber, raw, $1/2$ cup slices | 7 |
| figs, raw, 2 medium | 32 |
| grapefruit, raw, white, $1/2$ medium | 20 |
| lemon, raw, 1 medium | 13 |
| okra, raw, $1/2$ cup | 12 |
| olive oil, 1 tablespoon | 30 |
| onion, raw, $1/2$ cup | 12 |
| orange, navel, 1 medium | 34 |
| peaches, raw, 1 medium | 9 |
| pear, raw, 1 medium | 13 |
| pecans, dried, 1 oz. | 31 |
| pomegranate, Japanese, raw, 1 medium | 26 |
| pumpkin, raw, $1/2$ cup | 7 |
| soybean oil, 1 tablespoon | 34 |
| tomato, red, raw, 1 medium | 9 |
| walnut oil, 1 tablespoon | 24 |
| walnuts, English/Persian, dried, 1 oz. | 31 |
| yams, raw, $1/2$ cup | 8 |

# Supplementation of Phytochemicals

Even though new phytochemicals are being discovered each day, there is still much to be learned about the potential beneficial effect on disease. Many health food manufacturers have begun to market phytochemicals in supplement form: examples include garlic and broccoli pills, as well as supplements that contain polyphenols and isoflavones. It is premature at this time to be selling synthetically made phytochemicals because we know so little about their beneficial and possibly harmful effects. Many questions are still unanswered.

It is unclear whether these substances protect against disease once extracted from plants and incorporated into pill form. Often the pill forms of these substances contain very little or none of the proposed active ingredient. The amount that is beneficial is not known; neither is the effect of megadoses (more is not always better). It may be dangerous for people to "treat" themselves with these substances. Furthermore, there are thousands of other substances in plants that have not been identified that may work in conjunction with the phytochemical of interest that a supplement would not provide.

Given the current lack of knowledge about the effects of phytochemicals, it is best to get these substances from the foods we eat versus taking a pill form. Eating a variety of foods, including fruits, vegetables, grains, and legumes each day will ensure this.

# CHAPTER 4

# Cooking for Cancer Prevention

**N**ow that you know why and how to make improvements in your diet, let's get cooking! While the recipes here aim to follow the guidelines we've given you, keep in mind that the two words you hear so often relative to diet are *balance* and *moderation*. This means that your diet can include a dish, meal, or even a full day of indulgence that can be balanced out by improvements in the next meal or day. For example, some nutritious low-calorie items, such as Sautéed Spinach with Garlic (page 179), with 43 percent of its calories derived from fat, is almost double our recommended 20 to 25 percent range. When you look more closely, the recipe contains just 4 grams of fat per serving (just over a teaspoon), and when combined with a whole balanced meal, the percentage of calories from fat will fall within the suggested range. The same is true for Master Chef Andre Soltner's succulent Roast Baby Chicken (page 240; 51 percent calories from fat); but combined with Gianni Scappin's Smashed Orange-scented Sweet Potatoes (page 251), a serving of broccoli, a whole wheat roll, and finished with Charlie Trotter's Warm Mango and Yanni Pear Soup with Fruit Sorbets (page 279), your entire meal will balance with respect to fat and nutrients. And don't limit the holiday menus to special occasions; the same flexibility should be applied to them, as none are so complicated or indulgent that they shouldn't be part of your regular repertoire.

The range of enormously talented chefs who have provided recipes for this book proves that healthy eating and great taste are not mutually exclusive. Some chefs have provided recipes from their restaurants (encouraging news for those who try to maintain a healthy diet when dining out). If you visit Daniel Boulud at his Restaurant Daniel or

Michael Chiarello at Tra Vigna during the summer months, you are likely to see their Summer Vegetable Casserole with Basil and Black Olives (page 121) and Lentil and Shelling Bean Stew (page 196), respectively, on the menu. Many chefs have also provided us with the inside scoop—a recipe from a rare day of cooking at home.

If you are unsure about putting all of the information together and making it work, consider this: the chefs who have successfully submitted recipes that are low in fat and high in cancer-protective nutrients were provided with the following guidelines:

**1.** Remember ease of preparation—skill level, time, and equipment—for the home cook.

**2.** Use colorful fruits and/or vegetables.

**3.** Limit added fat to approximately 1/2 to 1 teaspoon per serving for appetizers, side dishes, or accompaniments, and 1 teaspoon per serving for entrées and desserts.

**4.** Choose from all types of whole grains and legumes.

**5.** Consider incorporating soybeans or soy products.

**6.** If your recipe includes meat, select leaner cuts, game, or poultry.

**7.** Select from all types of fish and shellfish.

**8.** Use fresh herbs and seasonings whenever possible.

Using this limited amount of information the chefs almost unanimously met the specifications. In all cases the recipes have been tested and in some instances *slightly* modified for nutrient profile or ease of preparation in the home kitchen. With all of this information at your fingertips, you can do it too!

The nutritional analyses and commentary on recipes serve to further your knowledge of the composition of foods—important for decision making when shopping, cooking, and dining out. The phytochemical lists include some very complicated words that you will likely be hearing a lot more about in the future. Our goal in including them with recipes is not to overwhelm you, but to demonstrate that a lot of these protective compounds are probably already in your diet, and we invite you to review the chapter on phytochemicals for more information about these potentially life-saving compounds.

Successful cooks, whether professional or in the home, have a few things in common. They read recipes in their entirety first, have all ingredients on hand and "prepped" before beginning, and make minor adaptations when necessary with regard to cooking facilities, equipment, and ingredient availability. The shopping and equipment lists will help you get your kitchen organized for healthy and tasty cooking. So, there you have it! You are on your way to making delicious meals for optimal health.

# Ingredients for Healthy Cooking

It is much easier to prepare a healthy meal on a busy day when you already have the basic ingredients on hand. Here's a shopping list to work from: not every food is absolutely necessary; this is a sample of balance and variety in food choices.

## DAIRY

"lite" 1 percent soy milk (or 1 percent or skim cow's milk)
low-fat cheese (soy cheese or any other type with less than 3 grams of fat per ounce)
low-fat or fat-free sour cream
low-fat or nonfat yogurt (also soy-based yogurts)

## FRESH PRODUCE

citrus fruits: grapefruits, lemons, limes, oranges
cruciferous vegetables: broccoli, Brussels sprouts, cabbage, cauliflower, kohlrabi, rutabagas, turnips
green leafy vegetables: collard, dandelion, turnip and mustard greens, kale, mesclun, spinach, Swiss chard, watercress
fresh herbs: basil, cilantro, oregano, parsley, rosemary, sage, tarragon, thyme
onion family: chives, garlic, garlic head, leeks, onions, shallots
Other deep-green, orange, red, and yellow produce (rich in vitamins A and/or C, carotenes, and other phytochemicals): apricots; seasonal berries; carrots; cherries; chiles; melons (all types); peppers (all types); potatoes (sweet and white); tomatoes; tropical fruit such as mangos; kiwi; and papaya; peaches; winter and summer squash

## MEAT/FISH/POULTRY

chicken: skinless breast, skinless boneless thigh meat, ground chicken (ask your butcher to grind skinless breast meat to help keep fat low)
beef: flank steak, choice or select top, bottom or eye round (trimmed), chuck
turkey: skinless breast meat
game: skinless duck or quail breast, rabbit, venison, elk, ostrich
lamb: trimmed leg
pork: trimmed center loin or tenderloin, extra-lean ham
fish: any fish, particularly those rich in omega-3 fatty acids (see page 35)

## FATS AND OILS

butter (store frozen to keep fresh for its limited uses)

canola oil

nut, flavored, or spice- or herb-infused oils (walnut, chili, rosemary, etc.)—a little bit goes a long way with flavor

extra virgin olive oil

sesame oil (dark or light)

# The Kitchen Cupboard

## CANNED GOODS

beans: an assortment such as chickpeas, black beans, Great Northern, kidney, and pinto

whole tomatoes*

tomato paste*

stewed tomatoes*

soups, low-fat, low-sodium (bean, vegetable, or other broth-based soups that can be further enriched with fresh vegetables)

## DRIED FRUIT

apricots

cranberries

currants

raisins

## GRAINS, CEREALS, DRIED LEGUMES

barley (a good way to add texture and fiber to soup; a rice substitute for risotto)

beans, dried: black beans, chickpeas, red beans, white beans

bread: rye, multigrain, whole wheat, flaxseed, pita, walnut raisin

breakfast cereals, hot and cold (look for one with more than 3 grams of fiber per serving and less than 2 to 3 grams of fat)

bulgur (fine-ground bulgur cooks quickly and is a good source of fiber)

couscous, whole wheat: quick-cooking and easy to prepare; a great base to top with any type of lean stewed meat or vegetables

cracked wheat (great for high-fiber salads such as tabbouleh)

*Processed tomatoes have more of the phytochemical lycopene—a powerful antioxidant—than fresh tomatoes.

crackers (low-fat, whole-grain)

flaxseed: whole or ground (a tasty way to increase nutrients and fiber in baked goods)

flour: all-purpose, low-fat soy, whole wheat

lentils: red and green

pasta, dry: all types and shapes

polenta (fine-ground cornmeal cooks quickly and makes a nice change from the usual starch)

rice, brown and long-grain (other good selections to have around include arborio, an Italian short-grain rice; wild; and basmati rices)

tortillas (whole wheat, fat-free)

## DRIED SPICES AND HERBS**

| | |
|---|---|
| bay leaves | nutmeg |
| cayenne | oregano |
| chili powder | paprika |
| cloves | peppercorns (white and black) |
| coriander seed | rosemary (dried) |
| cumin, ground | tarragon |
| curry powder | thyme (dried) |
| fennel seed | turmeric |
| ginger | |

## BASICS

baking powder
baking soda
cornstarch
kosher or coarse salt
sea salt
sugar (brown, white, granulated, and powdered)
vanilla extract

## CONDIMENTS

capers
catsup*

*Processed tomatoes have more of the phytochemical lycopene—a powerful antioxidant—than fresh tomatoes.

**Dried herbs and spices lose their potency and flavor over time, so buy small containers when possible.

Dijon mustard or other flavored mustards
dried mushrooms, such as porcini or morels
honey
maple syrup
olives
tahini (sesame paste)
tamari or soy sauce
vinegars (an assortment of types and flavors is useful)
Worcestershire sauce

## FROZEN FOODS

all-natural, low-fat soy products (frozen soy burgers, sausages, bacon, and hot dogs can provide a quick and healthy protein source; soy burgers can be ground and substituted for ground beef in recipes; soy sausages can be eaten plain or added to soups, stews, or casseroles)

fruit: berries (great for savory or dessert sauces or sorbets)

vegetables: broccoli, corn, Brussels sprouts, spinach, winter squash, or vegetable combinations (plain vegetables, not in the form of soufflés or with sauces)

## HOMEMADE GOODS

defatted stocks or broths such as beef, chicken, mushroom, or vegetable, stored frozen in small 2- to 4-cup portions make healthy cooking easier

sauces and soups (when preparing healthy sauces or soups, double or triple the recipe and freeze in small containers—a low-fat tomato sauce, for instance, can be used in a variety of recipes)

---

- Though fresh vegetables taste terrific, don't hesitate to buy frozen vegetables; in many cases they are nutritionally equivalent.
- Buy bags of frozen fruits and vegetables instead of boxes—it is easier to store leftovers for another use.
- Fruits and vegetables bought in season not only taste better, but are cheaper.
- Try bulk shopping; depending on your family size, you can buy larger portions of your favorite grains, cereals, beans, or dried fruits.

# Kitchen Equipment for Healthy Cooking

ESSENTIAL

2 nonstick skillets (8- and 14-inch), preferably with a metal handle that allows transfer from stove to oven

nonstick sauté pan (12- or 14-inch) with a lid

2-quart pot with a lid

6-quart pot with a lid

roasting pan, preferably nonstick

One or two 9 × 12-inch nonstick cookie sheets

bottle opener

can opener

colander

food processor

blender (by whipping air into sauces and vinaigrettes, a smooth texture is achieved without adding fat; also great for fruit smoothies)

grater (grating cheese allows you to spread it out more evenly and therefore use less; also good for zesting citrus or shredding vegetables)

1 large fork

chef's knife (8-, 10-, or 12-inch)

paring knife

serrated knife (for bread, tomatoes, vegetable terrines)

2 wooden spoons

kitchen scale

slotted and solid kitchen spoons

2 ladles (2-oz. and 4-oz.)

2 spatulas (metal and for nonstick cookware)

rubber spatula

measuring cups and measuring spoons

plastic containers with lids (useful for storing and freezing batches of soups, sauces, stews, and leftovers)

pot holders

2 strainers (medium and fine, for straining sauces, soups, fruit purees, and coulis)

salad spinner (useful for both salad greens, herbs, and other washed vegetables)

stainless-steel mixing bowls

steamer basket

wire whisk

wooden and/or plastic cutting board

vegetable peeler

## HELPFUL

4-quart pot with a lid

12-quart stockpot

mandoline (Used for chopping, mandolines can save a lot of time when a large amount of slicing is required. They make vegetables more attractive, and the thinner slices shorten cooking time, preserving nutrients. Mandolines are usually sold with a variety of blades for thin slicing and julienne and french-fry cutting. Inexpensive, good-quality plastic mandolines are available at most culinary stores.)

kitchen tongs

electric mixer

hand blender

4-, 6-, and/or 8-oz. ramekins (perfect for low-fat puddings, soufflés, and molds)

terrine mold (great for making vegetable terrines; the possible vegetable, herb, and seasoning combinations are limitless).

nonstick loaf pan for low-fat fruit and vegetable quick breads, meat, poultry, or fish loafs

nonstick muffin pans

cast-iron pan* (Once well seasoned, there is usually no need to add more fat, even when sautéing a delicate meat. A properly seasoned pan has been treated with enough oil to permeate the relatively porous metal. After a pan has been seasoned, it should be wiped clean rather than washed to maintain its protective seal.)

pastry rings (great for making low-fat tarts using fresh fruits with phyllo dough crust)

slicing and boning knives

---

Pans with heavy bottoms (usually from a copper core that conducts and distributes heat well) allow you to sauté vegetables for long periods without browning (unless desired) or burning. This technique is called "sweating" and is important for concentrating and extracting maximum flavor.

---

*To season a cast-iron pan: Rinse a new cast-iron pan in warm sudsy water. Dry thoroughly, then pour a small amount of oil into the pan. Using a paper towel or a kitchen rag, spread it evenly on the bottom and sides of the pan. Place the pan in an oven preheated to 350° F for one to two hours. Let cool. Repeat the process. After use, do not wash a cast-iron pan with dish soap. Instead, scrub with an abrasive sponge, dry, rub with a small amount of oil, then dry over heat on the stove.

# General Tips for Healthy Cooking

How much should you worry about cancer risk from pesticide residues, food additives, or even natural carcinogens in food? In 1996, a twenty-member panel of the National Research Council confirmed that cancer-causing substances, both natural and synthetic, exist in foods, but their potential to cause cancer is minimal when compared with overconsumption of calories and fat. Obesity and diets high in fat and saturated fat are much more strongly linked to cancer. Many fruits and vegetables have natural carcinogens that do not pose a risk of cancer unless eaten in enormous amounts. In addition, any cancer risk from fruits and vegetables is far outweighed by their anticarcinogenic compounds—vitamins, minerals, and phytochemicals. Still, there are steps you can take to further minimize the amounts of cancer-causing compounds in food and from cooking.

## Cooking

To prevent or limit formation of carcinogenic compounds during cooking, take some of the following steps:

- Trim all excess fat from meat and remove the skin from poultry. This limits the amount of fat that drips during grilling, reducing, or charring.
- Marinate meat, fish, poultry, or vegetables, but wipe them off before grilling.
- Precook (microwave, poach, or roast) chicken or pork before placing on the grill, limiting high heat contact and charring. (This will also help to ensure that bacteria that can cause food-borne illnesses is killed.)
- Do not use juices that are released from the cooked meat once it has been taken off the grill.
- When grilling, cook food at least 6 inches above the heat source.
- If charring occurs, do not eat the burned portions.
- Don't use mesquite; it produces very high heat that can cause charring.
- If drippings from fat create a lot of smoke, remove food from the grill or reduce heat.
- Serve grilled foods with vitamin C–rich foods. Try tomato salads, fruit or vegetable salsas, chutneys or relishes, or orange and red onion salad.
- Steam foods sealed in foil wrap over the grill.
- Brush vegetables with a little oil to prevent sticking to the grill and burning.
- Slice vegetables less than 2 inches thick to reduce cooking time on the grill or precook slightly by roasting.
- Limit or avoid fried foods.

## Minimizing Pesticide Residues

- Rinse all fruits and vegetables thoroughly to remove dirt, bacteria, and any surface residues from pesticides. If you use a small amount of mild detergent to help remove pesticides, be sure to rinse thoroughly, otherwise chemicals not meant for consumption will be left behind.
- Peel vegetables with wax-coated skins, such as apples, cucumbers, and eggplant, but do not peel all vegetables because fiber as well as other nutrients are concentrated in or near the skin. Also, seasonal produce is less likely to be coated with wax.
- Use a scrub brush for potatoes, sweet potatoes, carrots, zucchini, or summer squash when you plan to eat the skin.
- Chop or tear vegetables with nonuniform shapes and curvatures, such as broccoli, cauliflower, spinach, or lettuce leaves, before rinsing.
- Discard outer leaves of the head of salad vegetables like cabbage or lettuce.
- Root vegetables (grown under the ground) accumulate more pesticides than those grown aboveground, so consider buying organic root vegetables.
- Eat a variety of foods to minimize your exposure to pesticides.
- Try to eat locally grown produce when it is in season.
- Buy some or all "certified organic" produce.

## Minimizing Food Additives

- Food additives are put in during processing, so eat minimally processed foods which have more fiber, vitamins, minerals, and phytochemicals.
- Limit use of "instant" and quick-cooking products.
- Limit convenience products or meals with seasoning packs, such as rices and other packages that say "just add . . ."
- Limit commercial sweets and snack foods. Select fruit or some other form of whole food instead.
- Look for animal products such as dairy or meat with labels that indicate they're from animals not treated with antibiotics or hormones.

## Organic Foods

The term *organic* on foods or food labels means that the product was grown without synthetic fertilizers, pesticides, herbicides, or fungicides. The Organic Foods Production Act passed in 1990 promises national certification and a standardized definition of organic foods. At present, the federal government has yet to devise a legal definition for organic, and more than thirty states currently have legislation pending about their own organic standards and labeling. Private organizations operate and regulate in other states, but there are many different standards for regulating "certified organic" foods. In almost all cases, there is some form of regulation process intact to assure that the food was grown consistent with the standards of the state's legislature or that of private governing groups. The National Organic Program is creating a uniform definition for organic and setting up a nationwide system to certify producers. It may go into effect in 1997. Expedient implementation of the 1990 legislation will benefit not only consumers, but also reputable farmers who comply with their local established organic farming codes.

There have been concerns about pesticides and drug residues present in livestock and poultry. To date, no studies demonstrate detrimental effects. Still, many people choose to buy meat and poultry from producers who do not expose their animals to hormones or antibiotics and who feed their animals organic grains. Products are available at many supermarkets, butcher shops, specialty markets, and through mail order.

There is no legal definition for "free range." It generally means that the animal was allowed to roam and forage for food rather than being completely confined. Although free-range does not assure that the animal is fed grains devoid of antibiotics, pesticides, or other chemicals, their relative freedom of movement makes them better exercised than their commercial counterparts, and therefore free-range products generally contain less fat. Because free-range animals spend more time outside and have liberty to forage, they can be more prone to salmonella. As with all poultry, be sure to cook meat completely (165° F internal temperature).

Even though scientific evidence does not support that pesticide residues are highly causative factors associated with incidence of cancer, there are still some very good reasons to buy organic foods:

- Reduction in intake of pesticides and fertilizers. Even though under the best of circumstances organic food is not completely free of pesticides, the amounts that can be detected are generally trace.
- Many people think organic foods taste better.
- This type of farming replenishes the soil and helps to protect the water supply.

When not to buy organic:

- Buying exclusively organic foods limits the variety of fruits and vegetables in your diet.
- The expense may limit your consumption of fruits and vegetables.

# Cooking with Olive Oil

By increasing public awareness of the variety of uses and health benefits of olive oil, the International Olive Oil Council (IOOC), an intergovernmental agency, is largely responsible for the increase in consumption seen in the last decade. Part of the IOOC's education campaign is informing consumers about the different classifications of olive oil. Having an understanding of the different types of olive oil will help you in selecting and using this flavorful and healthful type of fat.

**1.** "Extra Virgin Olive Oil" and "Virgin Olive Oil." Virgin olive oil is obtained from the fruit of the olive tree solely by mechanical or other physical means under conditions that do not lead to deterioration of the oil. This oil does not undergo any treatment other then washing, decantation, centrifugation, and filtration.

The two kinds of virgin olive oil sold in the United States are "extra virgin olive oil" and "virgin olive oil," the latter being a very small part of the market. These oils differ in terms of flavor, aroma, color, and acidity level. Extra virgin olive oil is described as having the perfect balance of these characteristics. To be labeled extra virgin olive oil, its acidity must not exceed 1 percent (1 gram per 100 grams). Virgin olive oil can contain up to 3.3 percent acidity, but industry practice in the producing countries is to keep levels under 2 percent.

Extra virgin olive oils share many of the same characteristics, however they do vary in taste. Many nuances contribute to the diversity of flavors, color, and aromas found in olive oil. Connoisseurs generally categorize olive oil flavors as mild (delicate, light, or "buttery"); semi-fruity (stronger, with more taste of the olive); and fruity (oil with a full-blown olive flavor). The best way to become familiar with the wide range of olive oil flavors is to taste as many of them as possible. One very cost-effective way is to split up a number of large bottles of different oils with friends.

**2.** What is now called "olive oil" is defined as the blend of refined olive oil with virgin olive oil. The blend of refined olive oil and virgin olive oil may bear on the label, beneath its designation, the term "pure" or "100% pure." The addition of virgin olive oil adds "fruitiness," color, aroma, and certain basic elements, especially alpha-tocopherol (vitamin E). The amount of virgin olive oil added varies from one producer to another and depends on the desired flavor the producer is trying to create.

For heavy-duty, high-heat cooking, it's probably best to use olive oil as it is less rich in volatile compounds that disappear with heat and may "perfume" your kitchen. It has the same fatty acid content as virgin olive oil and this is what gives it such good resistance to high temperatures It is also less expensive than virgin olive oils.

**3.** "Olive Pomace Oil." Pomace is the portion of the olive that remains after pressing or centrifuge operations remove the oil and water. Additional oil can be extracted from the olive pomace with the use of solvents. This oil is then refined to produce a product that has no specific taste, color, or solvents. To produce a product that is acceptable to consumers, this oil is then blended with virgin olive oil. As with olive oil, the relative proportions of virgin olive oil and oil extracted from the pomace are determined by the individual manufacturer. The percentage of virgin olive oil is usually quite low. The final product is called "olive pomace oil." It is produced at a lower cost than olive oil because pomace, the starting material, does not have nearly the value of olives that are used for pressing into oil. Olive pomace oil, like olive oil, can be used for high-heat cooking.*

Studies indicate that a Mediterranean diet low in saturated fats such as butter, lard, and animal fats, but rich in monounsaturated fats such as olive oil, in addition to grains, fruits, and vegetables, helps keep the artery clogging LDL ("bad cholesterol") low while maintaining healthful levels of HDL ("good cholesterol"). HDL has a preventive effect on cardiovascular illness because it may help to eliminate the LDL from the blood by carrying it to the liver. In addition, many medical researchers and nutritionists agree that olive oil is a good source of vitamin E, which may protect against cancer and heart disease. Olive oil also contains other compounds that are being investigated for their potential to lower risk of cancer.

*Information provided by the International Olive Oil Council.

# CHAPTER 5

# Recipes

**H**ere are more than a hundred recipes that will make delicious, healthful eating a day-to-day reality. Included are everything from savory side dishes and appetizers to main meals, even holiday menus. The recipes cover everything from hearty stews to light summer salads, from no-fuss broccoli casserole to a very special Christmas duck. Concocted by the top chefs in America, these recipes will start the most basic cook on the road to preparing fresh, easy, and healthful meals. Recipes not attributed to a particular chef have been created by Laura Pensiero, Strang nutritional consultant and French Culinary Institute-trained chef.

Nutritional analysis for each recipe was performed using a widely accepted software application. Sources of nutrition information are believed to be reliable and accurate, including but not limited to the original manufacturers and the United States Department of Agriculture. Although computerized nutritional analysis provides an accurate approximation of nutrients, the values are just that—an approximation.

Within each recipe reference is made to the amount of nutrients provided compared to the Daily Values (DV).* For instance, if a serving provides 30 percent of the DV for vitamin C, this has been calculated based on the reference value of 60 mg for vitamin C. The following are the basis for the Daily Reference Values (DRVs) for other nutrients highlighted in the recipes that follow:

| | | |
|---|---:|---|
| Vitamin A | 1,000 | RE |
| Vitamin C | 60 | mg |
| Calcium | 1,000 | mg |
| Vitamin D | 400 | IU |

*For more information about Daily Values, see pages 78 to 80.

| Vitamin E | 30 | IU |
| Folate | 400 | mcg |
| Dietary fiber | 25 | gm |

- Nutrient levels are rounded to the nearest whole number.
- When total fat is less than 0.5 gram, it is considered a trace amount and represented by 0. If you try to calculate the percentage of calories from fat, carbohydrate, or protein using the rounded numbers, your results will not always match ours.
- Comments about the levels of selenium and omega-3 fatty acids are expressed as "potentially good" or "potentially very good" sources of these nutrients because these values are dependent on other factors and nutritional database information is not complete.

In circumstances in which total fat may seem high (as a percentage of calories), keep the following in mind:

- Total grams of fat as it relates to your goal for the day. For example, a low-calorie, low-fat vinaigrette may contain 30 calories and only 2 grams of fat (much less than a classic vinaigrette), but the percentage of calories from fat is 60 percent.
- The type of fat. In many cases the fat source is predominantly monounsaturated fatty acids, such as canola or olive oil which contain linolenic and/or omega-3 fatty acids, which may have a protective role in the prevention of cancer.
- The total nutrient profile of the menu item. Rather than focus on the goal of keeping everything you eat at less than 20 to 25 percent of calories from fat, put more emphasis on getting a wide variety of the nutrients and phytochemicals that play a significant role in promoting good health.
- Put the menu item in context with other accompaniments or, better yet, your total intake for the day or the week.

# APPETIZERS AND SIDES

## ❧ *Healthy Hummus* ❧
## *with Toasted Pita Chips*

### 12 SERVINGS

* *Use hummus instead of mayonnaise as a sandwich spread to lower your fat intake, or serve with crackers or crusty bread.*

### Hummus

| | |
|---|---|
| 1 1/2 cups chickpeas, cooked, or canned, drained (see Notes) | 1/2 cup 1% cottage cheese (see Notes) |
| 2 garlic cloves or 1 head roasted garlic (page 178) | 1 small potato (about 5 ounces), cooked and peeled (see Notes) |
| 1/4 cup tahini (see Notes) | 1/4 teaspoon ground cumin |
| 1/3 cup water | 1/8 teaspoon cayenne |
| 2 teaspoons lemon juice | salt |

### Pita Chips

| | |
|---|---|
| 6 whole wheat pitas, halved horizontally and cut into quarters | 1 tablespoon olive oil |
| | salt |
| | pinch cayenne |

To prepare the hummus, combine all ingredients in the bowl of a food processor and puree until smooth.

To prepare the toasted pita chips, preheat the oven to 375 degrees F.

Place the pita wedges in a large bowl. Drizzle the oil over the pita pieces, sprinkle with salt and cayenne, and then toss with your hands to evenly mix. Spread the seasoned pita wedges in a single layer on a baking sheet and bake for 6 to 8 minutes, until golden brown and crisp; be careful not to burn. Serve on a platter with a bowl of hummus in the center.

*Notes:* To cook dried chickpeas, soak them in water to cover for 4 hours; change the water 2 to 3 times. Drain and place in a saucepan, cover with water, and add a bay leaf (1 to 2 celery stalks, a carrot, and half of a large onion may also be added for more flavor).

Bring to a boil and then reduce to a gentle simmer. Cook until the beans are tender but firm, 2 to 2½ hours, adding more water as necessary so that the beans are always covered. Drain and use in a recipe or as an addition to soups and salads.

Tahini is toasted sesame seed paste.

For a nondairy version, substitute 2 ounces of lite silken tofu for the cottage cheese.

To bake the potato, scrub the potato and pat dry, then prick the skin several times with a fork. Bake directly on the oven rack at 375 degrees F for about 50 minutes, depending on the size of the potato. The potato is done when it gives when gently squeezed. To microwave the potato, scrub, dry, prick the potato skin, and cook at high power. The time will depend on the size of the potato and the power of the microwave.

---

- The addition of roasted garlic not only adds flavor and creaminess, but also provides cancer-protective allium compounds.
- Sesame seeds (toasted and ground for tahini) are a good source of the following cancer-protective compounds: inositol or phytic acid, protease inhibitors, plant sterols, and isoflavones.
- The addition of baked potato provides a fat-free creaminess to this recipe and also bolsters the potassium and vitamin C content.
- A good source of fiber.

---

**Per serving of Healthy Hummus (3 tablespoons):**

| calories | protein | carbohydrates | fat | cholesterol | dietary fiber | saturated fat |
|---|---|---|---|---|---|---|
| 105 | 4 Gm | 14 Gm | 4 Gm | 0 mg | 3 Gm | 1 Gm |

**Per serving of Toasted Pita Chips (4 chips):**

| calories | protein | carbohydrates | fat | cholesterol | dietary fiber | saturated fat |
|---|---|---|---|---|---|---|
| 95 | 3 Gm | 17 Gm | 2 Gm | 0 mg | 3 Gm | 0 Gm |

**Per serving of Healthy Hummus with Toasted Pita Chips:**

| calories | protein | carbohydrates | fat | cholesterol | dietary fiber | saturated fat |
|---|---|---|---|---|---|---|
| 200 | 7 Gm | 32 Gm | 6 Gm | 0 mg | 6 Gm | 1 Gm |

**% of Calories:** 62% carbohydrate, 13% protein, 25% fat

### Major Sources of Potential Cancer Fighters

**Phytochemicals**: capsaicin, phytic acids, plant polyphenols (flavonoids, isoflavones, phenolic acids), plant sterols, protease inhibitors, terpenes (monoterpenes)

# ✤ *Roasted Eggplant Dip* ✤

8 SERVINGS

• *This low-fat, phytochemical-rich spread is terrific with toasted pita chips (see Healthy Hummus, page 115) or can replace mayonnaise as a zesty sandwich spread.*

| | |
|---|---|
| 1 medium eggplant (about 20 ounces), halved lengthwise | 1/2 cup 1% cottage cheese |
| 1 teaspoon olive oil | 2 tablespoons tahini (see Note) |
| 1 head roasted garlic | 1/8 teaspoon cayenne |
| 1 medium potato (about 6 ounces), cooked (baked or microwaved) | 1 teaspoon lemon juice |
| | 1 tablespoon sesame oil |
| | 1/3 teaspoon salt |

Preheat the oven to 350 degrees F.

Brush the flesh of the halved eggplant with the olive oil. Place on a nonstick baking pan, flat side down, and roast for 20 to 30 minutes. Turn over and continue roasting for approximately 20 minutes. Remove from the oven and let cool.

Scoop the pulp from the skin of the eggplant and place into the bowl of a food processor. Add the flesh of the roasted garlic and the potato and puree. Then add the cottage cheese, tahini, cayenne, and lemon juice and puree again until smooth. With the motor running, drizzle in the sesame oil. Season to taste with salt and transfer to an attractive serving bowl.

*Note:* Tahini is toasted sesame seed paste. If you do not eat dairy, silken tofu substitutes well for cottage cheese.

---

• The addition of potato not only adds a fat-free creaminess to this dip, but also enriches it with vitamin C.
• Although not particularly rich in vitamins, eggplant contains flavonoids such as quercetin that act as antioxidants and help to boost cancer-fighting enzymes.

---

**Per serving:**

| calories | protein | carbohydrates | fat | cholesterol | dietary fiber | saturated fat |
|---|---|---|---|---|---|---|
| 110 | 4 Gm | 15 Gm | 4 Gm | 1 mg | 2 Gm | 1 Gm |

**% of Calories:** 50% carbohydrate, 15% protein, 35% fat

### Major Sources of Potential Cancer Fighters

**Phytochemicals:** allium compounds, plant polyphenols (flavonoids, phenolic acids), phytic acids, plant sterols, terpenes (monoterpenes)

# ❦ Fricassee of Young ❦ Vegetables in Tomato Consommé

Wayne Nish, March, New York, New York

### 4 SERVINGS

•   *This vegetarian dish is one of the most popular appetizer's at Wayne Nish's March Restaurant. He suggests that you make it in the summer when the selection of fresh vegetables are at their peak. If you make it late in the summer, you will be able to find fresh aromatic black truffles.*

1   tablespoon extra virgin olive oil
1/4   cup butternut or acorn squash (about 1 1/2 ounces), peeled and diced into small cubes
1   cup vegetable stock or broth or water
4   tender young green string beans, cut into 1/2-inch lengths
4   tender young yellow wax beans, cut into 1/4-inch lengths
2   young, flat Romano beans (about 1 ounce), cut into 1/4-inch lengths
1   handful zucchini (about 1 ounce), julienned
1   handful yellow squash (about 1 ounce), julienned
1   garlic clove, minced
    sea salt to season
6   thin asparagus tips (about 1 ounce), 1 1/2 inches long

1/4   cup sweet peas (about 1 1/2 ounces)
3   red pear tomatoes (about 2 ounces) or other small sweet red tomatoes, cut in half
3   yellow pear tomatoes (about 2 ounces) or other small sweet yellow tomatoes, cut in half
6   squash blossoms (about 1/2 ounce)
1/2   teaspoon sweet butter
1   small black truffle (about 1/4 ounce), finely chopped (optional)
1 1/2   tablespoons chopped fresh mixed herbs (equal amounts of chervil, chives, parsley, tarragon, and basil)
4   fresh thyme sprigs

Preheat an 8-inch nonstick sauté pan and add the olive oil and butternut squash. Cook over low heat for 2 minutes. Add the stock or broth, all of the cut beans and squashes, and the garlic and season to taste with salt. Simmer for 4 minutes; the vegetables should be tender but not soft.

Add the asparagus, peas, tomatoes, and squash blossoms and stir well. Cook for 1 minute more. Add the butter, chopped truffle, if using, and the mixed herbs. The fricassee is ready to serve when the fragrance of the herbs and truffles is full, about 1 to 2 minutes. Adjust the seasoning, if necessary, with a pinch of salt. Remove the vegetables with a slotted spoon to a plate to keep warm. Reduce the liquid in the pan to $1/2$ cup.

To assemble, neatly pile the vegetables in equal amounts in 4 soup bowls and drizzle the sauce over the top of each. Garnish with fresh thyme sprigs and serve immediately.

> • Each serving provides 15% of the DV for vitamin A and more than 25% for vitamin C.

**Per serving:**

| calories | protein | carbohydrates | fat | cholesterol | dietary fiber | saturated fat |
|---|---|---|---|---|---|---|
| 74 | 3 Gm | 8 Gm | 4 Gm | 1 mg | 2 Gm | 1 Gm |

**% of Calories**: 38% carbohydrate, 13% protein, 49% fat

**Major Sources of Potential Cancer Fighters**
**Phytochemicals**: plant polyphenols (flavonoids, phenolic acids), plant sterols, terpenes (carotenoids, monoterpenes)

# ❧ *Pastina Risotto with White* ❧ *Beans and Baby Clams*

Nick Morfogen, Maxaluna, Boca Raton, Florida

8 SERVINGS

• *The perfect warm appetizer for lunch or a brunch buffet. Or serve in the center of the table for a family-style meal.*

• *Serve with toasted bread rounds that have been rubbed with garlic.*

## Pastina

1   cup clam broth or
    vegetable stock
$1/2$   medium onion
    (about 2 ounces), diced
2   teaspoons minced garlic
2   tablespoons olive oil
1   cup pastina (see Notes)
$1/2$   cup white wine

$1^1/2$   cups cooked white beans,
    well drained (about 10 ounces),
    or canned beans, drained
    salt and freshly ground
    black pepper
$1/4$   cup unseasoned bread
    crumbs

*Clams*

|   |   |   |   |
|---|---|---|---|
| 1 | tablespoon olive oil |   | salt and pepper |
| 1 | tablespoon minced garlic | 1/2 | cup chopped tomatoes |
| 1 | tablespoon chopped fresh basil |   | (about 1 medium) |
| 1 | tablespoon chopped fresh oregano | 1/4 | cup clam juice |
| 2 | pounds clams (little necks or |   | or broth (see Notes) |
|   | manillas), rinsed |   |   |
| 1/4 | cup vermouth |   |   |

Pastina cooks quickly, so have all ingredients on hand once you begin preparation. To make the pastina, in a small saucepan, combine the clam broth and 1 cup pastina plus 2 tablespoons water, bring to a boil, and then reduce the heat to low.

In a medium, heavy, oven-safe saucepan, sauté the onion and garlic in the olive oil over medium heat for 2 to 3 minutes, until tender. Add the pastina and stir with a wooden spoon to evenly coat with oil. Add the white wine and cook, while stirring, until all the wine is absorbed or cooked off, less than 1 minute. Add one-third of the clam juice–water mixture to the sauté pan and reserve the remaining two-thirds. Maintain a low simmer at medium-low heat and stir frequently.

To cook the clams, in a large nonstick sauté pan, heat the olive oil over high heat. Add the garlic and cook until it just turns golden, then reduce the heat to medium, stir in the herbs, and continue to cook for another minute. Do not burn garlic. Add the clams, remaining clam juice, and vermouth, season with salt and pepper, and bring to a boil. Cover, and after less than 1 minute, begin to transfer the opened clams to a clean bowl. Add the tomatoes to the clam juice–vermouth mixture left in the sauté pan, and reduce the liquid over high heat until the volume is halved.

Preheat the oven to 425 degrees F.

Add the cooking liquid from the clams, the white beans, and another one-third of the clam juice–water mixture to the saucepan with the pastina. Continue stirring until all liquid is absorbed, about 5 minutes, then add the remaining one-third of the clam juice–water mixture. It should be somewhat soupy at this point and the pasta should be al dente. Season to taste with salt and pepper.

Place the clams, with the open end facing upward, over the pastina. Sprinkle with the bread crumbs and place in the oven until the mixture is bubbly and lightly browned. Place the pan over a pot holder or a heavy kitchen towel in the middle of the table. Have oyster forks and spoons available.

*Notes:* Pastina means "tiny dough" and refers to any very small pasta shape. Available at supermarkets.

Clam juice is available at most supermarkets.

- Clams are a potentially good source of selenium.
- Each serving provides 15% of the DV for vitamin C.
- White beans provide fiber (17% of the DV per serving), as well as many of the same protective phytochemicals found in soybeans.

**Per serving:**

| calories | protein | carbohydrates | fat | cholesterol | dietary fiber | saturated fat |
|----------|---------|---------------|-----|-------------|---------------|---------------|
| 234 | 10 Gm | 29 Gm | 6 Gm | 7 mg | 3 Gm | 1 Gm |

**% of Calories**: 50% carbohydrate, 16% protein, 23% fat, 10% alcohol

**Major Sources of Potential Cancer Fighters**

**Phytochemicals**: allium compounds, phytic acids, plant polyphenols (flavonoids, phenolic acids), protease inhibitors, terpenes (carotenoids, monoterpenes)

# ❧ Summer Vegetable Casserole ❧ with Basil and Black Olives

Daniel Boulud, Restaurant Daniel, New York, New York
From *Cooking with Daniel Boulud*, Random House, 1993.

### 4 SERVINGS

2 tablespoons olive oil
salt and freshly ground
black pepper

1 large sweet red pepper (about
7 ounces), quartered lengthwise,
stems and seeds discarded

1 small zucchini (about 5 ounces),
ends trimmed and cut
lengthwise into thin slices

1 small eggplant (about 14 ounces),
ends trimmed, peeled, and cut
horizontally into thin slices

16 to 20 wax beans, ends trimmed
and cut into 1/2-inch segments

3 ears fresh corn, husks and
silk removed

1/4 cup small black olives (Niçoise)

1 celery heart (about 1 ounce),
cut into 1/4-inch slices (reserve
the small yellow leaves for
garnish)

2 medium tomatoes (about 8
ounces), split, cored, seeded,
and cut into 1/8-inch dice

3 scallions, white part only,
finely sliced

1 small European hothouse cucumber
(about 4 ounces), peeled, split
lengthwise, seeded, and cut into
1/4-inch dice (use domestic
if unavailable)

1    bunch watercress (about 2 ounces)
     leaves only
3    basil sprigs, leaves only, coarsely
     chopped
     juice of 2 lemons
6 to 8 drops Tabasco

1    bunch arugula (about 3 ounces),
     leaves only
6    round radishes (about 3 ounces),
     stems and rootlets trimmed,
     very thinly sliced

Preheat the broiler.

Brush a nonstick baking sheet or shallow roasting pan (large enough to hold each of the vegetables in a single layer) with 1/2 teaspoon of the olive oil and sprinkle with salt and pepper. Place the red pepper skin side up in the broiler and broil until the skin turns black, 8 to 10 minutes. Transfer the red pepper to a plate and cool. When cool, rub off the burnt skin with a paper towel and set the pepper slices aside.

Wipe off the baking sheet with a paper towel. Brush it with 1/2 teaspoon of the olive oil and sprinkle with salt and pepper. Place the zucchini and eggplant slices tightly side by side on the sheet. Brush the top of the slices with 2 teaspoons of olive oil and season with a pinch each of salt and pepper. Broil for 7 to 8 minutes or until lightly brown. Turn the slices over and broil for another 5 to 7 minutes. When done, remove from the pan and set aside to cool.

Bring 3 quarts water with 1/2 tablespoon salt to a boil in a large pot over medium heat. Add the wax beans and boil for 8 to 10 minutes or until very tender. Remove the beans with a slotted spoon to a colander and cool.

Add the corn on the cob to the same boiling water used for the beans and boil for 4 to 5 minutes. Drain and set aside to cool. When cool, remove the kernels from the cob. Discard the cobs and set the corn kernels aside.

Place the black olives in a resealable plastic bag and seal. Lightly pound with a mallet or rolling pin. Remove the olives and pit them. Cut the pitted olives into small pieces and set aside.

When ready to serve, in a large bowl, combine the wax beans, corn kernels, celery heart, tomatoes, scallions, cucumber, half of the Niçoise olives, the watercress, basil, juice of 1 lemon, 1 tablespoon olive oil, the salt, and Tabasco. Toss well and taste for seasoning.

Form a ring around the edge of a round casserole by alternating the zucchini and eggplant slices. Fill the center of the ring with the corn mixture. Place a tight bunch of arugula leaves in the center of the corn mixture. Arrange the red pepper strips around the arugula on top of the corn mixture and place the radish slices over and around the arugula on top of the corn mixture. Sprinkle the whole dish with the remaining chopped black olives, celery leaves, and a pinch of salt and pepper. Drizzle the remaining lemon juice over the top and serve at room temperature.

- Peppers, tomatoes, and watercress are all rich in vitamin C—each serving of this delicious casserole provides 95% of the DV.
- Contains more than 15% of the DVs for vitamin A and folate.
- A good source of fiber—16% of the DV per serving.

*Per serving:*

| calories | protein | carbohydrates | fat | cholesterol | dietary fiber | saturated fat |
|----------|---------|---------------|-----|-------------|---------------|---------------|
| 224 | 4 Gm | 22 Gm | 15 Gm | 0 mg | 4 Gm | 2 Gm |

**% of Calories**: 37% carbohydrate, 7% protein, 56% fat

**Major Sources of Potential Cancer Fighters**

**Phytochemicals**: allium compounds, glucosinolates, plant polyphenols (flavonoids, phenolic acids), plant sterols, terpenes (carotenoids, monoterpenes, triterpenes)

# ↓ Timbale of Salmon Tartare ↓ with Avocado and Lemon Oil

Casadio Luca, Bice Ristorante, New York, New York

4 SERVINGS

- *Serve as a first course for brunch, lunch, or dinner.*
- *Top toasted bread rounds with salmon tartare for a delicious and attractive appetizer.*

## Salmon

8  ounces sashimi-quality salmon, raw skin and gray part removed, diced (see Notes)

1  tablespoon snipped fresh chives

1/2  tablespoon chopped fresh dill

1  tablespoon minced shallots

1/4  fresh jalapeño pepper, seeded and minced

1/2  tablespoon canola oil

2  teaspoons lemon juice

salt and freshly ground pepper

## Garnish

1  teaspoon lemon oil (see Notes)

1/2  teaspoon canola oil

1  avocado (about 6 ounces), peeled, pitted, and diced

1  hard-cooked egg, white and yolk separated and finely chopped

2  tablespoons snipped chives

Lemon oil is a natural essence or oils extracted from the peel. Available at most supermarkets and gourmet specialty stores.

To prepare the salmon, in a medium bowl, combine all ingredients for the salmon and season with salt and pepper (the salmon is not smoked, so season generously). Stir gently to combine all ingredients and pack the salmon tartare into 4 timbale molds. Refrigerate.

In a small bowl, whisk together the lemon and canola oils. Unmold the salmon onto the center of 4 plates (tap the bottom of each mold and run a small paring knife around the edges, if necessary, to release). Sprinkle the avocado around each salmon mold, followed by the chopped egg whites and egg yolks. Garnish with the chives and drizzle with the oil mixture.

*Notes:* Salmon should be kept cold, especially when cutting.

---

- Although relatively high in percentage of calories from fat, the fat sources are predominantly monounsaturated (more than 60%), including potentially protective omega-3 fatty acids.
- Salmon is a potentially good source of selenium.
- The natural oils found in the peel of lemon and other citrus fruits contain limonene, a phytochemical that may help your body dispose of carcinogens.

---

*Per serving:*

| calories | protein | carbohydrates | fat | cholesterol | dietary fiber | saturated fat |
|---|---|---|---|---|---|---|
| 164 | 13 Gm | 2 Gm | 12 Gm | 62 mg | 1 Gm | 2 Gm |

**% of Calories**: 5% carbohydrate, 32% protein, 63% fat

### Major Sources of Potential Cancer Fighters

**Phytochemicals**: allium compounds, capsaicin, plant polyphenols (flavonoids), terpenes (monoterpenes; limonene; triterpenes)

# ❧ *Portobello Mushroom–* ❧ *stuffed Chiles Rellenos*

Miles Angelo, Caribou Club, Aspen, Colorado

6 SERVINGS

### Chiles Rellenos

3 large corn cobs or 1¹/₂ cups
   (6 ounces) frozen corn,
   thawed and drained

6 medium poblano chiles
   (about 5 ounces)

1¹/₂ pounds portobello mushrooms,
   brushed with a moist cloth,
   stems and underside gills
   removed

juice from 1 lemon

1 tablespoon olive oil

¹/₂ teaspoon salt

¹/₂ teaspoon white pepper

4 ounces queso blanco, grated
   (1 cup; see Notes)

¹/₂ bunch cilantro, chopped

### Chimayo Chile Sauce

6 chimayo chiles (or New
   Mexican chiles), seeded and
   stemmed (see Notes)

1 small yellow onion
   (about 2 ounces), sliced

2 garlic cloves

2 cups water

1 bay leaf

   salt

To cook the corn, heat 4 quarts of water and the ears of corn in a large pot. Bring to a boil and cook for 6 to 8 minutes. Drain and let cool.

To roast the chiles, preheat the broiler. Rub the peppers with a small amount of olive oil (less than ¹/₂ teaspoon) and place in an oven-safe skillet under the broiler. Using kitchen tongs, rotate the peppers to assure even cooking (browning) on all sides. Remove the peppers from the oven, place in a bowl, and cover with foil or plastic wrap so that steam helps to loosen the skins. When cool, remove the skins, seeds, and stems. Set aside.

To prepare the filling, in a medium bowl, marinate the mushrooms in the lemon juice, olive oil, ¹/₄ teaspoon salt, and ¹/₄ teaspoon white pepper for at least 20 minutes. Meanwhile, cut the sweet corn from the cob and place it in a small bowl with the queso blanco.

Grill the mushrooms over medium heat until tender (or roast on a nonstick baking pan for 7 to 8 minutes at 400 degrees F); remove from the grill and cool. Cut the mushrooms into medium cubes and add to the corn-queso mixture. Season with the cilantro and the remaining salt and white pepper. Mix to combine and set aside.

To prepare the sauce, combine all ingredients, except the salt, in a saucepan and bring to a boil. Reduce the heat and simmer for 10 minutes. Turn off the heat, remove the bay leaf, and let cool slightly. Transfer to the bowl of a food processor or blender and puree until very smooth; add a little water if necessary to thin to a sauce consistency. Strain through a fine mesh strainer into a small bowl and season to taste with salt.

To stuff the chiles, bring 2 cups of water to a boil in a pot with a steamer insert. Lightly season the inside and outside of each poblano. Fill each with the mushroom mixture and then wrap individually in plastic wrap, twisting the ends to form a seal. Place the chiles in the steamer insert and steam, covered, for 8 to 10 minutes. Carefully remove the chiles and set aside to cool slightly. When they are cool enough to handle, gently unwrap the plastic. Spoon the chimayo chile sauce on plates and place the chiles on top. Drizzle a little more sauce over the chiles.

*Notes:* Substitute ancho chiles for less heat and a more smoky flavor.

You can use low-fat white Cheddar, Monterey Jack, or soy versions of either instead of queso blanco.

---

- Capsaicin, found in chile peppers, may help to neutralize carcinogens.
- Chile peppers are very good sources of vitamin C; each serving provides more than 25% of the DV.
- Although corn does not contain substantial amounts of vitamins, it derives its color from the carotenoid lutein, a potent antioxidant.
- Mushrooms are a potentially good source of selenium.

---

*Per serving:*

| calories | protein | carbohydrates | fat | cholesterol | dietary fiber | saturated fat |
|---|---|---|---|---|---|---|
| 123 | 11 Gm | 10 Gm | 4 Gm | 7 mg | 5 Gm | 1 Gm |

**% of Calories**: 32% carbohydrate, 36% protein, 32% fat

### Major Sources of Potential Cancer Fighters

**Phytochemicals**: allium compounds, capsaicin, plant polyphenols (flavonoids, phenolic acids), terpenes (carotenoids, monoterpenes)

# ❧ *Roasted Tomato and Mint Salsa* ❧

Jerry Traunfeld, The Herbfarm, Fall City, Washington

4 SERVINGS

• *Jerry suggests using this high-flavor, nutrient-rich condiment for grilled or roasted meat, fish, or poultry.*

| | |
|---|---|
| 10 plum or medium tomatoes (1½ pounds), stemmed and halved | ¼ cup shredded mint leaves |
| 1 tablespoon olive oil | 1½ tablespoons red wine vinegar |
| 2 tablespoons red onion, minced | salt to taste |
| ½ jalapeño pepper, seeded and minced | |

Preheat the oven to 450 degrees F.

In a large bowl, toss the tomatoes in the olive oil. Arrange them on a wire rack, cut side down, and place the rack on a baking pan. Roast the tomatoes for 10 to 15 minutes, or until they start to brown. Remove from the oven and let cool.

Dice the tomatoes coarsely. Toss them in a bowl with the remaining ingredients. Let the salsa sit for at least 1 hour to blend the flavors.

---

• Tomatoes and tomato products are a great source of the carotenoid lycopene, a powerful cancer fighter.
• Mint contains monoterpenes, phytochemicals of the terpene class, which may help bolster cancer-fighting enzymes.
• One serving provides 60% of the DV for vitamin C.

---

**Per serving:**

| calories | protein | carbohydrates | fat | cholesterol | dietary fiber | saturated fat |
|---|---|---|---|---|---|---|
| 72 | 1 Gm | 9 Gm | 4 Gm | 0 mg | 2 Gm | 1 Gm |

**% of Calories**: 50% carbohydrate, 6% protein, 44% fat

### Major Sources of Potential Cancer Fighters

**Phytochemicals**: allium compounds, plant polyphenols (flavonoids, phenolic acids), plant sterols, terpenes (carotenoids, monoterpenes)

# ↯ *Tomato-Basil Sauce* ↯

MAKES 2 CUPS (1 SERVING = ½ CUP)

- *Double or triple this recipe, put in small containers, and freeze. You will have a quick and healthy tomato sauce for a busy day.*

| | |
|---|---|
| 2 pounds plum tomatoes (10 to 12) | ½ cup fresh basil, leaves cut into long strips |
| 1 tablespoon olive oil | salt and pepper |
| 2 garlic cloves, crushed | |
| 1 small onion (about 4 ounces), thinly sliced | |

To peel and seed the tomatoes, cut a shallow **X** into the bottom of the tomatoes and drop into boiling water for 20 to 30 seconds. Remove the skins and put in a bowl of ice water. Peel off the skins. Slice the tomatoes in half horizontally. Gently squeeze the halves over a bowl to force out the seeds.

Use your fingers to remove any remaining seeds. Discard the seeds, chop the tomatoes, and reserve.

Heat the olive oil over high heat in medium nonstick skillet. Add the crushed garlic and cook until lightly browned, then add the onion and cook over medium-high heat until limp, about 5 minutes, stirring often.

Add the reserved tomatoes and bring to a simmer. Cook, uncovered, over medium heat, stirring occasionally, for 35 minutes, until the sauce thickens.

Stir in the chopped basil, season with salt and pepper, and simmer for 2 to 3 minutes.

---

- Contains the carotenoids lycopene and beta-carotene; both are powerful antioxidants.
- One serving provides 60% of the DV for vitamin C and more than 10% for vitamin A.
- A good source of fiber.

---

**Per serving of Tomato-Basil Sauce (½ cup):**

| calories | protein | carbohydrates | fat | cholesterol | dietary fiber | saturated fat |
|---|---|---|---|---|---|---|
| 93 | 3 Gm | 14 Gm | 4 Gm | 0 mg | 3 Gm | 1 Gm |

**Per serving of Tomato-Basil Sauce with 8 ounces of cooked pasta:**

| calories | protein | carbohydrates | fat | cholesterol | dietary fiber | saturated fat |
|---|---|---|---|---|---|---|
| 422 | 13 Gm | 79 Gm | 6 Gm | 0 mg | 5 Gm | 1 Gm |

**% of Calories**: 75% carbohydrate, 12% protein, 13% fat

**Major Sources of Potential Cancer Fighters**
**Phytochemicals**: allium compounds, plant polyphenols (flavonoids, phenolic acids), plant sterols, phytic acids, terpenes (carotenoids, monoterpenes)

# ✔ *Venetian Pepperonata* ✔

Francesco Antonucci, Co-Owner/Executive Chef, Remi Restaurants, New York, New York, Santa Monica, California, Tel Aviv, Israel
Adapted from *Venetian Taste*, Abbeville Press, 1995.

4 SERVINGS

• *Francesco recommends serving this tasty Venetian pepperonata as a sauce for pasta, an accompaniment for fish, or a topping for polenta.*

| | |
|---|---|
| 1 large eggplant (about 18 ounces) | 1 medium zucchini (about 6 ounces), sliced 1/4 inch thick |
| 2 tablespoons extra virgin olive oil | |
| 1 large red onion (about 8 ounces), sliced 1/4 inch thick | 1 cup canned plum tomatoes, drained and crushed |
| 2 garlic cloves, peeled | salt and pepper |
| 2 large sweet red peppers (about 1 pound), seeded and cut into julienne strips | handful of fresh basil leaves, slivered |

Quarter the eggplant and cut away the flesh to within 1/2 inch of the skin. Save the center of the eggplant for another use and cut the skin in slivers about 1/4 inch wide. Set aside.

Heat the olive oil in a large, heavy skillet. Add the onion and garlic and sauté over medium heat, stirring, until the onion is golden, about 15 minutes. Add the peppers and sauté another 10 to 15 minutes. Add the eggplant and zucchini. Continue to sauté another 15 to 20 minutes, adjusting the heat, if necessary, to prevent browning or burning.

Stir in the tomatoes and cook another few minutes, then season with salt and pepper, stir in the basil, and serve.

---

• One serving provides 100% of the DV for vitamin C. By weight, peppers have two to three times the amount of vitamin C as citrus fruit. Green, yellow, and red bell peppers and chile peppers are also great sources of beta-carotene as well as other carotenoids.
• High in fiber—24% of the DV per serving.

*Per serving:*

| calories | protein | carbohydrates | fat | cholesterol | dietary fiber | saturated fat |
|---|---|---|---|---|---|---|
| 150 | 4 Gm | 20 Gm | 7 Gm | 0 mg | 6 Gm | 1 Gm |

*Per serving of Venetian Pepperonata with 8 ounces of cooked pasta:*

| calories | protein | carbohydrates | fat | cholesterol | dietary fiber | saturated fat |
|---|---|---|---|---|---|---|
| 469 | 14 Gm | 84 Gm | 9 Gm | 0 mg | 9 Gm | 1 Gm |

**% of Calories**: 71% carbohydrate, 12% protein, 17% fat

**Major Sources of Potential Cancer Fighters**

**Phytochemicals**: allium compounds, plant polyphenols (flavonoids, phenolic acids), plant sterols, terpenes (carotenoids, monoterpenes)

## Cooking Tips

*When a recipe just calls for olive oil, how do you know what kind to use?*

Let your own taste preferences be your guide, but temper it by the end result you want. As a general rule, cook with olive oil and season or drizzle with extra virgin after food is cooked.

Light and delicate dishes like poached or sautéed fish, chicken, or veal, or perhaps mild-flavored soups, may be better served by a milder, less fruity olive oil. Full-flavored robust dishes such as hearty stews, soups, or tomato-based sauces welcome a more fruity, flavorful olive oil, as do steamed vegetables and salads.

For roasted, barbecued, and braised dishes that require high temperature or prolonged cooking, it is probably best to use olive oil (or even olive pomace oil) because it is less rich in the volatile compounds that evaporate with heat. Equally important, it has the same health benefits as virgin olive oils, and is less expensive.

## Olive Oil and Frying

Because olive oil is stable at high temperature, you can fry, sauté, stir fry, and deep fry in olive oil. You can even filter olive oil after frying and use it again. Standard olive oil is the best for these forms of high-heat cooking.

## Olive Oil and Baking

- Olive oil, a monounsaturated fat, has a small fat crystal which yields even, fine-textured baked goods.
- Using olive oil in baking dramatically cuts the cholesterol and saturated fat in baked goods.

- Baking with olive oil produces lighter, tastier baked goods than butter and allows the flavor of the other ingredients to come through with more clarity.
- Olive oil contains tocopherols (vitamin E) that act as emulsifiers producing a smooth, homogenous batter that results in baked goods with a moist and tender crumb.
- Tocopherols also have antioxidant properties that retard staling and result in a fresher product.

Olive oil is particularly suited to the baking of carrot, chocolate, spice and fruit cakes; cookie bars; brownies; graham cracker, nut, or cookie crusts; corn bread or sticks and other quick breads, muffins, and biscuits; pancakes, blinis, and crepes; and flat breads and pizzas.

## Baking Conversions

Using olive oil in baked goods often allows for use of less fat. Here are some conversions for recipes:

| Butter/Margarine | Olive Oil |
|---|---|
| 1 teaspoon | $3/4$ teaspoon |
| 1 tablespoon | $2^1/4$ teaspoons |
| 2 tablespoons | $1^1/2$ tablespoons |
| $1/4$ cup | 3 tablespoons |
| $1/3$ cup | $1/4$ cup |
| $1/2$ cup | $1/4$ cup plus 2 tablespoons |
| $2/3$ cup | $1/2$ cup |
| $3/4$ cup | $1/2$ cup plus 1 tablespoon |
| 1 cup | $3/4$ cup |

For more information call the toll-free Olive Oil Hotline at (800) 232-6548 or send a self-addressed stamped, business size envelope to:

International Olive Oil Council
JAF Station, Box 2197
New York, NY 10116
(800) 232-Olive Oil

# SOUPS AND STOCKS

# ❧ *Black Bean Soup* ❧

Jimmy Sneed, The Frog and the Redneck, Richmond, Virginia

6 SERVINGS

• *Serve with a tossed green salad for lunch or dinner. Garnish with grilled or seared shrimp or scallops.*

• *Double the batch and freeze in small containers for a quick, high-fiber meal on a busy day.*

| | | | |
|---|---|---|---|
| 1 | pound dried black beans | 3 | garlic cloves, minced |
| 1 | tablespoon olive oil | 1 | bay leaf |
| 2 | medium carrots (about 6 ounces), peeled and diced | 4 | cups chicken stock (page 147 or 148), vegetable stock (page 146), or low-sodium canned |
| 2 | medium celery stalks (about 4 ounces), diced | | salt and pepper |
| 1 | medium onion (about 5 ounces), diced | 3 | scallions, chopped |
| 1 | large red bell pepper (about 7 ounces), seeded and diced | 4 | tablespoons low-fat sour cream |

In a medium bowl, soak the black beans in water to cover for 4 to 6 hours. Change the water 2 to 3 times. Drain and set aside.

In a large, heavy saucepan, heat the olive oil. Add the carrots, celery, onion, and red pepper and sauté over medium-high heat, without browning, until tender, about 10 minutes. Add the garlic and cook for 2 to 3 minutes, then add the drained beans, bay leaf, and stock. Simmer, covered, until the beans are tender enough to be easily crushed between two fingers, about 45 minutes. Remove the bay leaf and puree in a blender or food processor until smooth. If you want a more chunky texture, puree only half of the beans and vegetables and return them to the saucepan. Season to taste with salt and pepper. Serve in soup bowls and garnish with the chopped scallions and low-fat sour cream.

---

• Black beans contain isoflavones, which may lower the risk of breast and other types of cancer. They are also high in fiber and folate: this dish provides 50% of the DVs for both.
• One serving provides 85% of the DV for vitamin A and more than 50% for vitamin C.

*Per serving:*

| calories | protein | carbohydrates | fat | cholesterol | dietary fiber | saturated fat |
|----------|---------|---------------|-----|-------------|---------------|---------------|
| 232 | 13 Gm | 36 Gm | 4 Gm | 7 mg | 12 Gm | 1 Gm |

**% of Calories**: 63% carbohydrate, 22% protein, 15% fat

### Major Sources of Potential Cancer Fighters

**Phytochemicals**: allium compounds, phytic acids, plant polyphenols (flavonoids, isoflavones), protease inhibitors, terpenes (carotenoids, monoterpenes)

# ❧ *Butternut Squash Soup* ❧

Maria Helm, PlumpJack Cafe, San Francisco, California

4 SERVINGS

- *Makes a delicious, low-fat, nutrient-packed meal or first course.*
- *Other seasoning ideas include grated ginger, curry and diced apple, or curry and ancho chile.*

1 medium onion (about 5 ounces), chopped
1 tablespoon olive oil
4 sage leaves, finely chopped
1 tablespoon honey
1 medium butternut squash (about 2 pounds), peeled, halved, seeded, and cut into 1-inch chunks

6 cups chicken stock (page 147 or 148), vegetable stock (page 146), low-sodium canned broth or water
salt and pepper
1/2 cup 1% or soy milk (optional; see Note)

Sauté the onion in olive oil over moderate heat until slightly golden, about 10 minutes. Add the squash, sage, and honey and sauté until the honey bubbles.

Add the stock and simmer until the squash is tender when pierced with a knife, 30 to 35 minutes. Let cool slightly, and blend in food processor or blender until smooth. Return to the saucepan, if using milk, add and bring to a boil, and season with salt and pepper. Remove from the heat and serve.

*Note:* Soy milk is found at some supermarkets and most health food stores. It adds both creaminess and soy nutrients and phytochemicals.

- Butternut squash is among the richest dietary sources of beta-carotene. One serving of this soup has enough beta-carotene to provide more than 100% of the DV for vitamin A.
- Rich in vitamin C, this soup provides about 40% of the DV per serving.

*Per serving:*

| calories | protein | carbohydrates | fat | cholesterol | dietary fiber | saturated fat |
|----------|---------|---------------|-----|-------------|---------------|---------------|
| 152 | 6 Gm | 22 Gm | 5 Gm | 16 mg | 2 Gm | 1 Gm |

**% of Calories**: 53% carbohydrate, 15% protein, 32% fat

### Major Sources of Potential Cancer Fighters

**Phytochemicals**: allium compounds, plant polyphenols (flavonoids), terpenes (carotenoids, monoterpenes)

# ❧ Cauliflower Soup ❧

Francesco Antonucci, Remi Restaurants, New York, New York; Santa Monica, California; Tel Aviv, Israel
Adapted from *Venetian Taste*, Abbeville Press, 1995.

## 4 SERVINGS

- *"In Venice we have big soups, simple soups," says Francesco. "This is a good example."*
- *Serve hot or at room temperature.*

1 tablespoon olive oil
1 small onion (about 4 ounces), chopped
1 leek, white part only, chopped (about 2 ounces)
1 medium baking potato (about 6 ounces), peeled and coarsely chopped
1 small head cauliflower (about 20 ounces), core removed and coarsely chopped

1 anchovy fillet, rinsed and chopped
8 cups cold water
  salt and freshly ground white pepper
4 3-inch rounds of Italian country bread
1 garlic clove, crushed

Heat the olive oil in a large, heavy saucepan. Add the onion and leek and sauté slowly until they are tender but not brown, about 12 minutes.

Add the potato, cauliflower, anchovy, and water. Bring to a gentle simmer and cook, uncovered, for 1 hour. Allow the soup to cool briefly, then puree it in a blender or food processor. You may have to do this in two batches.

Return the soup to the saucepan, bring it to a simmer, and season with salt and white pepper.

Five minutes before serving, rub the bread rounds with the garlic and toast them until they are golden. Serve them alongside the soup.

---

- Cauliflower, a member of the cruciferous vegetable family, contains cancer-fighting phytochemicals, and is rich in vitamin C: one serving of this soup provides more than 100% of the DV.
- Anchovy adds omega-3 fatty acids and a subtle dimension to the flavor of this soup.
- A good source of fiber.

---

**Per serving:**

| calories | protein | carbohydrates | fat | cholesterol | dietary fiber | saturated fat |
|---|---|---|---|---|---|---|
| 152 | 5 Gm | 24 Gm | 4 Gm | 0 mg | 3 Gm | <1 Gm |

**% of Calories**: 63% carbohydrate, 12% protein, 25% fat

**Major Sources of Potential Cancer Fighters**

**Phytochemicals**: allium compounds, glucosinolates, omega-3 fatty acids, plant polyphenols (flavonoids, phenolic acids)

# ✤ Gazpacho ✤

Martin Saylor, The Lafayette at the Hay-Adams Hotel, Washington, D.C.

8 SERVINGS

- *This soup is ideal for a summer lunch or first course. Best of all, it's easy to prepare (under 30 minutes) and is full of flavor and helps keep those vegetable servings high.*

| | |
|---|---|
| 2 medium yellow bell peppers (about 12 ounces) | 16 ounces low-sodium tomato juice |
| 2 medium red bell peppers (about 14 ounces) | 1 tablespoon olive oil |
| 5 medium tomatoes (about 1 pound) | 2 medium cucumbers (about 1½ pounds), peeled, seeded, and diced |
| | 1 jalapeño pepper, seeded and diced |

1    shallot, minced
1    garlic clove, minced
     juice of 1 lime
3    scallions, thinly sliced

3    tablespoons chopped fresh cilantro
3    tablespoons chopped fresh basil
     salt and pepper

To roast the peppers, preheat the broiler. Rub the peppers with a small amount of olive oil (less than $1/4$ teaspoon), and place in an oven-safe skillet under the broiler. Using kitchen tongs, rotate the peppers to assure even cooking (browning) on all sides. Remove the peppers from the oven, place in a bowl, and cover with foil or plastic wrap so that steam helps to loosen the skins. When cool, remove the skins, seeds, and stems. Dice the peppers and set aside.

To peel and seed the tomatoes, bring 2 quarts of water to a boil in a large pot. Cut the core from the tomatoes with a paring knife and plunge them into boiling water for 30 seconds. Remove with a slotted spoon and immediately immerse in ice water until cool. Use a knife to gently peel the skin, which should be discarded. Slice the tomatoes in half and gently squeeze to force out the seeds. Use your fingers to remove any remaining seeds. Discard the seeds, chop the tomatoes, and set aside.

In a large bowl, combine all ingredients and season to taste with salt and pepper. Serve chilled.

---

- One serving provides more than 250% of the DV for vitamin C.
- Tomatoes and tomato products contain the carotenoid lycopene, a potent antioxidant. Peppers and tomatoes contain plant polyphenols that may act as blocking agents against cancer.
- A good source of fiber.

---

*Per serving:*

| calories | protein | carbohydrates | fat | cholesterol | dietary fiber | saturated fat |
|----------|---------|---------------|-----|-------------|---------------|---------------|
| 86 | 3 Gm | 14 Gm | 2 Gm | 0 mg | 3 Gm | 0 Gm |

**% of Calories**: 65% carbohydrate, 14% protein, 21% fat

### Major Sources of Potential Cancer Fighters
**Phytochemicals**: allium compounds, plant polyphenols (flavonoids, phenolic acids), plant sterols, protease inhibitors, terpenes (carotenoids, monoterpenes)

# ❧ *Ratatouille Soup* ❧

Michael Romano, Union Square Café, New York, New York
From *Union Square Café Cookbook*, HarperCollins Publishers, 1994.

### 4 SERVINGS

- *Serve this delicious year-round soup hot or cold.*
- *If you are trying to use up all of those summer garden vegetables, prepare a large batch and can or freeze in small containers.*

| | |
|---|---|
| 2 pounds ripe tomatoes (about 6 medium or 10 to 12 plum tomatoes) | 2 tablespoons fresh basil leaves, rinsed and sliced, plus 4 to 6 sprigs for garnish |
| 2 tablespoons olive oil | 1 teaspoon minced fresh thyme leaves |
| 1/3 cup chopped red onion (1 small) | 2 cups vegetable stock (page 146), chicken stock (page 147 or 148), or low-sodium canned broth |
| 1 teaspoon minced garlic | |
| 3/4 cup chopped zucchini (4 ounces) | |
| 3/4 cup peeled and chopped eggplant (3 ounces) | pinch cayenne |
| 3/4 cup chopped red bell pepper (4 ounces) | 1 teaspoon kosher salt |
| | 1/8 teaspoon freshly ground pepper |

Bring 2 quarts of water to a boil in a large pot. Cut the core from the tomatoes with a paring knife and plunge them into boiling water for 30 seconds. Remove with a slotted spoon and immediately immerse in ice water until cool. Use a knife to gently peel the skin, which should be discarded. Cut the tomatoes in half crosswise and squeeze them gently over a mesh strainer to separate the seeds from the juice. Reserve the juice. Gently flatten the tomato halves on a cutting board and coarsely chop into 1-inch pieces. Place the chopped tomatoes and the reserved juice in a bowl and set aside.

Heat the olive oil over medium heat in a 3-quart saucepan. Add the onion and garlic and cook for 1 minute. Stir in the zucchini, eggplant, and red pepper, sautéing until softened but not browned, about 5 minutes.

Add the tomatoes and their juice, the basil, thyme, stock, cayenne, salt, and pepper. Bring to a boil, lower the heat to a simmer, cover, and cook until soft, about 15 minutes.

Carefully pour the hot soup into a blender or food processor and puree until smooth. Serve hot or chilled with a sprig of fresh basil as a garnish.

- One serving provides three times the DV for vitamin C and enough carotenoids to supply 20% of the DV for vitamin A.
- A good source of fiber.

*Per serving:*

| calories | protein | carbohydrates | fat | cholesterol | dietary fiber | saturated fat |
|----------|---------|---------------|-----|-------------|---------------|---------------|
| 130 | 3 Gm | 19 Gm | 5 Gm | 0 mg | 4 Gm | 1 Gm |

**% of Calories**: 60% carbohydrate, 10% protein, 30% fat

### Major Sources of Potential Cancer Fighters
**Phytochemicals**: allium compounds, capsaicin, plant polyphenols (flavonoids, phenolic acids), plant sterols, terpenes (carotenoids, monoterpenes)

# ❧ *Roasted Pumpkin Soup* ❧

RoxSand Scocos, RoxSand's Restaurant & Bar, Phoenix, Arizona

#### 4 SERVINGS

• *Roasting vegetables before adding them to a soup creates a unique, rich flavor. Use this technique with other vegetables to replace pumpkin, such as butternut squash, turnips, or celery root.*

| | |
|---|---|
| 1 **small pumpkin** (about 1¹/₂ pounds), peeled, seeded, and cut into large pieces (approximately 2¹/₂ cups) | 1 **tablespoon olive oil** |
| | 4 **fresh rosemary sprigs** |
| | 3 **fresh thyme sprigs** |
| 2 **large onions** (about 14 ounces), cut into large pieces | 6 **cups vegetable stock** (page 146), chicken stock (page 147 or 148), low-sodium canned broth or water |
| 6 **garlic cloves**, peeled and crushed | |
| 2 **large potatoes** (about 1 pound), peeled and cut into medium-size chunks | salt and pepper |

Preheat the oven to 375 degrees F.

In a large bowl, combine the pumpkin, onions, garlic, and potatoes. Toss with the olive oil and fresh herbs and then spread out in a single layer on a nonstick baking pan. Roast for 50 minutes, stirring halfway through, until all vegetables are tender and lightly browned. Transfer to a saucepan and cover with the stock. Stir and bring to a boil. Lower the temperature and simmer until the flavors meld, about 15 minutes. Turn off the heat and let cool slightly. Remove the stems of fresh herbs and puree the soup in a food processor or blender. Return the puree to the saucepan and season to taste with salt and pepper. Heat to a simmer and adjust the seasoning. If a thinner consistency is de-sired, add more stock or water.

- Winter squash such as pumpkin provides substantial amounts of beta-carotene.
- Rich in vitamins A and C, this soup provides 65% and 50% of the DVs, respectively.
- Rosemary contains carnosol, a cancer-fighting phytochemical.
- A good source of fiber.

**Per serving:**

| calories | protein | carbohydrates | fat | cholesterol | dietary fiber | saturated fat |
|----------|---------|---------------|-----|-------------|---------------|---------------|
| 206 | 5 Gm | 38 Gm | 4 Gm | 0 mg | 4 Gm | 1 Gm |

**% of Calories:** 73% carbohydrate, 9% protein, 18% fat

### Major Sources of Potential Cancer Fighters

**Phytochemicals:** allium compounds, plant polyphenols (flavonoids), plant sterols, terpenes (carotenoids, carnosol, monoterpenes)

# ✢ *Leek and Potato Soup* ✢

#### 4 SERVINGS

- *Serve this broth-based soup chunky or pureed. Add 1/2 cup of 2% cow's milk or soy milk to the puree to lighten the color and add creaminess. Serve hot or chilled.*

| | |
|---|---|
| 4 medium leeks, white part only (about 10 ounces) | 2 large potatoes (about 1 pound), peeled and cubed |
| 2 teaspoons canola oil | salt and white pepper |
| 1 teaspoon unsalted butter | |
| 1 garlic clove, minced | |
| 5 cups chicken stock (page 147 or 148), vegetable stock (page 146), low-sodium canned broth, or water | |

To clean the leeks, slice them in half lengthwise, leaving the root end intact, and place under running water. Run your fingers through the leaves to remove any dirt.

Heat the canola oil and butter in a medium saucepan. Sauté the leeks over moderate heat for at least 15 minutes, stirring frequently; do not brown. (This step is essential to con-centrate the flavor and bring out the natural sweetness of the leeks, so be patient.) Add the garlic and cook for another minute, then add the chicken broth and potatoes. Bring the mixture to a boil, reduce the heat, and simmer for 20 minutes or until the potato chunks are tender when pierced with a knife. Season to taste with salt and white pepper and serve.

> - Leeks are rich in allium compounds, vitamin C, and folate (if the green part is used). They are generally considered a good source of selenium; however, amounts depend on the soil in which they are grown.
> - Potatoes are also high in vitamin C; combined with leeks they provide more than 25% of the DV per serving.

***Per serving:***

| calories | protein | carbohydrates | fat | cholesterol | dietary fiber | saturated fat |
|---|---|---|---|---|---|---|
| 209 | 9 Gm | 32 Gm | 5 Gm | 3 mg | 2 Gm | 1 Gm |

**% of Calories**: 61% carbohydrate, 17% protein, 22% fat

**Major Sources of Potential Cancer Fighters**
**Phytochemicals**: allium compounds, plant polyphenols (flavonoids, phenolic acids)

# ❧ *Spinach and Potato Cream Soup* ❧

## 6 SERVINGS

- *Depending on season and preference, substitute escarole, kale, or broccoli rabe for the spinach.*
- *Make a large batch and freeze in small containers for a quick vegetable serving.*

| | |
|---|---|
| 2 teaspoons olive oil | 2 medium potatoes (about 14 ounces), peeled and cubed |
| 1 large onion (about 8 ounces), chopped | 20 ounces fresh spinach, rinsed |
| 2 garlic cloves, peeled and crushed | 2 teaspoons salt |
| 4 medium carrots (about 12 ounces), peeled and sliced | 1/4 teaspoon black pepper |
| 5 cups water, chicken stock (page 147 or 148), or low-sodium canned broth | 1 cup skim milk (see Note) |

Heat the olive oil in a 6-quart saucepan and sauté the onion, garlic, and carrots over medium-high heat for at least 15 minutes; stir frequently. (This initial sauté releases the flavor of the vegetables, so be patient, adjust the temperature as necessary to prevent browning, and wait to add the liquid.)

Add the water or stock and potatoes and bring to a boil. Reduce the heat, cover, and simmer until the potato chunks and carrots are very tender when pierced with a knife, 30 to 35 minutes.

Add the spinach to the saucepan; push down slightly, if necessary, so that you can place the lid on the pot. Cook for 2 to 3 minutes, until the spinach is completely wilted, then remove from the heat and let cool slightly.

Puree in a food processor or blender (it will take two to three batches) until very smooth. Return the pureed soup to the saucepan, heat to a simmer, and season with salt and pepper. Stir in the skim milk for a creamier texture.

*Note:* You can substitute 1% soy milk or ¹/₂ cup creamed, silken tofu for skim milk.

---

- This carotenoid blend from both dark-green and orange sources (carrots and spinach), provides enough beta-carotene to supply 200% of the DV for vitamin A.
- One serving of this soup provides more than 90% of the DV for vitamin C and 60% for folate.
- High in fiber—35% of the DV per serving.

---

**Per serving:**

| calories | protein | carbohydrates | fat | cholesterol | dietary fiber | saturated fat |
|----------|---------|---------------|-----|-------------|---------------|---------------|
| 171 | 7 Gm | 29 Gm | 3 Gm | 0 mg | 7 Gm | 0 Gm |

**% of Calories:** 67% carbohydrate, 17% protein, 16% fat

**Major Sources of Potential Cancer Fighters**
**Phytochemicals:** allium compounds, phytic acids, plant polyphenols (flavonoids, phenolic acids), plant sterols, terpenes (carotenoids, monoterpenes)

# ❧ *Winter Vegetable Soup (Ribollita)* ❧

8 SERVINGS

- *This traditional Tuscan soup is flavorful and hearty, making a nutrient-rich winter meal by itself.*

| | |
|---|---|
| 3 cups cooked chickpeas or 3 cups canned, drained (see Note) | 2 garlic cloves, peeled and crushed<br>3 medium celery stalks (about 7 ounces), chopped |

3  medium carrots (about
      9 ounces), peeled and chopped
1  large red onion (about
      8 ounces), peeled and chopped
2  tablespoons olive oil
2  bunches Swiss chard (about
      2 pounds), cleaned
1/2  head Napa or Savoy cabbage
      (about 20 ounces)
1/4  cup chopped Italian parsley

2  fresh rosemary sprigs (leave on stem)
1  can (14 1/2 ounces)
      plum tomatoes, drained
6  cups boiling water, chicken stock
      (page 147 or 148), or low-sodium
      canned broth
5  ounces stale bread, such as
      semolina or baguette, sliced
      (about 3/4 loaf)
   salt and pepper

In a large saucepan, over medium-low heat, sauté the garlic, celery, carrots, and onion in the olive oil for about 20 minutes; stir often so that the vegetables do not brown.

Cut out the tough, triangular inner core of the Swiss chard leaves and slice into 1/4- to 1/2-inch slices. Add to the vegetables in the saucepan. Tear the Swiss chard leaves and set aside.

Cut out the triangular core of the 1/2 cabbage head, then discard. Place the cabbage, flat side down, on a cutting board. With a large chef's knife, slice at close intervals down the cabbage, forming long, ribbonlike strips. Set aside with the Swiss chard leaves.

Add the parsley, rosemary sprigs, and tomatoes to the saucepan and cook at a low simmer for 15 more minutes. Add the cabbage and Swiss chard leaves, half of the chickpeas, and enough boiling water or chicken stock to cover. Simmer for 20 minutes.

Puree the remaining chickpeas in a food processor and add to the soup with just enough boiling water or stock to keep the soup liquid. Remove the rosemary sprigs and add the bread slices. Add more liquid if necessary, but keep in mind that the soup should have a very thick "stewlike" consistency. Season with salt and pepper to taste.

*Note:* To cook dried chickpeas, soak them in water to cover for 4 hours; change the water 2 to 3 times. Drain and place in a saucepan with water to cover (do not add salt). Bring to a boil and then reduce to a gentle simmer. Cook until the beans are tender but firm, 2 to 2 1/2 hours.

---

- Chickpeas add fiber, flavor, and a creamy consistency with minimal fat. They also contain phytoestrogens.
- Rich in cancer-protective vitamins A, C, and folate: one serving provides more than 120%, 100%, and 40% of the DVs, respectively.
- Cabbage, a member of the cruciferous family of vegetables, contains glucosinolates, powerful inducers of protective enzymes.
- High in fiber; each serving provides 25% of the DV.

*Per serving:*

| calories | protein | carbohydrates | fat | cholesterol | dietary fiber | saturated fat |
|----------|---------|---------------|-----|-------------|---------------|---------------|
| 250 | 11 Gm | 41 Gm | 5 Gm | 0 mg | 6 Gm | 1 Gm |

**% of Calories**: 65% carbohydrate, 17% protein, 18% fat

**Major Sources of Potential Cancer Fighters**
**Phytochemicals**: allium compounds, glucosinolates, plant polyphenols (flavonoids, phenolic acids), plant sterols, protease inhibitors, terpenes (carotenoids, carnosol, monoterpenes)

# ↯ *Tomato Bread Soup* ↯

Michael Otsuka, Chasen's, Beverly Hills, California

6 SERVINGS

• *A perfect soup for any time, especially when you are trying to use up all of those perfectly ripe tomatoes at the end of the summer.*

• *Serve hot or at room temperature.*

| | | | |
|---|---|---|---|
| 3 | pounds ripe tomatoes (about 12 medium) | 1 | bunch fresh basil (about 3 ounces), leaves picked and cut into long strips, stems reserved |
| 2 | tablespoons olive oil | | |
| 3 | garlic cloves, peeled and crushed | | |
| 2 | large leeks, white part plus a little green (about 10 ounces), rinsed thoroughly and roughly chopped | 3 | bay leaves |
| | | 1/2 | cup white wine |
| | | 4 | cups chicken stock (page 147 or 148), vegetable stock (page 146), or low-sodium canned broth or water |
| 1 | medium onion (about 6 ounces), sliced | | |
| 1 | large carrot (about 4 ounces), chopped | | salt and pepper |
| 2 | medium celery stalks (about 4 ounces), chopped | 4 | ounces bread, cut into small cubes (about 1/3 Italian semolina loaf or 1/2 medium French baguette) |
| 3 | fresh thyme sprigs | 1/3 | cup Parmesan cheese, grated |

To peel and seed the tomatoes, bring 2 quarts of water to a boil in a large pot. Cut the core from the tomatoes with a paring knife, cut a shallow **X** into the bottom of the tomatoes, and plunge them into boiling water for 30 seconds. Remove with a slotted spoon and immediately immerse in ice water until cool. Use a knife to gently peel the skin, which should be discarded. Slice the tomatoes in half and gently squeeze to force out the seeds. Use your fingers to remove any remaining seeds. Discard the seeds, chop the tomatoes, and set aside.

In a large, heavy saucepan (at least 4 quarts) heat the olive oil and add the garlic, leeks, onion, carrot, and celery. Sauté over medium heat until the vegetables are tender and slightly wilted, about 15 minutes. Do not allow the vegetables to brown.

Place the thyme, basil stems, and bay leaves inside a square of cheesecloth and tie up to form a little pouch. Add this to the vegetables along with the tomatoes and white wine. Cook on medium-high heat until most of wine evaporates, about 2 minutes. Add the chicken stock and bring to a boil, then reduce the heat and simmer for 25 minutes. Remove the cloth bag, pressing it between two spoons to extract maximum flavor, and discard.

Carefully puree the soup in small batches in a food processor. Return to the saucepan and season to taste with salt and pepper. (To this point, the soup may be prepared up to 2 days in advance.)

Preheat the oven to 375 degrees F.

Place the bread cubes in a single layer on a baking sheet and place in the oven until they are toasted and dried out, 12 to 15 minutes.

Toss the croutons with the basil leaves and divide them among 6 soup bowls. In a saucepan, heat the soup until it's very hot, adjust the seasoning with salt and pepper, if necessary, and ladle into the bowls. Sprinkle Parmesan over the top of each bowl and serve.

---

- Tomatoes and tomato products are made red by the carotenoid lycopene, a potent antioxidant.
- The combination of carrots, leeks, and tomatoes provides more than 65% of the DV for vitamin A, 90% of the DV for vitamin C, more than 20% of the DV for folate per serving.
- High in fiber—20% of the DV per serving.

---

**Per serving:**

| calories | protein | carbohydrates | fat | cholesterol | dietary fiber | saturated fat |
|----------|---------|---------------|-----|-------------|---------------|---------------|
| 261 | 11 Gm | 34 Gm | 9 Gm | 4 mg | 5 Gm | 2 Gm |

**% of Calories**: 52% carbohydrate, 17% protein, 31% fat

### Major Sources of Potential Cancer Fighters

**Phytochemicals**: allium compounds, plant polyphenols (flavonoids, phenolic acids), plant sterols, terpenes (carotenoids, monoterpenes)

# ❧ *Miso Soup* ❧

## 4 TO 6 SERVINGS

- *There are many different types of miso, all with different intensities of flavor (see page 43). For soup, dark miso can be combined with water to make a broth or "tea" or enriched with vegetables.*

- *This healthy recipe freezes well; make a large batch and store in small containers for easy defrosting and reheating.*

| | |
|---|---|
| 3 tablespoons dark miso paste | 1/2 teaspoon fresh ginger, grated |
| 2 teaspoons canola oil | 2 teaspoons rice wine or |
| 1 celery stalk (about 2 ounces), thinly sliced | sherry vinegar |
| 1 medium red onion (about 5 ounces), thinly sliced | 1 tablespoon tamari (Japanese soy sauce) |
| 1 garlic clove, crushed | salt and pepper |
| 1 medium carrot (about 3 ounces), peeled and thinly sliced | 2 teaspoons brown sugar |
| 2 cups shredded cabbage | 8 ounces extra-firm lite tofu, cut into small cubes |
| 1 cup mushrooms, cleaned and sliced | 2 scallions, thinly sliced, for garnish |

In a large bowl, dissolve the miso paste in 6 cups boiling water (follow package instructions, usually 1 tablespoon miso for 2 cups water); stir to combine well. Set aside.

Heat the canola oil in a large nonstick saucepan. Sauté the celery, onion, and garlic for 5 minutes over medium-high heat and then add the carrot, cabbage, and mushrooms. Continue cooking for 15 more minutes without browning; stir frequently. Add the ginger and miso-water mixture, bring to a boil, then reduce the heat so that the mixture simmers. Cook for 15 to 20 minutes, then season with the rice wine vinegar, tamari, salt and pepper, and brown sugar. Add the tofu 1 to 2 minutes before serving. Garnish with slices of scallions.

- This recipe contains three sources of soy: tofu, miso paste, and tamari. All can be found at most natural food stores as well as some supermarkets.
- By adding cooked adzuki beans, you can add texture and further increase the fiber and nutrient content.
- Each serving provides 110% of the DV for vitamin A and more than 25% for vitamin C.

*Per serving (based on 4 servings):*

| calories | protein | carbohydrates | fat | cholesterol | dietary fiber | saturated fat |
|----------|---------|---------------|-----|-------------|---------------|---------------|
| 125 | 8 Gm | 15 Gm | 4 Gm | 0 mg | 4 Gm | 0 Gm |

**% of Calories**: 48% carbohydrate, 25% protein, 27% fat

### Major Sources of Potential Cancer Fighters

**Phytochemicals**: allium compounds, glucosinolates, phytic acids, plant polyphenols (flavonoids, isoflavones), plant sterols, protease inhibitors, terpenes (carotenoids, monoterpenes, triterpenes)

# ✤ *Vegetable Stock* ✤

Diane Forley, Verbena, New York, New York

## 6 SERVINGS

- *Use stock as a low-calorie, low-fat base for sauces, soups, or stews.*
- *Freeze in 1-pint containers so that you have a healthy stock available whenever a recipe calls for it.*

| | |
|---|---|
| 3　medium celery stalks (about 6 ounces), cubed | 1　large fennel bulb (about 8 ounces), cubed |
| 2　large leeks, white part and a little green (about 5 ounces), halved, washed, and thinly sliced | 1　teaspoon olive oil |
| | 4　quarts water |
| | 2　medium onions (about 10 ounces), halved |
| 2　medium parsnips (about 5 ounces), peeled and cubed | 1　large plum tomato (about 3 ounces), quartered |
| 2　large carrots (about 6 ounces), peeled and cubed | salt |

In a large stockpot, sauté the celery, leeks, parsnips, carrots, and fennel in olive oil over medium-high heat until soft and translucent, about 15 minutes. Add the water and bring to a boil, then reduce the heat and simmer.

Slice the onions in half crosswise and rub with olive oil. Place the onions, cut side down, on a heated cast-iron pan or griddle and "brûlee" or "burn" them until they are a deep-brown color, about 3 minutes. Add the onions and the tomato to the rest of the vegetables.

Bring the stock to a boil, reduce the heat, and simmer for 1¹/₂ hours. Season with salt to taste and strain through a cheesecloth-lined colander into a large bowl.

---

**Per serving (1 cup):**

| calories | protein | carbohydrates | fat | cholesterol | dietary fiber | saturated fat |
|---|---|---|---|---|---|---|
| 20 | 1 Gm | 4 Gm | <1 Gm | 0 mg | 0 Gm | 0 Gm |

**% of Calories**: 68% carbohydrate, 11% protein, 21% fat

---

# ✙ *White Chicken Stock* ✙

### 2 QUARTS (1 SERVING = 1 CUP)

• *White chicken stock can be used as a flavorful, low-calorie, low-fat base for soups, stews, and sauces.*

5 pounds chicken bones, as much
   skin and fat removed as possible
6 quarts cold water
2 medium onions (about 8 ounces),
   chopped
1 large carrot (about 4 ounces),
   washed and cut into large pieces

3 medium celery stalks (about
   5 ounces), cut into large pieces
1 bay leaf
1 fresh thyme sprig or
   1 teaspoon dried thyme
4 to 5 black peppercorns, whole

Rinse the chicken bones and place them in a large stockpot with the water. Bring to a full boil, uncovered, for 5 minutes, then reduce to a low boil for 1 hour. Using a fine mesh skimmer, remove any particles, foam, or fat that rise to the surface.

Add the onions, carrot, celery, bay leaf, thyme, and peppercorns. Keep the stock on a low boil, uncovered, for 3 to 4 hours.

Strain the stock through a fine strainer into a large bowl. You should have about 2 quarts of stock. If you have substantially more, boil until it reduces to about 2 quarts; if you have less, add water to bring the total volume to 3 quarts, then boil and reduce to 2 quarts.

Place the stock in a large container and cool in a sink of cold water. Cover and refrigerate for at least 12 hours. Skim off and discard any fat that has solidified on the surface. Keep refrigerated for 3 to 4 days or store in small containers in the freezer.

---

Almost all fat can be removed by chilling the stock overnight and removing the hardened fat the next day.

*Per serving (1 cup):*

| calories | protein | carbohydrates | fat | cholesterol | dietary fiber | saturated fat |
|----------|---------|---------------|-----|-------------|---------------|---------------|
| 33 | 4 Gm | 2 Gm | 1 Gm | 0 mg | 0 Gm | 0 Gm |

**% of Calories**: 24% carbohydrate, 49% protein, 27% fat

# ❧ *Brown Chicken Stock* ❧

## 2 QUARTS (1 SERVING = 1 CUP)

• *It is always good to have brown chicken stock on hand (frozen in pint containers) for whenever a recipe calls for it. Use it as a low-calorie, low-fat base for sauces.*

5 pounds chicken bones, as much skin and fat removed as possible

2 large carrots (about 8 ounces), washed and cut into large pieces

2 medium onions (about 8 ounces), quartered

1 cup white wine

2 gallons cold water

3 medium celery stalks (about 5 ounces), cut into large pieces

1 bay leaf

2 fresh thyme sprigs or 1 teaspoon dried thyme

½ tablespoon tomato paste

Preheat the oven to 425 degrees F.

Spread out the bones in an even layer in a roasting pan and bake for 30 minutes, stirring occasionally so that they do not burn. During the last 10 minutes of roasting, add the carrots and onions. The bones and vegetables should be well browned.

Transfer the bones and vegetables to a large stockpot; use tongs or a slotted spoon to minimize the amount of fat transferred. Discard any fat in the roasting pan, then pour the wine into the pan. Bring to a boil on the stovetop and stir with a wooden spoon to dissolve the particles on the bottom of the roasting pan. Add these juices to the stockpot along with the water.

Bring the mixture to a boil, then reduce the heat and boil gently for 1 hour. Using a fine mesh skimmer, remove any particles, foam, or fat that rise to the surface.

Add the celery, bay leaf, thyme, and tomato paste. Keep the stock on a low boil, uncovered, for 4 to 5 hours.

Strain the stock through a fine strainer into a large bowl. You should have about 2 quarts of stock. If you have substantially more, boil until it reduces to about 2 quarts; if you have less, add water to bring the total volume to 3 quarts, then boil and reduce to 2 quarts.

Place the stock in a large container and cool in a sink of cold water. Cover and refrigerate for at least 12 hours. Skim off and discard any fat that has solidified on the surface. Keep refrigerated for 3 to 4 days or store in small containers in the freezer.

| **Per serving (1 cup):** | | | | | | |
|---|---|---|---|---|---|---|
| calories | protein | carbohydrates | fat | cholesterol | dietary fiber | saturated fat |
| 33 | 5 Gm | 1 Gm | 1 Gm | 0 mg | 0 Gm | 0 Gm |

**% of Calories**: 13% carbohydrate, 60% protein, 27% fat

# ❧ *Fish Stock* ❧

2 QUARTS (1 SERVING = $1/2$ CUP)

•  *Fish stock can be used to make sauces, soups, bisques, risottos, or other dishes that include seafood or shellfish. Fish stock is also a flavorful liquid for poaching fish.*

| | | | |
|---|---|---|---|
| 4 | quarts cold water | 3 to 4 | parsley stems |
| 4 | pounds fish bones (snapper, striped bass, grouper, or halibut) | 1 | cup mushrooms (about $2^1/2$ ounces), chopped |
| 1 | cup white wine | 1 | fresh thyme sprig or |
| 2 | strips lemon zest | | $1/2$ teaspoon dried thyme |
| 1 | bay leaf | | |

Combine all ingredients in a large stockpot and bring slowly to a simmer. Using a fine mesh skimmer, remove any particles or foam that rise to the surface.

Simmer, uncovered, for 30 to 40 minutes, then strain and cool in a large container in a sink of cold water. Cover and refrigerate for 3 days or store in small containers in the freezer.

| **Per serving (1/2 cup):** | | | | | | |
|---|---|---|---|---|---|---|
| calories | protein | carbohydrates | fat | cholesterol | dietary fiber | saturated fat |
| 16 | 2 Gm | 1 Gm | <1 Gm | 0 mg | 0 Gm | 0 Gm |

**% of Calories**: 25% carbohydrate, 50% protein, 25% fat

# ✔ *Root Vegetable Broth* ✔
# *(Potage Maigre aux Racines)*

Andre Soltner, The French Culinary Institute, New York, New York

6 SERVINGS

• *Andre suggests cooking julienned or finely diced vegetables, rice, pastina, or risotto in this flavorful broth.*

| | | | |
|---|---|---|---|
| 1 | cup lentils<br>salt and pepper | 1 | medium onion (about<br>5 ounces), diced |
| 1 | tablespoon olive oil | 1 | large celery stalk (about |
| 2 to 3 | medium carrots, peeled and<br>diced (1 to 1½ cups diced) | | 2 ounces), diced |
| 1 | medium leek, white part only<br>(about 1½ ounces), diced | 1 | bunch Italian parsley sprigs<br>(about 1 ounce) |

Thoroughly wash the lentils under cold running water. Cook them slowly for 45 minutes in 2 quarts of simmering water seasoned with salt and pepper, then let stand in cooking liquid for at least 5 minutes.

Pour the cooking liquid through cheesecloth and set aside. Do not press the lentils against the cloth—the liquid will become cloudy. Reserve the lentils for another use, perhaps a salad.

Heat the olive oil in a medium saucepan and gently sauté the carrots, leek, onion, and celery over medium heat until golden brown. Add the reserved liquid and the parsley. Adjust the seasoning with salt and pepper, if necessary, and bring to a boil. Cook, uncovered, at a low simmer for 1 hour.

Line a colander with a moistened cloth napkin (not cheesecloth) and pour the broth through it.

| **Per serving:** | | | | | | |
|---|---|---|---|---|---|---|
| calories | protein | carbohydrates | fat | cholesterol | dietary fiber | saturated fat |
| 38 | 1 Gm | 4 Gm | 2 Gm | 11 mg | 0 Gm | <1 Gm |

**% of Calories**: 42% carbohydrate, 11% protein, 47% fat

# SALADS

## ❧ *Roasted Garlic Caesar Salad* ❧ *with Focaccia Croutons*

Gianni Scappin, Maximillian, New York, New York;
Trattoria alla Pesa, Mason Vicentino, Veneto, Italy

4 SERVINGS

• In Gianni's recipe, roasted garlic contributes subtle flavor and creaminess to this dressing, as well as protective allium compounds. He remarks that roasted garlic replaces raw eggs and most of the oil, emulsifying the dressing and making it healthier and longer lasting. The same serving size of traditional Caesar salad provides almost double the calories (approximately 580), and more than four times the amount of fat (50 grams).

### Caesar Dressing

MAKES ³/₄ CUP

| | |
|---|---|
| 3 medium heads garlic | 1 tablespoon Dijon mustard |
| 1 shallot, peeled and sliced | 3 whole anchovy fillets (see Notes) |
| 1 tablespoon sherry vinegar | pinch cayenne |
| ¹/₈ cup chicken stock or water | 1 teaspoon dried oregano |
| juice of 1 lemon | 2 tablespoons olive oil |
| 1 teaspoon Worcestershire sauce | salt and freshly ground pepper |

### Romaine Salad with Croutons

| | |
|---|---|
| 1 large slice focaccia, cut into ¹/₂-inch cubes (see Notes) | salt and freshly ground pepper |
| 1 teaspoon olive oil | 1 large head romaine lettuce (about 1¹/₂ pounds; see Notes) |
| 1 tablespoon minced fresh rosemary | ¹/₃ cup grated Parmesan cheese |

Preheat the oven to 325 degrees F. Follow the procedure for roasting garlic on page 178.

To prepare the croutons, increase the oven temperature to 375 degrees F. Toss the focaccia cubes, olive oil, rosemary, salt, and pepper in a mixing bowl. Spread out evenly on a baking sheet and bake until lightly toasted, about 10 minutes. Cool.

To prepare the Caesar dressing, in the bowl of a food processor or blender, squeeze the roasted garlic from the cloves. Add the remaining ingredients except olive oil. Blend well. With the machine running, gradually add the oil. Adjust the seasoning with salt and freshly ground pepper.

Place the romaine "hearts" in a large bowl. Add half of the croutons and dressing. Toss to combine. Divide among 4 salad plates and sprinkle with the cheese and remaining croutons.

*Notes:* You can increase or decrease amount of anchovies depending on your taste preference or that of your guests.

Be sure to use the inner crispy "hearts" of the romaine and the firm center of each leaf You can substitute half of a 1-day-old baguette, or 2 slices of any other bread.

---

- Garlic is a potentially good source of selenium.
- Romaine lettuce is a good source of vitamins A, C, and folate (as well as other B vitamins), providing more than 45%, 85%, and 60% of the DVs, respectively.
- High in fiber—20% of the DV per serving.

---

*Per serving of Caesar Dressing (2 tablespoons):*

| calories | protein | carbohydrates | fat | cholesterol | dietary fiber | saturated fat |
|---|---|---|---|---|---|---|
| 38 | 1 Gm | 4 Gm | 2 Gm | 1 mg | 0 Gm | 1 Gm |

*Per serving of Roasted Garlic Caesar Salad with Focaccia Croutons:*

| calories | protein | carbohydrates | fat | cholesterol | dietary fiber | saturated fat |
|---|---|---|---|---|---|---|
| 232 | 11 Gm | 32 Gm | 7 Gm | 7 mg | 5 Gm | 2 Gm |

**% of Calories**: 55% carbohydrate, 19% protein, 26% fat

### Major Sources of Potential Cancer Fighters
**Phytochemicals**: allium compounds, omega-3 fatty acids, plant polyphenols (flavonoids, phenolic acids), plant sterols, terpenes (carotenoids, carnosol)

---

# ❧ Red Onion, Grapefruit, and Tomato Salad ❧

Jacques Pépin, Dean of Special Studies, The French Culinary Institute, New York, New York

6 SERVINGS

Reprinted from *Jacques Pépin's Simple and Healthy Cooking*, copyright 1994 by Jacques Pépin. Permission granted by Rodale Press, Inc., Emmaus, PA 18098. For ordering information, please call 1 (800) 848-4735.

- *A refreshing salad for any season. The classic sherry vinaigrette serves well for many other salads.*

## Red Onion, Grapefruit, and Tomato Salad

3 medium tomatoes (about 1 pound)

1 large Ruby Red grapefruit (about 1 pound)

1 medium red onion (6 ounces), peeled and cut into 1/4-inch dice

1/3 cup fresh basil leaves, sliced into long, thin strips

1 bunch watercress (about 2 ounces), well rinsed

### Sherry Vinaigrette

MAKES ABOUT 1/4 CUP

2 tablespoons extra virgin olive oil

1 tablespoon sherry vinegar

1/2 teaspoon salt

1/4 teaspoon freshly ground black pepper

To peel and seed the tomatoes, bring 2 quarts of water to a boil in a large pot. Cut the core from the tomatoes with a paring knife, make an X at their base, and plunge them into boiling water for 30 seconds. Remove with a slotted spoon and immediately immerse in ice water until cool. Use a knife to gently peel the skin, which should be discarded. Slice the tomatoes in half and gently squeeze to force out the seeds. Use your fingers to remove any remaining seeds. Discard the seeds and cut the tomatoes into 1-inch pieces. Set aside.

Using a sharp knife, peel the grapefruit, removing all the skin and the underlying white pith so the flesh of the fruit is totally exposed. Then cut between the membranes on each side of every segment and remove the flesh in wedgelike pieces. Cut each grapefruit wedge in half and place the pieces in a large bowl. Then, holding the membranes over the bowl, squeeze them over the grapefruit flesh to extract any remaining juice before discarding them. (You should have about 1 cup of grapefruit flesh and 3 tablespoons of juice.)

Add the tomatoes, onion, and basil to the bowl. Mix well.

To make the sherry vinaigrette, mix the oil, vinegar, salt, and pepper in a small bowl. Toss with the grapefruit mixture.

Cut the bottom 2 inches of stems from the watercress and discard. Wash and thoroughly dry the rest of the bunch. Arrange the watercress attractively around the periphery of a platter and mound the salad in the center.

---

- Ruby Red grapefruits and tomatoes are made red by the carotenoid lycopene, a potent antioxidant. Together with watercress, they provide 65% of the DV for vitamin C per serving.
- Red onions are good sources of the flavonoids quercetin and rutin, which act as blocking agents against cancer.

*Per serving of Sherry Vinaigrette (1 tbsp):*

| calories | protein | carbohydrates | fat | cholesterol | dietary fiber | saturated fat |
|---|---|---|---|---|---|---|
| 51 | 0 Gm | 0 Gm | 6 Gm | 0 Gm | 0 Gm | 0 Gm |

*Per serving of Red Onion, Grapefruit, and Tomato Salad with Sherry Vinaigrette:*

| calories | protein | carbohydrates | fat | cholesterol | dietary fiber | saturated fat |
|---|---|---|---|---|---|---|
| 106 | 2 Gm | 11 Gm | 6 Gm | 0 mg | 2 Gm | 0 Gm |

**% of Calories**: 42% carbohydrate, 8% protein, 50% fat

### Major Sources of Potential Cancer Fighters

**Phytochemicals**: allium compounds, plant polyphenols (flavonoids, phenolic acids), plant sterols, terpenes (carotenoids, monoterpenes, triterpenes)

# ❧ *Asparagus Salad with Black Truffles* ❧

Roberto Donna, Galileo, Washington, D.C.

4 SERVINGS

•  *Serve this flavorful spring or summer salad alone with crusty bread or followed by a simply prepared grilled fish course, such as sea bass, tuna, salmon, or swordfish.*

| | | | |
|---|---|---|---|
| 4 | ounces Vidalia onions or shallots | 1 | tablespoon olive oil |
| 1 | teaspoon olive oil | | salt and pepper |
| 1 | ounce black truffles, julienned | 20 | fresh asparagus stalks |
| 2 | tablespoons balsamic vinegar | | (about 20 ounces) |
| 2 | tablespoons chicken stock (page 147 or 148) or water | | |

To roast the onions, preheat the oven to 375 degrees F. Toss the unpeeled onions with the olive oil and place them in a single layer in a small baking dish. Add a little water or broth to the bottom of the pan, and bake until tender when pierced with a knife, 30 to 40 minutes. Let cool slightly, cut in half, and remove the skins.

Slice the roasted onions lengthwise as thinly as possible and place in a bowl with the truffles. Add the balsamic vinegar, chicken stock or water, and olive oil. Stir with a fork to combine. Adjust the seasoning with salt and pepper. Cover and let rest for at least 4 hours (refrigerate if stock is used). The black truffles will release their flavor into the vinaigrette.

Rinse the asparagus. If their stems are tough, peel them with a vegetable peeler. In a skillet, steam the asparagus in 1/3 cup water until just tender. Place them on an attractive serving platter and top with the vinaigrette. They are best served when still warm.

- Low in calories, asparagus is a great source of folate, providing 35% of the DV per serving in this recipe, and a good source of vitamin C and carotenoids.
- Truffles, grown under the earth, are a potentially good source of selenium.
- A good source of fiber.

---

*Per serving:*

| calories | protein | carbohydrates | fat | cholesterol | dietary fiber | saturated fat |
|---|---|---|---|---|---|---|
| 88 | 5 Gm | 8 Gm | 4 Gm | 0 mg | 3 Gm | 1 Gm |

**% of Calories**: 37% carbohydrate, 21% protein, 42% fat

**Major Sources of Potential Cancer Fighters**

**Phytochemicals**: allium compounds, plant polyphenols (flavonoids), plant sterols, terpenes (carotenoids)

# ❦ *Black-eyed Pea–Texmati Rice* ❦ *Salad with Organic Greens*

Dean Fearing, The Mansion on Turtle Creek, Dallas, Texas

## 6 SERVINGS

- *This salad can be made quickly and offers a variety of flavors, textures, and cancer-preventive nutrients and phytochemicals.*

| | |
|---|---|
| 2 cups cooked black-eyed peas or canned, drained (see Notes) | 2 teaspoons chopped fresh thyme leaves |
| 2 cups cooked texmati rice (see Notes) | 2 tablespoons chopped cilantro |
| 1 cup tomatoes, diced | 2 tablespoons chopped basil |
| 1/2 cup zucchini (1/2 small zucchini), diced | 2 canned chipotle chiles, chopped (see Notes) |
| 1/4 cup shallots (about 2), minced | 2 tablespoons malt vinegar |
| 2 tablespoons minced garlic | 1 tablespoon lemon juice |
| 1/4 cup scallions (about 3), white part only, cut into thin slices | 1/4 cup extra virgin olive oil |
| | salt |
| | 3 cups organic mesclun mix |

In a medium bowl, combine all ingredients, except the mesclun, and mix well. Allow to marinate for at least 2 hours. Place ¹/₂ cup of mesclun on each plate and top with the black-eyed pea–rice salad.

*Notes:* To cook dried black-eyed peas, soak them in water to cover for 4 hours; change the water 2 to 3 times. Drain and place in a saucepan with water to cover and cook for 45 minutes, or until tender but firm.

Texmati rice is a cross between American long-grain rice and basmati rice. Like basmati rice it has a fragrant aroma and a slightly nutty taste. It is found at most supermarkets.

Chipotle chiles are dried, smoked jalapeño peppers. They have a rich flavor and their hotness is mellowed by the smoking process. They are available at some supermarkets and gourmet specialty stores.

---

- Each serving provides more than 10% of the DV for vitamin A, 30% for vitamin C, and 20% for folate.
- Texmati rice is a good source of fiber and a potentially good source of selenium.
- High in fiber—20% of the DV per serving.

---

**Per serving:**

| calories | protein | carbohydrates | fat | cholesterol | dietary fiber | saturated fat |
|---|---|---|---|---|---|---|
| 225 | 5 Gm | 30 Gm | 10 Gm | 0 mg | 5 Gm | 2 Gm |

**% of Calories**: 53% carbohydrate, 8% protein, 39% fat

**Major Sources of Potential Cancer Fighters**

**Phytochemicals**: allium compounds, phytic acids, plant polyphenols (flavonoids, phenolic acids), protease inhibitors, terpenes (carotenoids, monoterpenes)

---

# ❧ Curried Whole Wheat ❧ Couscous Summer Salad

Charlie Trotter, Charlie Trotter's, Chicago, Illinois

4 SERVINGS

- *Serve alone as a light summer salad or surrounded by seared shrimp or scallops.*

| | | |
|---|---|---|
| 2 | cups chicken stock (page 147 or 148) | ¹/₂ teaspoon paprika |
| 1 | teaspoon curry powder | ¹/₄ teaspoon cayenne |

1    cup whole wheat couscous (see Notes)
1    leek, white part only, thinly sliced
1    tablespoon butter
¼    cup wax beans, cleaned and
     blanched, cut on the bias
¼    inch (see Notes)
¼    cup green beans, cleaned and
     blanched, cut on the bias
     ¼ inch (see Notes)

¼    cup fresh peas, cleaned and
     blanched (see Notes)
¼    cup fresh corn kernels, cleaned
     and blanched (see Notes)
     juice of 1 lime plus grated zest
     salt and pepper

Place the chicken stock into a saucepan and whisk in the spices. Add the couscous and bring to a boil, reduce the heat, and simmer for 1 minute. Remove from the heat and let sit, covered, for 10 to 15 minutes. Fluff with a fork. Let cool.

Sauté the leek in the butter until soft and golden. Add all other cut vegetables to the skillet and heat for 2 to 3 minutes, adding lime juice and zest at the end. Fold the vegetables into the couscous. Season with salt and pepper.

*Notes:* A staple of North African cuisine, couscous is granular semolina (very small pieces of pasta). Like pasta it cooks very quickly and is a great starch choice for a busy day. It serves well as a bed for vegetables and/or a moderate portion of meat, fish, or poultry (usually stewed or braised), a last-minute addition to soups, stews, or porridge, or a dessert sweetened with milk and fruit. Easy to find, couscous is available at most supermarkets.

You can substitute frozen, thawed, and drained vegetables. To cut on the bias means to slice at an angle. These cuts are more decorative and produce more surface area, potentially cutting the cooking time.

- Look for whole wheat couscous; it is less processed and contains more fiber, protein, B vitamins, and minerals, such as iron and magnesium.
- Using the peel of citrus (or zest) in cooking is encouraged; not only does it lend aroma and flavor, but also contains limonene, a phytochemical that may help your body to dispose of carcinogens.
- Curry powder contains curcumin, a plant polyphenol that lends yellow color and acts as an antioxidant; it may also play a role as a cancer-blocking agent.
- High in fiber—25% of the DV per serving.

**Per serving:**

| calories | protein | carbohydrates | fat | cholesterol | dietary fiber | saturated fat |
| --- | --- | --- | --- | --- | --- | --- |
| 233 | 8 Gm | 44 Gm | 3 Gm | 5 mg | 6 Gm | 2 Gm |

**% of Calories**: 76% carbohydrate, 14% protein, 10% fat

# ✷ Brown Turkey Figs, French Melon, ✷ and Persimmon with Arugula, Wild Watercress, and Black Pepper– Vanilla Bean Vinaigrette

Charlie Trotter, Charlie Trotter's, Chicago, Illinois

4 SERVINGS

- *This salad is a wonderful balance of flavors, textures, and colors.*
- *Try the Black Pepper–Vanilla Bean Vinaigrette with other types of slightly bitter greens.*

### Black Pepper–Vanilla Bean Vinaigrette

MAKES 1/4 CUP

| | |
|---|---|
| 2 teaspoons rice wine vinegar | 1/2 vanilla bean, cut in half lengthwise, beans in center scraped out, and pod discarded |
| 1 teaspoon lime juice | |
| 3 tablespoons canola oil | |
| 1/2 tablespoon cracked black pepper | |
| salt | |

### Salad

| | |
|---|---|
| 2 brown turkey or any ripe figs (about 3 1/2 ounces) | 2 cups arugula or any slightly bitter green (about 1 1/2 ounces) |
| 2 persimmons or papayas (about 5 ounces) | 2 cups wild or domestic watercress (about 2 ounces) |
| 1 French melon or cantaloupe (about 2 1/2 pounds) | |

To make the vinaigrette, combine the vinegar and lime juice in a small bowl. Slowly whisk in the canola oil and add the black pepper and vanilla scrapings. Season to taste with salt.

Cut each fig into 6 wedges and set aside. Peel the persimmons and cut into 12 wedges, removing the seeds. Set aside. Cut the melon in half and remove the seeds. Using a paring knife, peel away the skin. Slice the melon into 16 thin slices.

Place the arugula and watercress in a bowl and gently toss with the vinaigrette. Season to taste with salt.

In the center of each plate, place a mound of dressed greens. Place 3 wedges of the figs, 4 slices of the melon, and 3 wedges of the persimmon decoratively on top of the greens.

---

- Each serving provides more than 100% of the DV for vitamin A and 20% for vitamin C.
- A good source of fiber.

---

*Per serving of Black Pepper–Vanilla Bean Vinaigrette (1 tablespoon):*

| calories | protein | carbohydrates | fat | cholesterol | dietary fiber | saturated fat |
|----------|---------|---------------|-------|-------------|---------------|---------------|
| 96 | 0 Gm | 1 Gm | 10 Gm | 0 mg | 0 Gm | 1 Gm |

*Per serving of salad tossed with vinaigrette:*

| calories | protein | carbohydrates | fat | cholesterol | dietary fiber | saturated fat |
|----------|---------|---------------|-------|-------------|---------------|---------------|
| 247 | 4 Gm | 33 Gm | 11 Gm | 0 mg | 5 Gm | 2 Gm |

**% of Calories**: 53% carbohydrate, 6% protein, 40% fat

**Major Sources of Potential Cancer Fighters**

**Phytochemicals**: capsaicin, plant polyphenols (flavonoids, phenolic acids), plant sterols, terpenes (carotenoids)

# ✣ *Warm Pasta Vegetable Salad* ✣

Michael Chiarello, Tra Vigne, St. Helena, California

8 SERVINGS

- *Michael prefers the blended flavors of pasta salad when served warm. The "pan-made" vinaigrette and vegetables can be cooked ahead of time, but he recommends cooking the pasta at the last minute so that it is hot when mixed with the vinaigrette.*

• *Use other vegetables, such asparagus or fresh baby peas, when they are in season.*
*Roasted peppers are available year-round and are a perfect addition to this recipe.*

| | | | | |
|---|---|---|---|---|
| 1 | pound broccoli (1 small head) | 3 | tablespoons herb vinegar, |
| 3 | tablespoons extra virgin olive oil | | preferably flavored with |
| 2 | tablespoons finely chopped garlic | | oregano (see Note) |
| 1/4 | teaspoon New Mexican red | 2 | medium tomatoes (about 8 |
| | pepper flakes or crushed | | ounces), cut into large chunks |
| | red pepper flakes | 2 | tablespoons finely chopped |
| 1 | tablespoon finely chopped | | Italian parsley |
| | fresh thyme leaves | 1 | pound uncooked fusilli pasta |
| | salt and freshly ground pepper | 1/2 | cup freshly grated Parmesan |
| 2 | cups chicken stock (page 147 or 148) | | cheese |
| | or low-sodium canned chicken broth | | |
| 3 | small zucchini (about 1 pound), | | |
| | sliced into 1/4-inch-thick rounds | | |

Bring a large pot of salted water to a boil.

Separate the broccoli into florets. Using a vegetable peeler, peel the stems down to the light-green, tender core, then slice into thin rounds on the diagonal. Reserve the florets and stems separately.

Heat 1 tablespoon of olive oil in a large nonstick sauté pan until almost smoking. Add the garlic and sauté until light brown, moving the pan off and on the heat to regulate temperature and prevent burning. Add the red pepper flakes and thyme. Stir. Add the broccoli florets and sauté about 1 minute. Season with salt and pepper.

Add the chicken stock to the sauté pan and bring to a boil. Cook until the broccoli is half cooked, about 3 minutes. Add the broccoli stems and zucchini and cook until tender, but still firm, about another 3 minutes. Using a handheld strainer or a slotted spoon, skim the vegetables from the pan and reserve on a baking sheet to cool.

Bring the cooking liquid to a boil and boil until it thickens and reduces to about 1/2 to 3/4 cup. Stir in the vinegar and then add the tomatoes, allowing the tomatoes to warm for about 1 minute; do not cook them. Season to taste with salt and pepper. Add the remaining olive oil and parsley. Mix well.

While the sauce is reducing, add the pasta to the boiling water and cook until al dente, 9 to 10 minutes. Drain well and transfer to a serving bowl. Immediately add the vinaigrette, vegetables, and half of the cheese. Sprinkle with the remaining cheese and serve warm.

*Note:* Herb-infused vinegars can be found at many supermarkets and gourmet specialty stores.

- Broccoli is a near-perfect vegetable; it is rich in protective vitamins and minerals. Combined with other vegetables in this dish, it provides more than 110% of the DV for vitamin C, 20% for vitamin A and folate, and more than 10% for calcium. Broccoli is also a member of the cruciferous vegetable family, and contains cancer-fighting phytochemicals.
- Broccoli, zucchini, garlic, and pasta are all potentially good sources of selenium.
- A good source of fiber.

*Per serving:*

| calories | protein | carbohydrates | fat | cholesterol | dietary fiber | saturated fat |
|----------|---------|---------------|-----|-------------|---------------|---------------|
| 320 | 13 Gm | 50 Gm | 8 Gm | 7 mg | 4 Gm | 2 Gm |

**% of Calories**: 61% carbohydrate, 16% protein, 23% fat

**Major Sources of Potential Cancer Fighters**

**Phytochemicals**: allium compounds, glucosinolates, phytic acids, plant polyphenols (flavonoids, phenolic acids), plant sterols, terpenes (carotenoids, monoterpenes)

# ❧ *Healthy Tuna Salad* ❧

4 SERVINGS

- *Serve as a side salad or between pieces of multigrain or rye bread with fresh tomato slices.*

7 ounces canned white albacore
   tuna, water-packed
3/4 cup carrots, peeled and shredded
1 cup broccoli (3 ounces), cut
   into small florets
1 small red onion (about
   2 ounces), diced
1 medium celery stalk
   (about 2 ounces), chopped

1 teaspoon grated lemon zest
1/2 cup 1% cottage cheese
   (see Note)
2 tablespoons low-fat
   mayonnaise (see Note)
   freshly ground pepper to taste

Drain the tuna. In a medium bowl, mix it with the remaining ingredients.

*Note:* You can substitute creamed silken tofu for the cottage cheese and a low-fat tofu-based mayonnaise for the low-fat mayonnaise.

- One serving provides more than 40% of the DV for vitamin C, and enough carotenoids to supply 60% of the DV for vitamin A.
- Tuna is a lean protein source that is a potentially good source of selenium and protective omega-3 fatty acids.

*Per serving:*

| calories | protein | carbohydrates | fat | cholesterol | dietary fiber | saturated fat |
|----------|---------|---------------|-----|-------------|---------------|---------------|
| 120 | 17 Gm | 6 Gm | 3 Gm | 16 mg | 2 Gm | 1 Gm |

**% of Calories**: 22% carbohydrate, 58% protein, 20% fat

**Major Sources of Potential Cancer Fighters**

**Phytochemicals**: allium compounds, glucosinolates, omega-3 fatty acids, plant polyphenols (flavonoids), plant sterols, terpenes (carotenoids; monoterpenes; limonenes; triterpenes)

# ❧ *Cherimoya-Avocado Salad* ❧ *with Crispy Chinese Chicken*

Norman Van Aken, NORMAN'S, Coral Gables, Florida

4 SERVINGS

- *A light dinner for any season.*
- *For a vegetarian first course, prepare only the Cherimoya-Avocado Salad with Passion Fruit Vinaigrette.*

## Chicken and Marinade

3 tablespoons light soy sauce

1 teaspoon Chinese five-spice powder (see Notes)

2 garlic cloves, minced

1 inch gingerroot, peeled and minced

1 Scotch bonnet chile or jalapeño pepper, seeded and minced

3 tablespoons honey

1 tablespoon sesame oil

4 split chicken breasts (about 1 1/2 pounds), boneless with skin on (remove after cooking)

salt and pepper

1/4 cup cashews, roasted until crisp (optional)

### Passion Fruit Vinaigrette

MAKES 1/2 CUP (1 SERVING = 1 TABLESPOON)

1/4 cup passion fruit juice, strained
1 teaspoon honey
1 teaspoon light soy sauce

    salt and cracked black
      pepper
1/4 cup canola oil

### Salad

1 ripe cherimoya (about 18 ounces),
   peeled, seeds discarded, and
   fruit cut into bite-size cubes
   (1 cup; see Notes)
1/2 ripe avocado (about 10 ounces),
   peeled, pitted, and cut into
   bite-size pieces

3 to 4 cups mixed greens
      (about 3 ounces)

To prepare the marinade, in a medium bowl combine the soy sauce, five-spice powder, garlic, ginger, chile, honey, and sesame oil. Mix well and add the chicken breasts, rolling them in the marinade to evenly coat. Cover the bowl and refrigerate.

Toast the cashews in a skillet on the stovetop or spread them out on a baking sheet and toast them in the oven at 400 degrees F for 4 to 6 minutes, until golden brown. Set aside.

To prepare the vinaigrette, in a small mixing bowl, combine the passion fruit juice, honey, soy sauce, and salt and pepper. Whisk in the canola oil. Set aside.

To prepare the salad, in a small bowl combine the cherimoya, avocado, and about 2 tablespoons of the vinaigrette. Toss together and chill, covered. (This can be done up to 1 hour in advance.)

Preheat the broiler or grill. When hot, remove the excess marinade from the chicken, season with salt and pepper, and cook, turning the pieces and adjusting the heat as needed to prevent burning or charring. Cook until the juices run clear when the meat is pierced with a fork. (Rather than cook the chicken completely on the grill, you can just mark it on both sides and then roast it in an oven preheated to 375 degrees F until cooked, 20 to 30 minutes.)

Toss the greens in a bowl with the remaining dressing. Mound the avocado and cherimoya salad at the top of a large plate.

Thinly slice the chicken and fan out next to the salad. Garnish with toasted cashews.

Notes: Chinese five-spice powder is a combination of cinnamon, cloves, fennel seed, star anise, and Szechuan peppercorns. Available at Asian markets and most supermarkets.

Cherimoya is also called a custard apple. This tropical fruit tastes like a delicate combination of apple, pineapple, papaya, and banana. Now grown in California, cherimoyas are available from November to May.

---

- Cherimoya, passion fruit, chile peppers, and salad greens all contain substantial amounts of vitamin C: combined, they provide 65% of the DV.
- This recipe is also rich in carotenoids, providing 25% of the DV of vitamin A.
- Mixed greens and avocado provide substantial amounts of folate: more than 25% of the DV per serving.
- High in fiber—more than 25% of the DV per serving.

---

*Per serving of Passion Fruit Vinaigrette (1 tablespoon):*

| calories | protein | carbohydrates | fat | cholesterol | dietary fiber | saturated fat |
|---|---|---|---|---|---|---|
| 95 | 0 Gm | 8 Gm | 7 Gm | 0 mg | 0 Gm | 0 Gm |

*Per serving of Cherimoya-Avocado Salad with Passion Fruit Vinaigrette:*

| calories | protein | carbohydrates | fat | cholesterol | dietary fiber | saturated fat |
|---|---|---|---|---|---|---|
| 366 | 5 Gm | 46 Gm | 18 Gm | 0 mg | 7 Gm | 2 Gm |

*Per serving of Cherimoya-Avocado Salad with Passion Fruit Vinaigrette and Crispy Chinese Chicken:*

| calories | protein | carbohydrates | fat | cholesterol | dietary fiber | saturated fat |
|---|---|---|---|---|---|---|
| 500 | 32 Gm | 48 Gm | 20 Gm | 73 mg | 7 Gm | 3 Gm |

**% of Calories**: 39% carbohydrate, 25% protein, 36% fat

**Major Sources of Potential Cancer Fighters**

**Phytochemicals**: capsaicin, plant polyphenols (flavonoids, phenolic acids), plant sterols, terpenes (carotenoids, triterpenes)

---

# ✌ *Scallops and Lima Bean Salad* ✌

Lidia Bastianich, Felidia/Becco/Frico Bar, New York, New York

### 4 SERVINGS

- *This salad is easy to prepare and makes a perfect light lunch or first course.*

| | | | |
|---|---|---|---|
| 8 | ounces large sea scallops (approximately 8), sliced in half horizontally | | salt and pepper |
| | | 2 | teaspoons extra virgin olive oil |
| | | 1 | garlic clove, peeled and crushed |

| | pinch crushed red pepper flakes | 2 | teaspoons fresh lemon juice |
| 2 | cups lima beans, cooked or frozen (see Note) | 2 | tablespoons chopped fresh parsley |
| 1 | tablespoon olive oil | | |

Spread out the scallop slices in a single layer on a plate and season with salt and pepper.

In a nonstick skillet, heat 2 teaspoons of extra virgin olive oil and sauté the garlic over medium-high heat until golden. Remove the garlic, turn up the heat, and add the scallops and crushed red pepper. Sauté until lightly brown around the edges, turn over, and cook for 1 minute more.

Add the cooked, drained lima beans. Drizzle with the remaining olive oil and lemon juice and season with salt and pepper. Sprinkle with the parsley and serve.

*Note:* If frozen lima beans are used, thaw and drain the beans before adding to the skillet. To cook dried lima beans, soak 1¼ cups of beans in water to cover for 4 to 6 hours; change the water 2 to 3 times. Drain and place in a saucepan with 1 quart water to cover and bring to a boil. Simmer for 1 to 1½ hours, until tender.

---

- With a total fat content of less than 0.3 Gm per ounce, scallops are almost a "fat-free," high-quality protein source. In this salad, fat and flavor are added with extra virgin olive oil. The total fat content is still very low compared to total calories and the other nutritional merits of this entrée.
- Lima beans not only lend a nice texture contrast to this salad, but also are high in protein, fiber, folate and other B vitamins, phosphorus, calcium, iron, and potassium.

---

*Per serving:*

| calories | protein | carbohydrates | fat | cholesterol | dietary fiber | saturated fat |
|----------|---------|---------------|-----|-------------|---------------|---------------|
| 220 | 18 Gm | 24 Gm | 6 Gm | 20 mg | 7 Gm | 1 Gm |

**% of Calories**: 42% carbohydrate, 32% protein, 26% fat

### Major Sources of Potential Cancer Fighters

**Phytochemicals**: capsaicin, phytic acids, plant polyphenols (flavonoids, isoflavones), protease inhibitors, terpenes (monoterpenes)

# ❧ *Lobster Salad* ❧

Michael Mina, Aqua, San Francisco, California

4 SERVINGS

- *The perfect light summer lunch or first course to complement those perfectly ripe tomatoes.*
- *Use the vinaigrettes in any season to dress other salads.*

### Tomato Salad and Lobster Brochette

| | | | | |
|---|---|---|---|---|
| 2 | 1-pound lobsters | | | salt and pepper |
| 8 | 1-inch cubes of French bread | | 1 | head frisee (about 4 ounces; see Note) |
| 4 | red cherry tomatoes (about 2 ounces) | | 1 | bunch watercress (about 2 ounces), ends trimmed |
| 8 | basil leaves | | 1 | cup mixed greens (about 2 ounces) |
| 4 | yellow cherry tomatoes (about 2 ounces) | | | |
| 4 | medium ripe tomatoes (about 1 pound), cut into wedges | | | |

### Balsamic Vinaigrette

MAKES 1 CUP (1 SERVING = 1 TABLESPOON)

| | | | |
|---|---|---|---|
| 1/4 | cup balsamic vinegar | | salt and freshly ground pepper |
| 1 | shallot, minced | 2 | tablespoons extra virgin olive oil |

### Pinot Noir Vinaigrette

MAKES 1 CUP (1 SERVING = 1/2 TABLESPOON)

| | | | |
|---|---|---|---|
| 1 | cup Pinot Noir wine | 2 | shallots, minced |
| 6 | tablespoons sugar | 2 | tablespoons extra virgin olive oil |
| 6 | tablespoons red wine vinegar | | |

Preheat the oven to 400 degrees F.

To cook the lobsters, separate them into tails and claws. Cook the tails in boiling water for 3 1/2 minutes. Cook the claws for 4 minutes. When they are cool enough to handle, remove the claw meat from the shells. Split the tails in half lengthwise, then remove the meat from the tail. Set aside.

To prepare the balsamic vinaigrette, in a medium bowl combine the balsamic vinegar, shallot, and salt and pepper, mixing well. Whisk in the olive oil. Set aside.

To prepare the Pinot Noir vinaigrette, in a small saucepan combine all ingredients except the olive oil. Bring to a boil, reduce the heat, and simmer until the mixture reduces to about 1/4 cup and is somewhat syrupy, about 10 minutes. Set aside to cool. Whisk in the olive oil.

To prepare brochette, skewer 1 piece each of bread, tail meat, red cherry tomato, basil leaf, bread, yellow cherry tomato, basil leaf, lobster claw (in this order).

Place the lobster brochettes on the grill for 1 minute on each side, then transfer to a baking sheet pan and place in preheated oven for 1 minute. (If you skip the grill, roast in the oven for 3 minutes).

Place the tomato wedges around the perimeter of the plates; 8 per plate. Season with salt and pepper.

Toss the frisee, watercress, and mixed greens in 1/4 cup balsamic vinaigrette. Place in the center of the tomatoes.

Place the brochettes atop the dressed salads and drizzle each with 1/2 tablespoon Pinot Noir vinaigrette.

*Note:* A member of the chicory family, frisee has curly white-yellow leaves and a slightly bitter flavor that mixes well with other greens. It is available in fairly constant supply throughout the year at some supermarkets and green markets.

---

- Tomatoes and tomato products contain the carotenoid lycopene, a potent antioxidant. They, along with salad greens, are also rich in vitamins C and A, providing more than 40% and 85% of the DVs per serving, respectively.
- Green leafy vegetables tend to be rich in folate; in this dish, 25% of the DV is provided per serving.
- High in fiber—20% of the DV per serving.

---

*Per serving of Balsamic Vinaigrette (1 tablespoon):*

| calories | protein | carbohydrates | fat | cholesterol | dietary fiber | saturated fat |
|---|---|---|---|---|---|---|
| 94 | 0 Gm | 1 Gm | 10 Gm | 0 mg | 0 Gm | 1 Gm |

*Per serving of Pinot Noir Vinaigrette (1/2 tablespoon):*

| calories | protein | carbohydrates | fat | cholesterol | dietary fiber | saturated fat |
|---|---|---|---|---|---|---|
| 63 | 0 Gm | 4 Gm | 5 Gm | 0 mg | 0 Gm | 1 Gm |

*Per serving of Lobster Salad with Balsamic and Pinot Noir Vinaigrettes:*

| calories | protein | carbohydrates | fat | cholesterol | dietary fiber | saturated fat |
|---|---|---|---|---|---|---|
| 312 | 16 Gm | 25 Gm | 17 Gm | 41 mg | 5 Gm | 2 Gm |

**% of Calories**: 31% carbohydrate, 20% protein, 47% fat, 2% alcohol

> **Major Sources of Potential Cancer Fighters**
> **Phytochemicals:** allium compounds, plant polyphenols (flavonoids, phenolic acids), plant sterols, terpenes (carotenoids, monoterpenes)

# ❧ *Warm Salmon Salad with Capers* ❧

Adam Busby, Director of Culinary Programs, Dubrulle Culinary School,
Vancouver, British Columbia, Canada

### 4 SERVINGS

• *This warm, savory salad is terrific for a light lunch meal or first course that can be prepared in less than 20 minutes.*

## Vinaigrette

### MAKES 3/4 CUP (1 SERVING = 1 TABLESPOON)

| | | | |
|---|---|---|---|
| 1/2 | cup extra virgin olive oil | 1 | shallot, minced |
| 3 1/2 | tablespoons Chardonnay vinegar or any good-quality white wine vinegar | 1 | teaspoon sugar salt and pepper |

## Salmon

| | | | |
|---|---|---|---|
| 12 | slices (12 oz.) smoked salmon | 1 | teaspoon crushed black pepper |
| 2 | teaspoons extra virgin olive oil | 2 | tablespoons drained capers |

## Salad

| | | | |
|---|---|---|---|
| 2 | heads oak leaf lettuce (or red leaf), rinsed well and large leaves torn | 1 | bunch spinach (about 8 ounces), rinsed well, stems removed, and large leaves torn |

Preheat the broiler.

To prepare the vinaigrette, combine all ingredients in a blender and puree at the highest speed until smooth and frothy. Season to taste with salt and pepper and set aside.

To cook the salmon, preheat the broiler. Lay the salmon slices out on a baking sheet lined with foil. Lightly brush with olive oil in sets of 3 slices. Drizzle with the olive oil and sprinkle with crushed black pepper. Place the tray under the broiler until the salmon begins to turn pale pink, about 2 to 3 minutes depending on the thickness of the slices. Remove the baking pan from the oven and set aside.

In a large bowl, toss the well-rinsed and dried lettuce leaves and spinach with
¼ cup of the vinaigrette and then arrange the greens on 4 plates.

Using a spatula, carefully lift the salmon off the baking pan and fan 3 slices over the
dressed greens. Sprinkle the capers around and on top of the salmon.

---

- Salmon is a potentially good source of omega-3 fatty acids. It is also a potentially very
  good source of selenium.
- Each serving is rich in cancer-protective vitamins: 50% of the DV for vitamin A, 45% for
  vitamin C, and 35% for folate.
- A good source of fiber.

---

*Per serving of Vinaigrette (1 tablespoon):*

| calories | protein | carbohydrates | fat | cholesterol | dietary fiber | saturated fat |
|---|---|---|---|---|---|---|
| 76 | 0 Gm | 1 Gm | 8 Gm | 7 mg | 0 Gm | 1 Gm |

*Per serving of Warm Salmon Salad with Capers and Vinaigrette:*

| calories | protein | carbohydrates | fat | cholesterol | dietary fiber | saturated fat |
|---|---|---|---|---|---|---|
| 224 | 19 Gm | 5 Gm | 15 Gm | 44 mg | 3 Gm | 2 Gm |

**% of Calories**: 9% carbohydrate, 34% protein, 57% fat

### Major Sources of Potential Cancer Fighters

**Phytochemicals**: allium compounds, plant polyphenols (flavonoids, phenolic acids), terpenes (carotenoids)

---

# ❦ *Warm Shrimp and Barley Salad* ❦

Barbara Lynch, No. 9 Park, Boston, Massachusetts

4 SERVINGS

- *The perfect all-season lunch or light dinner.*

## Shrimp Salad

| | |
|---|---|
| 1 small eggplant (about 12 ounces) | ½ cup pearl barley |
| 1 tablespoon olive oil | 8 large tiger shrimp (about |
| 1 tablespoon chopped basil | 12 ounces), peeled, deveined, |
| 1 tablespoon chopped mint | and tail end left intact |
| 1 tablespoon chopped parsley | (save shrimp shells) |
| salt | 1 tablespoon lemon juice |
| 8 ripe plum tomatoes | 4 handfuls arugula |
| (about 20 ounces) | |

*Shrimp Oil*

MAKES 1/2 CUP (1 SERVING = 1/2 TABLESPOON)

|  |  |
|---|---|
| shrimp shells | salt and pepper |
| 1/2 cup olive oil |  |

Preheat the oven to 400 degrees F. Dice the eggplant into 1/4-inch dice and marinate with 1/2 tablespoon each of the olive oil, basil, mint, and parsley. Season the eggplant with salt and roast on a nonstick sheet tray for 10 to 12 minutes.

Slice the tomatoes in half lengthwise, remove the seeds and pulp, and discard. Cut the tomato halves into 1/4-inch dice. Set aside.

Place the barley in a saucepan with 2 1/2 cups water, season with salt, and bring to a boil. Reduce to a simmer and cook, covered, for 30 to 35 minutes, until almost all of the liquid has been absorbed. Let stand, covered, for 5 minutes.

To prepare the shrimp oil, place the shrimp shells and 1/2 cup oil in a small baking pan. Season with salt and pepper and bake at 400 degrees F for about 20 minutes. Strain through a fine mesh strainer.

In a large nonstick skillet, heat the remaining 1/2 tablespoon of oil. Season the shrimp with salt and pepper and place in very hot pan, searing for 2 minutes on each side. Turn off the heat and remove the shrimp from the pan. Add the lemon juice while stirring with a wooden spoon. Set aside.

Toss the shrimp, tomatoes, barley, eggplant, remaining herbs, remaining pan juices, and 2 tablespoons of shrimp oil together. Adjust the seasoning with salt and pepper to taste. Divide the arugula among 4 salad plates and serve the shrimp-barley salad over top.

---

- Tomatoes and arugula contribute vitamin C (almost 50% of the DV per serving) and carotenoids, such as the antioxidant lycopene and beta-carotene (more than 15% of the DV for vitamin A per serving).
- Shrimp and barley are potentially good sources of selenium.
- Like most minimally processed grains, barley provides inositol (phytic acid), which may have a variety of anticancer functions. Barley also contributes substantial fiber—this recipe provides 28% of the DV per serving.

---

*Per serving:*

| calories | protein | carbohydrates | fat | cholesterol | dietary fiber | saturated fat |
|---|---|---|---|---|---|---|
| 321 | 29 Gm | 39 Gm | 13 Gm | 128 mg | 7 Gm | 2 Gm |

**% of Calories**: 36% carbohydrate, 28% protein, 36% fat

### Major Sources of Potential Cancer Fighters

**Phytochemicals**: phytic acids, plant polyphenols (flavonoids, phenolic acids), plant sterols, protease inhibitors, terpenes (carotenoids, monoterpenes)

# VEGETABLES

## ✦ *Crispy Oven-roasted Vegetables* ✦

Gianni Scappin, Maximillian, New York, New York; Trattoria alla Pesa, Mason Vicentino, Veneto, Italy

#### 4 SERVINGS

• *Who said healthy cooking is only poaching and steaming? High-temperature roasting caramelizes the natural sugar in vegetables and concentrates flavor. The vegetable combinations are limitless—just be sure to cut vegetables according to their cooking times (small cubes for those that take a longer time to cook).*

• *Gianni recommends serving these vegetables warm with roasted or grilled meat or fish, or at room temperature on a buffet table for lunch or brunch.*

| | |
|---|---|
| 1 large bell pepper (about 8 ounces), seeded and cut into large pieces | 1 large red onion (about 8 ounces), peeled and cut into large pieces |
| 2 medium sweet potatoes (about 12 ounces), peeled and cut into medium-size cubes | 2 large carrots (about 7 ounces), peeled and cut into 1/2-inch-thick slices |
| 2 medium turnips (about 10 ounces), peeled and cut into medium to small cubes | 3 garlic cloves, peeled and crushed |
| | 3 fresh rosemary sprigs |
| 2 medium potatoes, preferably Yukon Gold (about 9 ounces), peeled and cut into medium-size cubes | 2 teaspoons olive oil |
| | salt and pepper |

Preheat the oven to 450 degrees F.

Place the vegetables into a large mixing bowl with the garlic and rosemary sprigs (on stem). Drizzle with the olive oil and toss the vegetables so that they are evenly coated. Spread in one even layer on a large nonstick baking pan. Sprinkle with salt and pepper and place in the oven. Roast for 20 minutes, or until they are golden brown, then turn them using a spatula safe for nonstick cookware. Lower the heat to 375 degrees F and continue roasting until the vegetables are crispy and browned and tender when pierced with a knife, about 15 minutes. Remove the rosemary sprigs and serve.

- One serving provides enough carotenoids to supply almost 200% of the DV for vitamin A and 100% of the DV for vitamin C, as well as significant amounts of folate and protective phytochemicals from the allium compounds and cruciferous families of vegetables.
- High in fiber—20% of the DV per serving.

*Per serving:*

| calories | protein | carbohydrates | fat | cholesterol | dietary fiber | saturated fat |
|---|---|---|---|---|---|---|
| 200 | 4 Gm | 41 Gm | 3 Gm | 0 mg | 5 Gm | 1 Gm |

**% of Calories**: 79% carbohydrate, 8% protein, 13% fat

### Major Sources of Potential Cancer Fighters

**Phytochemicals**: allium compounds, carnosol, glucosinolates, plant polyphenols (flavonoids, phenolic acids), plant sterols, terpenes (carotenoids, monoterpenes, triterpenes)

# ❧ Grilled Vegetables with ❧ Roasted Red Pepper Vinaigrette

## 4 SERVINGS

- *Serve with crusty multigrain bread to make a tasty summer lunch or a light and healthy first course for an evening menu.*
- *Use Roasted Red Pepper Vinaigrette to dress other salads.*

### Roasted Red Pepper Vinaigrette

#### MAKES 1½ CUPS

| | |
|---|---|
| 2 medium red bell peppers (about 11 ounces) | 1 garlic clove, crushed salt and freshly ground pepper |
| 2 tablespoons sherry vinegar | 1 tablespoon olive oil |

### Grilled Vegetables

| | |
|---|---|
| 2 medium carrots (about 7 ounces), cut diagonally into ¼-inch-thick slices and blanched in boiling water for 3 to 4 minutes, drained | 1 large red onion (about 7 ounces), quartered, with root intact to hold the slices together when grilling |
| 2 large yellow bell peppers (about 12 ounces), quartered lengthwise, stemmed, and seeded | |

2 medium red potatoes
(about 9 ounces), boiled until
just slightly undercooked,
sliced 1/4 inch thick
1 small fennel (about 1 pound),
long stems removed (save
feathery leaves for garnish),

bulb quartered with root
left intact
1 tablespoon olive oil
salt and freshly ground pepper

To prepare the vinaigrette, first roast the peppers. Rub the peppers with a small amount of olive oil (less than 1/4 teaspoon) and place in an oven-safe skillet under the broiler. Using kitchen tongs, rotate the peppers to assure even cooking, blistering on all sides. Remove the peppers from the oven, place in a bowl, and cover with foil or plastic wrap so that steam helps to loosen the skins. When cool, remove the skins, seeds, and stems.

Place the peppers, vinegar, 1/3 cup water, the garlic, salt, and pepper in the bowl of a food processor or blender and puree until very smooth. With the machine running, drizzle in the olive oil. Adjust the seasoning to taste with salt and pepper.

To grill the vegetables, heat the grill to medium temperature. Lightly brush the vegetables with the olive oil and season with salt and pepper. Place the vegetables on the grill and cook until they are at the desired tenderness and lightly brown. DO NOT CHAR! If the vegetables begin to brown faster than they are cooking, raise the grill higher above the heat, move the vegetables to a cooler area of the grill, or, if necessary, transfer the vegetables to a platter until the grill temperature lowers.

Spoon a pool of red pepper vinaigrette on the bottom of 4 salad plates. Arrange the vegetables decoratively on top, then drizzle with a little more vinaigrette. Garnish with reserved feathery fennel leaves.

---

One serving provides more than 80% of the DV for vitamin A, 250% of the DV for vitamin C, as well as many protective phytochemicals.

---

*Per serving of Roasted Red Pepper Vinaigrette (1/4 cup):*

| calories | protein | carbohydrates | fat | cholesterol | dietary fiber | saturated fat |
|---|---|---|---|---|---|---|
| 25 | 0 Gm | 1 Gm | 2 Gm | 0 mg | 0 Gm | 0 Gm |

*Per serving of Grilled Vegetables with Roasted Red Pepper Vinaigrette:*

| calories | protein | carbohydrates | fat | cholesterol | dietary fiber | saturated fat |
|---|---|---|---|---|---|---|
| 135 | 2 Gm | 19 Gm | 6 Gm | 0 mg | 2 Gm | 1 Gm |

**% of Calories**: 55% carbohydrate, 6% protein, 39% fat

# ❧ Roasted Parsnip and Rutabaga Ragout ❧

Charles Wiley, The Boulders, Carefree, Arizona

4 SERVINGS

• *When these vegetables are roasted at high temperatures, the natural sugar in them caramelizes and the flavors concentrate. The combinations of colors and flavors look and taste great.*

| | | | |
|---|---|---|---|
| 2 | Anaheim chiles | 1 | large red onion |
| 2 | large parsnips (about 9 ounces), peeled and cut into 1/2-inch pieces | | (about 7 ounces), peeled and cut into large pieces |
| 1 | small rutabaga (about 1 pound), peeled and cut into 1/2-inch pieces | 2 | teaspoons olive oil |
| | | | salt and pepper |
| 2 | Japanese eggplants (about 10 ounces), cut into 3/4-inch pieces | 2 | teaspoons fresh thyme leaves |
| | | 1/2 | cup tomatoes, diced (about 4 ounces or 1 medium tomato) |
| 1 | medium zucchini (about 5 ounces), cut into 3/4-inch slices | | |
| 1 | medium yellow squash (about 7 ounces), cut into 3/4-inch slices | | |

To roast the Anaheim chiles, preheat the broiler. Rub the peppers with a small amount of olive oil (less than 1/4 teaspoon) and place in an oven-safe skillet under the broiler. Using kitchen tongs, rotate the peppers to assure even cooking (browning) on all sides; the skins of the peppers should blister. Remove the peppers from the oven, place in a bowl, and cover with foil or plastic wrap so that steam helps to loosen the skins. When cool, remove the skins and seeds and dice. Set aside.

Preheat the oven to 500 degrees F.

Put the cut vegetables in a large bowl and toss with the olive oil, salt, and pepper. Transfer the vegetables to a large shallow baking pan (preferably nonstick). Roast for 10 minutes, then stir the vegetables, rotate the pan, and turn down the heat to 425 degrees.

Continue roasting for 45 minutes more, stirring the vegetables and rotating the pan occasionally for even browning.

Transfer the vegetables to a large serving bowl, add the thyme, tomatoes, and chiles, and stir. Serve warm or at room temperature.

---

- Parsnips and rutabagas are underused vegetables that contain moderate amounts of folate (more than 15% of the DV per serving is provided in this recipe) and substantial amounts of vitamin C; these vegetables, combined with tomatoes and zucchini, provide 50% of the DV for vitamin C per serving.
- Rutabagas are usually yellow in color and contain moderate amounts of beta-carotene. They also belong to the cruciferous family of vegetables and have protective phytochemicals.
- High in fiber—more than 20% of the DV per serving.

---

**Per serving:**

| calories | protein | carbohydrates | fat | cholesterol | dietary fiber | saturated fat |
|---|---|---|---|---|---|---|
| 137 | 3 Gm | 21 Gm | 5 Gm | 0 mg | 6 Gm | 1 Gm |

**% of Calories:** 61% carbohydrate, 8% protein, 31% fat

### Major Sources of Potential Cancer Fighters

**Phytochemicals:** allium compounds, glucosinolates, plant polyphenols (flavonoids, phenolic acids), terpenes (carotenoids, monoterpenes)

# ✤ Spicy Sweet Potato and Chestnut Gratin ✤

Charles Wiley, The Boulders, Carefree, Arizona

6 SERVINGS

- *This side dish is colorful and creamy. The sweet potatoes and maple syrup lend a sweetness that is balanced by the smokiness and slight spiciness of the ancho chiles.*

| | |
|---|---|
| 1 teaspoon olive oil | salt and pepper |
| 1 1/3 cups 1% milk | 3 medium leeks, white part only, thinly sliced |
| 1/4 cup maple syrup | |
| 3 garlic cloves, chopped | 1/2 cup roasted chestnuts, coarsely chopped (see Notes) |
| 2 ancho chiles, stems and seeds removed, torn into 1/2-inch pieces (see Notes) | 3/4 cup aged Monterey Jack cheese, grated (see Notes) |
| 2 large sweet potatoes (about 20 ounces), peeled and thinly sliced (see Notes) | 2 tablespoons chives, snipped |

Preheat the oven to 350 degrees F.

Evenly rub a 9 × 12-inch ovenproof casserole dish with olive oil. In a small saucepan, heat the milk and maple syrup. Remove from the heat, add the garlic and chiles, and let steep for 30 minutes. Puree in a blender.

Lay about one-third of the potato slices in a single layer in the casserole dish, overlapping slightly. Season with salt and pepper. Ladle one-third of the milk mixture over the potatoes. Sprinkle with one-third of the leeks and one-third of the chestnuts, then top with one-third of the cheese. Repeat this process two more times to form a 3-layer gratin.

Cover with foil and bake for 40 minutes. Uncover and bake for another 20 minutes, or until brown and bubbly. Let sit for 20 minutes. To serve, cut the gratin into squares or circles or spoon out of the casserole. Sprinkle with snipped chives before serving.

*Notes:* Ancho chiles are dried poblano peppers available at some supermarkets and most gourmet specialty stores. When soaked or steeped, they lend a rich smoky flavor to sauces and broths without too much heat.

Use a mandoline to slice sweet potatoes quickly and easily. A mandoline is a kitchen tool made of stainless steel or plastic; it has a variety of blades for thin slicing and julienning and french-fry cutting. Inexpensive, good-quality plastic mandolines are available at most culinary stores.

Chestnuts are available fresh from September to February. To roast them, use the tip of a knife to cut a small **X** in the flat side of their outer shell, then spread them out on a baking pan. Roast at 400 degrees F for 25 to 30 minutes, then let them cool slightly. The shells can be easily removed. Thaw frozen chestnuts and then roast them at 425 degrees F until they are lightly browned, about 15 to 20 minutes.

Soy Monterey Jack also works well and provides all of the phytochemicals found in soy products. Soy cheeses are available at some supermarkets and most natural food stores.

---

- Sweet potatoes are phenomenal sources of beta-carotene. This recipe contains enough to supply 130% of the DV for vitamin A.
- Sweet potatoes, leeks, chestnuts, and chiles combined contribute 40% of the DV for vitamin C per serving.
- The chiles provide capsaicin, which may block or neutralize carcinogens.
- Leeks, members of the allium compound family, provide allyl sulfides, which may boost cancer-fighting enzymes.
- Each serving provides 20% of the DV for calcium.

> **Per serving:**
>
> | calories | protein | carbohydrates | fat | cholesterol | dietary fiber | saturated fat |
> |----------|---------|---------------|-----|-------------|---------------|---------------|
> | 233 | 7 Gm | 38 Gm | 6 Gm | 17 mg | 1 Gm | 3 Gm |
>
> **% of Calories**: 65% carbohydrate, 12% protein, 23% fat
>
> **Major Sources of Potential Cancer Fighters**
> **Phytochemicals**: allium compounds, capsaicin, plant polyphenols (flavonoids), plant sterols, terpenes (carotenoids, monoterpenes)

# ❧ *No-Fuss Broccoli Soufflé* ❧

### 4 SERVINGS

• *Great for broccoli lovers, this untraditional "soufflé" is a good alternative for those who do not like broccoli "straight up." It provides two vegetable "servings" and a significant amount of protein without the fat.*

• *Prepare a larger soufflé and cut into wedges for a nutritious and easy family-style or brunch side dish.*

• *Because this puree freezes well, double or triple the recipe and store in small containers. Defrost and microwave for a quick, delicious serving of vegetables.*

• *This recipe works well with cauliflower, spinach, or Brussels sprouts: simply substitute the same amount of any of these vegetables for the broccoli.*

| | | | |
|---|---|---|---|
| 20 | ounces broccoli spears, frozen, thawed, and drained, or 1 large head, broken into florets, blanched until tender, and drained | 1/3 | cup grated Parmesan cheese |
| | | 1/4 | teaspoon cayenne |
| | | 1/3 | teaspoon salt |
| | | | freshly ground pepper |
| 4 | egg whites or 4 ounces nonfat pasteurized egg product | 1 | teaspoon olive oil or olive oil–based cooking spray |

Puree the broccoli in a food processor until no large chunks remain. Add the remaining ingredients, except the olive oil, and puree until very smooth.

Rub the interior of four 4- to 6-ounce ramekins (or small ceramic bowls) with olive oil to evenly coat. Fill with the broccoli mixture, then pat down and smooth out the surface with a rubber spatula so that it is flat and firmly packed.

Microwave individually for 6 to 8 minutes on high until the center is set and firm. Run a paring knife around the sides of the ramekins to loosen the soufflés for easy removal. Carefully invert each mold and serve hot or at room temperature.

*Notes:* For a lighter soufflé, whip the egg whites separately until soft peaks form. Fold the egg whites into the seasoned, pureed broccoli mixture and continue as directed.

For a creamier soufflé add 1 medium cooked potato (baked or microwaved) to the broccoli mixture, and puree until smooth.

---

- Broccoli is a near-perfect vegetable; it is rich in beta-carotene, vitamin A, vitamin C, folate, and calcium. It is also a member of the cruciferous vegetable family and contains cancer-fighting phytochemicals.
- Broccoli is a potentially good source of the cancer-protective mineral selenium.
- One serving provides almost 100% of the DV for vitamin C, 30% of the DV for vitamin A, and approximately 20% of the DVs for calcium and folate.
- A good source of fiber.

---

*Per serving:*

| calories | protein | carbohydrates | fat | cholesterol | dietary fiber | saturated fat |
|----------|---------|---------------|-----|-------------|---------------|---------------|
| 102 | 11 Gm | 8 Gm | 3 Gm | 5 mg | 4 Gm | 1 Gm |

**% of Calories**: 31% carbohydrate, 43% protein, 26% fat

**Major Sources of Potential Cancer Fighters**
**Phytochemicals**: capsaicin, glucosinolates, plant polyphenols (flavonoids), plant sterols, terpenes (carotenoids, monoterpenes)

# ❖ Roasted Garlic ❖

### 8 SERVINGS

- *The process of roasting mellows the flavor of garlic, allowing one to eat much greater amounts of this nutrient-rich allium vegetable.*
- *Squeeze the roasted garlic directly onto crusty bread or use in recipes for dips, sauces, and spreads to add flavor and creaminess.*

| | |
|---|---|
| 4   large garlic heads | chicken stock (page 147 or 148) |
| ½   cup water or defatted | or canned broth |
| | salt |

Preheat the oven to 325 degrees F.

Remove any loose papery skin from the garlic, but leave the heads intact. Using a large knife, slice off the top tips of all of the cloves, leaving the root end uncut.

Arrange the heads in a single layer in a small baking pan. Pour the water or chicken stock over the garlic heads and into the base of the pan and season with salt. Cover tightly with aluminum foil and oven-roast for 1 hour. Uncover and bake 15 minutes longer, adding more liquid, if necessary. When the garlic heads are cool enough to handle, squeeze the creamy roasted garlic paste out of their skins.

*Note:* An even easier method is to wrap trimmed garlic heads tightly in aluminum foil and roast at 350 degrees F for 1 hour and 15 minutes.

Garlic contains protective allium compounds and substantial amounts of vitamin C. In this recipe, more than 10% of the DV per serving.

*Per serving:*

| calories | protein | carbohydrates | fat | cholesterol | dietary fiber | saturated fat |
|---|---|---|---|---|---|---|
| 33 | 1 Gm | 7 Gm | 0 Gm | 0 mg | 0 Gm | 0 Gm |

**% of Calories:** 82% carbohydrate, 16% protein, 2% fat

**Major Sources of Potential Cancer Fighters**

**Phytochemicals:** allium compounds

# ❧ Sautéed Spinach with Garlic ❧

### 4 SERVINGS

• *This cooking method produces a quick and tasty spinach side dish. It can be applied to other leafy greens, such as Swiss chard, escarole, broccoli rabe, and beet or turnip greens.*

20  ounces fresh spinach,
    stems removed
1  tablespoon extra virgin olive oil

4  large garlic cloves, peeled,
    lightly crushed, and
    quartered lengthwise
    salt and pepper

Thoroughly rinse the spinach; do not dry completely.

Heat the olive oil in a large skillet. Add the garlic and cook over medium heat until the garlic is lightly golden; don't let the garlic get too brown or it will be bitter. Remove the garlic and set aside. Reserve the oil in the skillet.

Add the spinach, season with salt and pepper, and cover. When the spinach just wilts, remove it from the heat, drain, and transfer to plates or a platter, and top with the garlic.

- Spinach is exceptionally high in beta-carotene (110% of the DV for vitamin A per serving in this recipe) as well as other carotenoids, folate (more than 80% of the DV), vitamin C (more than 80% of the DV), and minerals such as calcium, iron, magnesium, and potassium. It is also high in protein when compared to other vegetables.
- A good source of fiber.

*Per serving:*

| calories | protein | carbohydrates | fat | cholesterol | dietary fiber | saturated fat |
|----------|---------|---------------|-----|-------------|---------------|---------------|
| 82 | 5 Gm | 7 Gm | 4 Gm | 0 mg | 4 Gm | 1 Gm |

**% of Calories**: 33% carbohydrate, 24% protein, 43% fat

**Major Sources of Potential Cancer Fighters**
**Phytochemicals**: allium compounds, terpenes (carotenoids)

# ✷ *Sicilian-style Cauliflower* ✷

### 4 SERVINGS

- *Serve hot or at room temperature for a convenient vegetable for lunch or dinner, or a delicious and easy vegetable for a buffet or brunch.*

| | |
|---|---|
| 1 large head cauliflower (2 pounds), core and outer leaves removed and discarded, florets broken into medium-size pieces | 1 1/2 tablespoons white wine vinegar |
| 3/4 cup cooked white beans or canned beans, drained | 1/4 cup chicken stock (page 147 or 148) or low-sodium canned broth |
| salt | 2 tablespoons olive oil |
| | 1/4 cup raisins |
| | 1/4 cup pine nuts |
| | 2 tablespoons chopped fresh parsley |
| | pinch crushed red pepper flakes |

Bring 4 quarts of salted water to a boil and blanch the cauliflower until tender but still firm, 8 to 10 minutes. Drain thoroughly and transfer to a large bowl.

In the bowl of a food processor, combine 1/4 cup of the white beans, the salt, vinegar, and chicken stock. Puree until very smooth, then, with the motor still running, drizzle in the olive oil. When well combined, add to the bowl with the cauliflower along with the remaining white beans, the raisins, pine nuts, parsley, and red pepper flakes. Toss well to combine. Adjust the seasoning with salt, if necessary.

Serve warm or at room temperature.

- Significant source of cancer-fighting phytochemicals, such as indoles and isothio-cyanates, found in cruciferous family.
- Each serving provides more than 45% of the DV for vitamin C.
- A good source of fiber.

**Per serving:**

| calories | protein | carbohydrates | fat | cholesterol | dietary fiber | saturated fat |
|----------|---------|---------------|-----|-------------|---------------|---------------|
| 108 | 4 Gm | 10 Gm | 6 Gm | 0 mg | 3 Gm | 1 Gm |

**% of Calories**: 38% carbohydrate, 14% protein, 48% fat

### Major Sources of Potential Cancer Fighters

**Phytochemicals**: allium compounds, glucosinolates, phytic acids, plant polyphenols (flavonoids), plant sterols, protease inhibitors, terpenes (carotenoids, monoterpenes)

## ❧ Sweet and Sour Cabbage ❧

### 6 SERVINGS

- *Makes a nutritious, colorful "bed" for fanned-out slices of Gianni Scappin's Marinated Pork Tenderloin, page 251, or slices of roasted chicken breast.*
- *Vegetarian topping ideas include soy sausages or a starch, such as mashed potatoes, or couscous served in a center well of the cabbage.*

| | | | |
|---|---|---|---|
| 1 | tablespoon olive oil | 2 | apples (about 10 ounces), peeled, cored, and cut into cubes |
| 2 | medium red onions (about 8 ounces), sliced | 1/2 | cup seedless raisins |
| 2 | garlic cloves, peeled and crushed | | salt |
| 2 | tablespoons sugar | | |
| 1/3 | cup rice wine vinegar | | |
| 1 | small red cabbage, triangular core removed and shredded (1 1/2 pounds shredded cabbage) | | |

Heat the olive oil in a medium nonstick (about 4-quart) saucepan. Add the onions and garlic and cook over low heat until limp, about 20 minutes. Add the sugar and turn up the heat, caramelizing the onions, about 2 to 3 minutes. Stir constantly with a wooden spoon to avoid overbrowning, sticking, or burning.

Stir in the rice wine vinegar. After most of the liquid has cooked off, add the cabbage and stir to thoroughly combine. Turn down the heat to low and cook, covered, for 1 hour. Stir occasionally and add water, 1 to 2 tablespoons at a time, if more liquid is necessary. During the last 15 minutes of cooking, add the apples and raisins. Season with salt to taste.

---

- Cabbage, like other members of the cruciferous vegetable family, contains glucosinolates, which act as antioxidants, promote protective enzymes, and inhibit the activity of other enzymes and hormones that may promote cancer.
- Contains protective enzyme–boosting allium compound vegetables: onions and garlic.
- One serving provides more than 70% of the DV for vitamin C and 15% of the DV for folate.
- High in fiber—20% of the DV per serving.

---

**Per serving:**

| calories | protein | carbohydrates | fat | cholesterol | dietary fiber | saturated fat |
|---|---|---|---|---|---|---|
| 162 | 3 Gm | 31 Gm | 3 Gm | 0 mg | 5 Gm | 0 Gm |

**% of Calories**: 77% carbohydrate, 7% protein, 16% fat

**Major Sources of Potential Cancer Fighters**

**Phytochemicals**: allium compounds, glucosinolates, indoles, plant polyphenols (flavonoids, isoflavones, phenolic acids), plant sterols, terpenes (carotenoids, monoterpenes)

# ❧ Tuscan-style Cannellini Beans ❧

Lidia Bastianich, Felidia/Becco/Frico Bar, New York, New York

6 SERVINGS

- *Can be served as a simple side dish (warm or at room temperature) with grilled meat or fish or as an appetizer, topping small toasted bread slices.*

| | | | |
|---|---|---|---|
| 1 | tablespoon olive oil | 3 | fresh sage leaves |
| 2 | garlic cloves, peeled and crushed | | salt and pepper |
| 3 | cups cooked cannellini beans | | pinch crushed red pepper |
| | or 3 cups canned, drained (see Note) | 2 | medium tomatoes (8 ounces), peeled, seeded, and diced |
| 1 | bay leaf | | |

In a large nonstick skillet, heat the olive oil and add the garlic. When the garlic turns golden brown, add the drained beans, bay leaf, sage leaves, and crushed red pepper to the skillet. Stir and sauté for 2 to 3 minutes, then add the tomatoes and season with salt and pepper. Cover and let simmer on medium-low heat for about 20 minutes to blend the flavors. Discard the sage leaves and crushed garlic before serving.

*Note:* To cook dried beans, soak them in water to cover for 4 hours; change the water 2 to 3 times. Drain and place in a medium saucepan, add the bay leaf, and cook until tender, about 1 hour.

---

- Tomatoes and tomato products are rich in vitamin C and contain the carotenoid lycopene, a potent antioxidant.
- Sage also contains phytochemicals that act as antioxidants.
- High in fiber—20% of the DV per serving.

---

*Per serving:*

| calories | protein | carbohydrates | fat | cholesterol | dietary fiber | saturated fat |
|---|---|---|---|---|---|---|
| 132 | 7 Gm | 21 Gm | 3 Gm | 0 mg | 5 Gm | 1 Gm |

**% of Calories**: 61% carbohydrate, 22% protein, 17% fat

### Major Sources of Potential Cancer Fighters

Phytochemicals: allium compounds, phytic acids, plant polyphenols (flavonoids, isoflavones, phenolic acids), plant sterols, protease inhibitors, terpenes (carotenoids, monoterpenes)

# VEGETARIAN ENTRÉES

## ❧ *Toasted Angel Hair Pasta* ❧
## *with Mushroom Broth*

Diane Forley, Verbena, New York, New York

4 SERVINGS

- *Toasting pasta gives it an earthy, nutty flavor that marries well with mushrooms.*
- *Use this mushroom broth in other recipes, such as a soup base or a broth for a risotto.*

### Mushroom Broth

| | | | | |
|---|---|---|---|---|
| 1 | pound white button mushrooms (about 6 cups), cleaned and halved or quartered if large | 6 | shallots, peeled |
| | | 2 | fresh thyme sprigs |
| 1/2 | head garlic, unpeeled and sliced crosswise | 1 | tablespoon olive oil |
| | | | salt and pepper |
| | | 10 | cups water |

### Toasted Pasta

| | | | | |
|---|---|---|---|---|
| 3/4 | pound uncooked angel hair pasta, broken in half | 1/4 | cup sliced shallots (2 medium) |
| 1 | tablespoon plus 1 teaspoon olive oil | 1 | cup sliced oyster mushrooms |
| | | | salt and pepper |
| 1 | garlic clove, minced | 1/4 | cup parsley leaves |
| | | 1 | tablespoon snipped chives |

Preheat the oven to 375 degrees F.

To prepare the mushroom broth, in a bowl, toss the mushrooms, garlic, shallots, and thyme with the olive oil and spread out evenly on a nonstick baking pan. Season with salt and pepper. Roast in the oven for 25 to 30 minutes, until the juice runs out and the mushrooms are well caramelized. Place the contents into a medium saucepan and cover with the water. Bring to a boil, reduce the heat, and cook at low boil for 20 minutes, or until reduced by half. Strain through a wire-meshed strainer into a medium bowl. Set aside.

While mushrooms are baking, prepare the toasted pasta, placing it on a large baking sheet and spreading it out as evenly as possible. Drizzle with 1 tablespoon of olive oil and, using your hands, toss to evenly coat. Bake in the oven at 375 degrees F until golden, 10 to 12 minutes (turn the sheet pan around halfway through baking). Remove from the oven and set aside.

Heat 1 teaspoon of olive oil in a medium saucepan (preferably nonstick). Over medium heat, sauté the garlic and shallots, without browning, for about 1 minute. Add the oyster mushrooms and cook for 3 to 4 minutes, stirring frequently. Turn up the heat and add the mushroom broth; when it boils, add the toasted pasta, cooking until al dente, about 5 minutes. Turn off the heat; season with salt and pepper, and add the parsley leaves and chives. Spoon into pasta bowls.

---

- Mushrooms contain significant amounts of B vitamins as well as copper and other minerals. They are also a potentially very good source of selenium.
- Mushrooms and parsley both contribute vitamin C, providing more than 15% of the DV per serving.
- A good source of fiber.

---

**Per serving of Mushroom Broth (1 cup):**

| calories | protein | carbohydrates | fat | cholesterol | dietary fiber | saturated fat |
|---|---|---|---|---|---|---|
| 39 | 1 Gm | 2 Gm | 3 Gm | 0 mg | 0 Gm | 0 Gm |

**Per serving of Toasted Angel Hair Pasta with Mushroom Broth:**

| calories | protein | carbohydrates | fat | cholesterol | dietary fiber | saturated fat |
|---|---|---|---|---|---|---|
| 412 | 13 Gm | 68 Gm | 10 Gm | 0 mg | 3 Gm | 1 Gm |

**% of Calories**: 66% carbohydrate, 13% protein, 21% fat

### Major Sources of Potential Cancer Fighters

**Phytochemicals**: allium compounds, phytic acids, plant polyphenols (flavonoids), terpenes (carotenoids, monoterpenes)

# ❧ Summer Vegetables in a Creamy Chile ❧ Cheese Sauce (Calabacitas con Queso)

Zarela Martinez, Zarela, New York, New York
Adapted from *Food from My Heart*, Macmillan, 1992.

### 4 SERVINGS

- *Serve as an appetizer (recipe provides 8 servings) with toasted pita chips (page 115), or as a vegetarian main course over rice or baked potatoes, or as a filling for steamed tortillas.*

1½   pounds zucchini (5 small, tender zucchini), scrubbed but not peeled and cut into ¼-inch dice
     salt and pepper
1    tablespoon olive oil
1    large garlic clove, minced
1    medium onion (about 5 ounces), finely chopped (about 1 cup)
1    large ripe, red tomato (about 7 ounces), chopped

2    cups fresh corn kernels cut from the cob, or 1 10-ounce package frozen corn, or 1 can (16 ounces) plain corn kernels, drained
2    poblano chiles, roasted, peeled, and finely chopped (see Notes)
1    5-ounce can evaporated skim milk
½    pound low-fat (not fat-free) white Cheddar cheese, diced (see Notes)

Place the zucchini in a medium saucepan with 1 cup water; season lightly with salt and pepper. Bring to a boil and simmer, covered, over medium heat for 2 minutes. Set aside without draining.

Heat the oil in a large nonstick skillet over high heat until hot but not smoking. Reduce the heat slightly and add the garlic and onion. Cook, stirring until the onion is translucent, about 2 minutes. Stir in the tomato and cook until its liquid is partly evaporated, about 5 minutes. Stir in the corn and poblanos and simmer 5 minutes more.

Add the zucchini and its cooking liquid along with the evaporated milk to the corn-chile mixture and bring to a boil. Reduce the heat to low, stir in the Cheddar, and cook just until it melts. Serve immediately.

*Notes:* Fresh poblano (or ancho) chiles are available at many supermarkets. Whole poblanos can also be purchased in 4- or 7-ounce cans and are very useful when fresh peppers are not available.

Try soy Cheddar cheese; it tastes great in cooked dishes and has all of the cancer-fighting phytochemicals found in soy. A variety of soy-based cheeses are available at some supermarkets and most natural food stores.

---

- One serving contains 40% of the DV for calcium if using soy Cheddar cheese and 75% with low-fat cheddar.
- Zucchini, tomato, and chiles all contribute substantial amounts of vitamin C: more than 40% of the DV is provided per serving. This recipe also contains 25% of the DV for vitamin A per serving.
- Moderate consumption of capsaicin, found in chile peppers, may help the body neutralize carcinogens.
- High in fiber—20% of the DV per serving.

**Per serving:**

| calories | protein | carbohydrates | fat | cholesterol | dietary fiber | saturated fat |
|---|---|---|---|---|---|---|
| 270 | 18 Gm | 31 Gm | 8 Gm | 0 mg | 5 Gm | 1 Gm |
| | | | (if soy Cheddar cheese is used) | (if soy Cheddar cheese is used) | | (if soy Cheddar cheese is used) |

**% of Calories**: 46% carbohydrate, 27% protein, 27% fat

### Major Sources of Potential Cancer Fighters

**Phytochemicals**: allium compounds, capsaicin, phytic acids*, plant polyphenols (flavonoids, isoflavones*, phenolic acids), plant sterols, protease inhibitors,* terpenes (carotenoids, triterpenes*)

# ❧ Fusilli with Cherry Tomatoes ❧

Lidia Bastianich, Felidia/Becco/Frico Bar, New York, New York

### 4 SERVINGS

• *A quick, easy entrée, first course, or side dish (recipe yields 6 servings) perfect with grilled or roasted chicken or fish.*

| | |
|---|---|
| 3 cups cherry tomatoes (about 1 pound), stems removed and halved | 1/4 teaspoon salt |
| | 1 pound dried fusilli |
| | 10 basil leaves |
| 2 tablespoons extra virgin olive oil | 4 tablespoons pecorino cheese, |
| 1/2 teaspoon crushed red pepper | grated (optional) |

In a large serving bowl, toss the tomatoes with the oil, crushed red pepper, and salt. Let marinate at room temperature for 20 minutes.

Cook the fusilli in a large pot of boiling salted water until al dente, 9 to 10 minutes. Drain the pasta, reserving 1/3 cup of the cooking water.

Stir the pasta water into the tomatoes and add the basil. Add the pasta and toss. Add the pecorino, tossing again, then serve.

---

- Pasta is a potentially good source of selenium.
- Tomatoes are rich in vitamins A and C, providing more than 10% and 50% of the DVs, respectively. They also contain the carotenoid lycopene, a powerful antioxidant.
- High in fiber.

---

*Present if soy Cheddar cheese is used.

*Per serving (based on 4 servings):*

| calories | protein | carbohydrates | fat | cholesterol | dietary fiber | saturated fat |
|----------|---------|---------------|-----|-------------|---------------|---------------|
| 565 | 21 Gm | 93 Gm | 12 Gm | 13 mg | 5 Gm | 4 Gm |

**% of Calories**: 66% carbohydrate, 15% protein, 19% fat

**Major Sources of Potential Cancer Fighters**

**Phytochemicals**: capsaicin, phytic acids, plant polyphenols (flavonoids, phenolic acids), plant sterols, terpenes (carotenoids, monoterpenes)

# ❧ *Farfalle with Asparagus and Peas* ❧

Marta Pulini, Corporate Chef, Toscorp., New York, New York

4 SERVINGS

• *Serve this light spring vegetable sauce with other pasta shapes, such as fusilli, penne, or cheese-stuffed tortellini or ravioli.*

| | | | |
|---|---|---|---|
| 1½ | cups peas, fresh or frozen | ½ | teaspoon salt |
| ½ | pound asparagus (1 small bunch), stem ends trimmed | ¼ | teaspoon pepper |
| 2 | medium shallots (about 2 ounces), finely chopped | 3 | tablespoons chopped Italian parsley |
| 2 | tablespoons olive oil | ¾ | pound dried farfalle or bow tie |
| 1 | teaspoon sugar | ¼ | cup Parmesan cheese, freshly grated |
| 1 | cup vegetable broth (page 146) or low-sodium, canned broth | | |

If using fresh peas, remove them from their shells. Trim the tough part of the stems of the asparagus. In a large saucepan, bring 5 quarts of salted water to a boil and cook the asparagus until tender but still firm. Using tongs, transfer the asparagus to an ice bath to cool them down quickly and maintain their bright color. If using fresh peas, place them in a steamer insert and drop them into the boiling water for 2 to 3 minutes, then transfer to a small bowl of ice water (separate from the asparagus). Reserve the cooking water at a low simmer to cook the pasta, adding more water if necessary. If using frozen peas, measure out 1½ cups and place them in a small strainer over a bowl to thaw.

Drain the vegetables and slice the tender part of the asparagus stems, reserving the tips separately.

In a medium nonstick sauté pan, sauté half of the shallots in 1 teaspoon of olive oil over medium-high heat for 2 minutes while stirring. Add the peas and sauté for 2 more minutes. Add the sugar, 1/2 cup broth, and season with salt and pepper. Bring to a boil, reduce the heat, and simmer for about 1 minute. Remove half of this mixture and puree in a food processor or blender with 2 tablespoons parsley, 1 tablespoon olive oil, and a little more broth if the sauce needs to be thinned slightly—it should be creamy and rather thick. In a medium bowl, combine the whole peas with the puree. Taste and adjust with salt, if necessary; reserve in a small bowl.

In a medium, heavy saucepan (preferably nonstick), sauté the remaining shallots in 2 teaspoons olive oil over medium-high heat until soft, about 2 minutes. Add the asparagus stems, season with salt and pepper, and continue to sauté. After 1 to 2 minutes, add the remaining 1/2 cup vegetable broth and bring to a simmer. When the asparagus are tender but not overcooked, add the asparagus tips and continue to simmer until they become tender, about 2 minutes.

Meanwhile, bring the water to a rolling boil and add the pasta. Cook until al dente, about 10 to 12 minutes, drain the pasta, and add to the saucepan along with the reserved pea sauce. Toss with the Parmesan and remaining chopped parsley.

---

- Peas, asparagus, and parsley all contribute folate, vitamin C, and carotenoids. This recipe provides more than 20% of the DV for folate, 30% of the DV for vitamin C, and enough carotenoids to supply more than 15% of the DV for vitamin A per serving.
- Aspargus contains plant sterols, which may suppress cancer growth.
- Pasta is a potentially good source of selenium.
- High in fiber—20% of the DV per serving.

---

*Per serving:*

| calories | protein | carbohydrates | fat | cholesterol | dietary fiber | saturated fat |
|----------|---------|---------------|-----|-------------|---------------|---------------|
| 465 | 17 Gm | 76 Gm | 10 Gm | 4 mg | 5 Gm | 2 Gm |

**% of Calories**: 66% carbohydrate, 15% protein, 19% fat

### Major Sources of Potential Cancer Fighters
**Phytochemicals**: allium compounds, plant polyphenols (flavonoids), protease inhibitors, terpenes (carotenoids, monoterpenes)

# ❦ *Cannelloni with Roasted* ❦ *Eggplant and Ricotta*

Roberto Donna, Galileo, Washington, D.C.

4 SERVINGS

• *Roberto has managed to create cannelloni with less than half of the fat of traditional cannelloni without sacrificing flavor.*

| | | | |
|---|---|---|---|
| 1 | large eggplant (about 20 ounces), roasted | 2 | garlic cloves, minced |
| 2 | teaspoons olive oil pinch cayenne | 1/4 | cup basil, chopped |
| | | 3/4 | cup fat-free sour cream salt and pepper |
| 4 | medium very ripe tomatoes (about 1 pound), peeled and seeded | 8 | 6 inch × 6 inch pasta squares |
| | | 2 | cups low-fat ricotta cheese |
| | | 1 | teaspoon marjoram |

Preheat the oven to 375 degrees F.

To roast the eggplant, halve the eggplant lengthwise, brush the flesh with olive oil, and sprinkle with cayenne. Place on a nonstick baking sheet, flat side down, and roast for 20 to 30 minutes. Turn over and continue roasting for approximately 20 more minutes. Remove from the oven and let cool. Scoop the pulp from the skin of the eggplant, place into a large bowl, and mash.

To prepare the sauce, bring 2 quarts of water to a boil in a large pot. Cut the core from the tomatoes with a paring knife, cut a shallow **X** into the bottom of the tomatoes, and plunge them into boiling water for 30 seconds. Remove with a slotted spoon and immediately immerse in ice water until cool. Use a knife to gently peel the skin, which should be discarded. Slice the tomatoes in half and gently squeeze to force out the seeds. Use your fingers to remove any remaining seeds. Discard the seeds and chop the tomatoes.

In a food processor or blender, puree the tomato. Transfer to a medium saucepan and add the garlic and basil. Bring to a boil, reduce the heat, and simmer for about 5 minutes. Turn off the heat, stir in 1/4 cup of fat-free sour cream, and season with salt and pepper.

Bring 5 quarts of salted water to a boil and cook the pasta until al dente, 6 to 8 minutes. Drain and reserve.

Add the ricotta, the remaining 1/2 cup fat-free sour cream, and the marjoram to the eggplant. Add salt and pepper and mix well. Divide the mixture between the pasta squares and roll them up. Place in a small, square, nonstick baking dish and bake for 15 minutes, until crisp.

Spoon some sauce onto 4 plates and place the cannelloni on top. Top the cannelloni with a little more sauce.

---

- Each serving provides more than 40% of the DV for vitamin C and 20% for vitamin A.
- High in fiber—22% of the DV per serving.

---

**Per serving:**

| calories | protein | carbohydrates | fat | cholesterol | dietary fiber | saturated fat |
|----------|---------|---------------|-----|-------------|---------------|---------------|
| 391 | 28 Gm | 54 Gm | 8 Gm | 22 mg | 6 Gm | 3 Gm |

**% of Calories**: 54% carbohydrate, 28% protein, 18% fat

**Major Sources of Potential Cancer Fighters**

**Phytochemicals**: allium compounds, plant polyphenols (flavonoids, phenolic acids), plant sterols, terpenes (carotenoids, monoterpenes)

# ✷ Curry Roasted Summer ✷ Vegetables over Basmati Rice

Nick Morfogen, Maxaluna, Boca Raton, Florida

6 SERVINGS

- *Nick serves these aromatic and delicious vegetables as a side dish or over grains such as basmati or brown rice, barley, couscous, or polenta.*

### Rice

| | | | |
|---|---|---|---|
| 1 1/2 | cups basmati rice | 1/2 | teaspoon butter |
| 1/2 | teaspoon salt | 2 | cardamom pods |

### Vegetables

| | | | |
|---|---|---|---|
| 12 | pearl onions (about 4 ounces), unpeeled, ends cut off | 2 | medium carrots (about 5 ounces), peeled and sliced diagonally |
| 1 | teaspoon olive oil | | |

2  medium potatoes (about
      10 ounces), peeled and quartered
1/2  pound green beans, split in
      half lengthwise and cut
      into 2-inch pieces
1  medium zucchini (about
      8 ounces), cut into large dice
12  asparagus (8 ounces), cut
      into 2-inch pieces
1  medium eggplant (about
      14 ounces), cut into large dice

1  tablespoon curry powder
   kosher salt and freshly ground
      white pepper
2  tablespoons extra virgin olive oil
2  teaspoons minced garlic
2  medium tomatoes
      (about 10 ounces), quartered
8  ounces vegetable stock (page 146)
      or low-sodium canned broth
12  basil leaves, sliced

In a medium bowl, soak the rice in warm water for 30 minutes; drain.

Preheat the oven to 450 degrees F. In a small bowl, toss the pearl onions with 1 teaspoon of olive oil and spread out in a small roasting pan. Place the pan in the oven and roast until tender, about 12 minutes. Allow to cool and then peel. Set aside.

In a saucepan, combine the soaked rice, 2 1/2 cups water, salt, butter, and cardamom. Heat to boiling over high heat, reduce the heat to low, and simmer gently, covered, for 15 minutes, or until the rice is light and fluffy and the water has been absorbed.

While the onions roast, place the carrots in a medium saucepan filled with cold salted water. Bring to a boil, then reduce the heat. When the carrots are almost cooked but still firm, after about 7 minutes, add the potatoes. Cook for 4 more minutes and add the green beans. After 2 minutes, drain the water from the vegetables and reserve in a large stainless-steel bowl.

Add the zucchini, asparagus, and eggplant to the bowl and sprinkle with curry powder and season with salt and white pepper. In a Dutch oven or oven-safe saucepan, heat 2 tablespoons of olive oil. When it is almost smoking, carefully add the seasoned vegetables. Shake the pan once or twice after 30 seconds, then place the pan into the oven. Cook for 10 minutes, then remove the pan from the oven and place it on the stove.

Stir in the garlic, tomatoes, vegetable stock, and basil. Bring this mixture to a boil, reduce the heat, and simmer for 2 to 3 minutes.

Spread out the rice on a serving platter and spoon the vegetables over the top. Pour the curry broth over the vegetables.

---

- One serving provides more than 100% of the DV for vitamin C, 85% for vitamin A, and 25% for folate.
- Curry powder contains curcumin, a plant polyphenol that lends yellow color and acts as an antioxidant; it may also play a role in blocking cancer at the initiation stage.
- High in fiber—more than one-third of the DV per serving.

**Per serving of Curry Roasted Summer Vegetables:**

| calories | protein | carbohydrates | fat | cholesterol | dietary fiber | saturated fat |
|---|---|---|---|---|---|---|
| 145 | 6 Gm | 31 Gm | 2 Gm | 0 mg | 7 Gm | 0 Gm |

**Per serving of Basmati Rice:**

| calories | protein | carbohydrates | fat | cholesterol | dietary fiber | saturated fat |
|---|---|---|---|---|---|---|
| 153 | 3 Gm | 33 Gm | 1 Gm | 0 mg | 2 Gm | 0 Gm |

**Per serving of Curry Roasted Summer Vegetables over Basmati Rice:**

| calories | protein | carbohydrates | fat | cholesterol | dietary fiber | saturated fat |
|---|---|---|---|---|---|---|
| 298 | 9 Gm | 64 Gm | 3 Gm | 0 mg | 9 Gm | 0 Gm |

**% of Calories**: 80% carbohydrate, 12% protein, 8% fat

### Major Sources of Potential Cancer Fighters

**Phytochemicals**: allium compounds, phytic acids, plant polyphenols (flavonoids, phenolic acids), plant sterols, terpenes (carotenoids, monoterpenes)

# ❧ Apple and Acorn Squash Risotto ❧

RoxSand Scocos, RoxSand's Restaurant & Bar, Phoenix, Arizona

4 SERVINGS (MAIN COURSE), 6 SERVINGS (FIRST COURSE)

- *The combination of apple and squash is both delicious and nutritious.*
- *To cut cooking time on a busy day, peel the squash, remove the seeds, cut into small cubes, and add directly to the risotto rather than first roasting.*

### Apple-Leek Broth

2  small leeks, white part only
(about 5 ounces),
cleaned and sliced thinly
1  teaspoon olive oil

3  fresh thyme sprigs
salt and pepper
3  cups fresh apple juice
or apple cider

### Risotto

1  acorn squash
(about 1½ pounds)
3  cups vegetable stock (page 146)
or low-sodium canned broth or
water, boiling

1  tablespoon olive oil
1  medium onion, finely chopped
2  Granny Smith apples (about
10 ounces), peeled, seeded,
and cut into small cubes

salt and pepper                          3    fresh thyme sprigs
1¹/₂   cups Italian Arborio rice


To prepare the apple-leek broth, in a small saucepan, sauté the leeks in the olive oil for 5 minutes; do not brown. Add the thyme sprigs and season with salt and pepper. Cook for another minute, then add the apple juice or cider. Heat just until it simmers, then remove from the heat and set aside.

To roast the squash, preheat the oven to 375 degrees F. Split the acorn squash into two halves, remove the seeds, and place in a small roasting pan. Add ¹/₂ cup water to the bottom of the pan and seal with aluminum foil. Roast for about 50 minutes, until very tender. Let cool slightly. Remove the pulp from the skin and set aside.

Combine the apple-leek broth and the vegetable stock in a medium saucepan, bring to a boil, and reduce the heat.

Heat the olive oil in a 4-quart saucepan with a heavy bottom. Sauté the onion for 3 to 4 minutes; do not brown. Add the apples and season with salt and pepper. Continue to sauté for another minute, then add the rice, squash, thyme sprigs, and 3 cups of simmering broth. Bring to a boil, then reduce the heat and simmer, stirring frequently, until the liquid is almost completely absorbed and the rice is just tender, about 18 to 20 minutes. Add more liquid, ¹/₃ cup at a time, if the rice absorbs all the liquid and needs to cook further. Adjust the seasoning with salt and pepper and serve.

- This recipe provides more than 25% of the DV for vitamins A and C per serving.
- Apples provide not only flavor and fiber, but also plant polyphenols that act as antioxidants, blocking agents against carcinogens.
- A good source of fiber.

*Per serving (based on 4 servings):*

| calories | protein | carbohydrates | fat | cholesterol | dietary fiber | saturated fat |
|---|---|---|---|---|---|---|
| 526 | 8 Gm | 110 Gm | 6 Gm | 0 mg | 4 Gm | 1 Gm |

**% of Calories**: 84% carbohydrate, 6% protein, 10% fat

**Major Sources of Potential Cancer Fighters**
**Phytochemicals**: allium compounds, plant polyphenols (flavonoids), plant sterols, terpenes (carotenoids, monoterpenes)

# ❧ *Green Chile Stew* ❧

Robert McGrath, Windows on the Green, Phoenix, Arizona

4 SERVINGS

- *Serve as a vegetarian entrée or with seared or roasted game or spicy roasted chicken.*

| | |
|---|---|
| 8 poblano chiles (see Notes) | ¹/₂ cup yellow hominy |
| 1 tablespoon extra virgin olive oil | ¹/₄ cup white hominy |
| ³/₄ cup carrots, peeled and cut into ¹/₄-inch dice | salt and freshly cracked black pepper |
| ¹/₂ cup yellow onion, chopped | ¹/₄ cup toasted pumpkin seeds |
| 3 garlic cloves, minced | |
| 2 cups hot vegetable broth (page 146) or low-sodium canned broth or water | |

To roast the poblano chiles, rub the peppers with a small amount of olive oil (less than ¹/₂ teaspoon) and place in an oven-safe skillet under the heated broiler. Using kitchen tongs, rotate the peppers to assure even cooking (browning) on all sides. Remove the peppers from the oven, place in a bowl, and cover with foil or plastic wrap so that steam helps to loosen the skins. When cool, remove the skins, seeds, and stems. Puree in a food processor or blender.

Heat the olive oil in a 2-quart saucepan (preferably nonstick) and sauté the carrots and onion over moderate heat until tender, about 10 minutes. Add the garlic and sauté for another minute, being careful not to burn it. Add the poblano puree, 1¹/₂ cups vegetable broth, and the hominy, then simmer over medium-low heat until the liquid has been absorbed and the hominy is cooked, about 15 minutes. Stir constantly and add more liquid and continue cooking if necessary. Season to taste with salt and pepper, top with the toasted pumpkin seeds, and serve.

*Notes:* Poblanos or anchos are long, dark-green chiles that have a distinctive smoky flavor and mild to moderate heat. They are relatively easy to find at supermarkets, especially during the summer and fall.

Cooking times and amount of liquid needed for the hominy will vary depending on the product.

---

- Capsaicin, found in chile peppers, may help the body neutralize carcinogens.
- Chile peppers are a very good source of vitamin C, providing more than 40% of the DV per serving.
- Each serving provides 110% of the DV for vitamin A.
- A good source of fiber.

*Per serving:*

| calories | protein | carbohydrates | fat | cholesterol | dietary fiber | saturated fat |
|---|---|---|---|---|---|---|
| 256 | 9 Gm | 36 Gm | 10 Gm | 0 mg | 4 Gm | 2 Gm |

**% of Calories**: 53% carbohydrate, 13% protein, 34% fat

### Major Sources of Potential Cancer Fighters
**Phytochemicals**: allium compounds, capsaicin, phytic acids, plant polyphenols (flavonoids, phenolic acids), protease inhibitors, terpenes (carotenoids, monoterpenes)

# ❧ *Lentil and Shelling Bean Stew* ❧

Michael Chiarello, Tra Vigna, St. Helena, California

4 SERVINGS

• *Michael Chiarello comments that the meaty flavor of lentils (particularly when smoked) makes a stew such as this a perfect vegetarian entrée. He originally created this recipe to pair with the beautiful medium-bodied red wines produced near his restaurant.*

• *Serve alone or as a bed for sausages or roasted fish, such as cod or halibut. (Soy sausages, browned, sliced, and added to the stew provide all of the protective benefits from soy protein as well as a spicy flavor kick without the fat. Also, try chicken or turkey sausages.) Roasted or grilled chicken also goes well with this lentil stew.*

2 tablespoons extra virgin olive oil
1 tablespoon finely chopped garlic
1 large onion (about 7 ounces), cut into 1/4-inch dice
2 medium carrots (about 6 ounces), cut into 1/4-inch dice
1 medium celery stalk (about 2 ounces), cut into 1/4-inch dice
1 tablespoon finely diced fresh thyme leaves
1 bay leaf

4 cups chicken stock (page 147 or 148) or low-sodium canned broth
1/2 pound dried green lentils (1 1/4 cups)
1 cup shelling beans (cranberry beans), removed from the pod and cooked (see Notes)
salt and freshly ground pepper
2 tablespoons sherry vinegar
2 tablespoons chopped fresh Italian parsley

Heat the oil in a large saucepan over medium-high heat until almost smoking. Add the garlic and sauté until light brown (be careful not to burn the garlic). Add the onion, carrots, and celery and sauté until they soften slightly, about 3 to 4 minutes. Lower the heat to medium and cook until the vegetables are soft, about 10 minutes. Add the thyme and bay leaf and stir to combine. Add 2¹/₂ cups stock, bring to a boil, and add the lentils. Lower the heat to a simmer, cover, and cook until the lentils are about half cooked, 15 minutes or so. Add more stock if necessary.

Add the cooked shelling beans to the lentils with 1 teaspoon salt and ¹/₂ teaspoon pepper. Add another ³/₄ to 1 cup stock. The consistency should be stewlike. Bring to a boil and simmer until the vegetables are tender, about 10 minutes. Remove and discard the bay leaf. Add the vinegar and remaining tablespoon of oil. Adjust the seasoning to taste with salt, pepper, and more vinegar if necessary. Ladle into 4 soup bowls and garnish with parsley.

*Notes:* Fresh shelling beans (or cranberry beans) must be removed from their large beige and red pods before cooking. The beans inside are pearl colored with red streaks and have a subtle nutty flavor. They are available fresh during the summer months and dried all year long. To cook fresh shelling beans, cover them with water, bring to a boil, reduce the heat, and simmer until tender, about 20 minutes. To cook dry shelling beans, soak the dried beans for 4 hours, changing the water 2 to 3 times. Drain, place in a saucepan, and cover with fresh water. Simmer for 1 hour or until tender.

Fresh fava beans, frozen lima beans or canned chickpeas (rinsed and drained) can be substituted for shelling beans (add during the last 5 minutes of cooking to prevent overcooking). Frozen peas may be added during the last 2 to 3 minutes of cooking.

Other fruit and vegetable additions could include diced roasted red peppers, chopped tomatoes, sautéed or roasted mushrooms, or even peeled and diced apples or pears.

Smoking (optional step): Preheat the grill and soak non-chemically-treated wood chips, preferably oak or apple. Spread the lentils and cooking liquid on a heavy baking sheet at least 2 inches deep. Add the wood chips to the coals, put the uncovered baking sheet on the grill, and cover the grill with its lid. Smoke for about 15 minutes, then remove the lentils from the grill and transfer to a bowl; refrigerate overnight. (The flavors will intensify and blend. However, the result is just as delicious if you cook the lentils in a saucepan.)

---

- Each serving provides 100% of the DV for vitamin A and more than 20% for vitamin C.
- Beans, particularly lentils, are very good sources of folate—more than 80% of the DV for folate is provided per serving.
- Lentils are a potentially good source of selenium.
- High in fiber—35% of the DV per serving.

**Per serving:**

| calories | protein | carbohydrates | fat | cholesterol | dietary fiber | saturated fat |
|----------|---------|---------------|-----|-------------|---------------|---------------|
| 320 | 19 Gm | 41 Gm | 9 Gm | 0 mg | 9 Gm | 2 Gm |

**% of Calories**: 51% carbohydrate, 24% protein, 25% fat

### Major Sources of Potential Cancer Fighters
**Phytochemicals**: allium compounds, glucosinolates, phytic acids, plant polyphenols (flavonoids, isoflavones), plant sterols, protease inhibitors, terpenes (carotenoids, monoterpenes)

# ✤ *Indian Spiced Vegetable Stew* ✤

## 4 SERVINGS

• *To make this into a protein-rich "one-pot meal" try adding chicken breast (cut into 2-inch-long strips and add during the last 10 minutes of cooking) or firm tofu cut into cubes (add 2 to 3 minutes before serving).*

• *A nice vegetable side served with grilled or seared fish, such as tuna, swordfish, salmon, or snapper.*

• *If you do not like Indian seasonings, omit them and use fresh herbs, such as thyme or basil.*

2 teaspoons olive oil

1 medium red onion (about 5 ounces), peeled and sliced

4 small carrots (about 7 ounces), peeled and sliced 1/4 inch thick

1/2 small jalapeño pepper, seeded and diced

1 garlic clove, peeled and crushed

1/4 teaspoon cumin seeds

1 teaspoon curry powder

1 teaspoon turmeric

1 medium head cauliflower, washed, core removed, and broken into medium-size florets or 18 ounces frozen cauliflower florets, thawed and drained

2 medium white potatoes (about 11 ounces; preferably Yukon Gold), peeled and cut into 1 1/2-inch cubes

1 medium sweet potato (about 6 ounces), peeled and cut into 1 1/2-inch cubes

14 1/2 ounces canned stewed tomatoes salt

1 cup canned chickpeas, drained

1 cup frozen peas

Heat the olive oil in a heavy 4-quart saucepan (preferably nonstick). Add the onion, carrots, jalapeño, and garlic. Sauté over medium-high heat until the onion slices are limp, about 10 minutes. Add the cumin and spices, stirring for about 1 minute to combine and release their flavors. Add the cauliflower, white and sweet potatoes, stewed tomatoes, and 3/4 cup water. Season with salt and stir to combine all ingredients. Bring to a boil, then reduce the heat and simmer for 20 minutes, covered, until all the vegetables are tender but firm. Add the chickpeas and peas 2 to 3 minutes before serving and adjust the seasoning with salt if necessary.

- One serving provides more than 100% of the DVs for vitamins C and A.
- Cauliflower belongs to the cruciferous family of vegetables and has protective phytochemicals.
- Curry and turmeric contain curcumin, a plant polyphenol that may provide many protective benefits.
- High in fiber—40% of the DV per serving.

**Per serving:**

| calories | protein | carbohydrates | fat | cholesterol | dietary fiber | saturated fat |
|----------|---------|---------------|-----|-------------|---------------|---------------|
| 262 | 10 Gm | 47 Gm | 4 Gm | 0 mg | 10 Gm | 0 Gm |

**% of Calories**: 72% carbohydrate, 15% protein, 13% fat

### Major Sources of Potential Cancer Fighters
**Phytochemicals**: allium compounds, capsaicin, glucosinolates, indoles, plant polyphenols (flavonoids, phenolic acids), plant sterols terpenes (carotenoids, monoterpenes)

# ❧ Shiitake Vegetable Chili ❧

## 6 SERVINGS

- *Serve as a main course with corn bread or over polenta, rice, or a baked potato, or as a side dish (recipe yields 8 appetizer servings).*
- *To increase both the protein and phytochemical content of this recipe, add 1 pound of firm "lite" tofu cut into medium cubes. Lean ground chicken or turkey breast or textured soy protein (see page 45) can also be used to boost protein (sauté the chicken or turkey before the vegetables).*
- *This recipe freezes well. Double or triple the recipe, transfer to small containers, and freeze for a convenient and healthy meal on a busy day.*

2 tablespoons olive oil

2 cups shiitake mushrooms (about 4 ounces), brushed clean and sliced into long strips

salt and pepper

1 large red onion (about 9 ounces), peeled and sliced

1 medium jalapeño pepper, seeded and diced

2 garlic cloves, peeled and minced

1 large red bell pepper (about 10 ounces), seeded and chopped

1 large green bell pepper (about 9 ounces), seeded and chopped

2 small zucchini squash (about 10 ounces), cut into 1/2-inch-thick slices

1 small eggplant (about 12 ounces), peeled and cut into 1/2-inch cubes

28 ounces canned plum tomatoes

4 fresh plum tomatoes (about 10 ounces), seeded and chopped

1 tablespoon tomato paste

1 teaspoon ground cumin

2 tablespoons chili powder

2 cups cooked black beans or canned black beans, drained and rinsed

1 1/2 cups fresh or frozen corn kernels

1/2 bunch fresh cilantro, washed and chopped or 1 bunch Italian parsley

Heat 1 tablespoon of olive oil in a large nonstick skillet. Add the mushrooms and sauté over high heat until brown on one side, then toss, season with salt and pepper, and continue cooking over high heat for 2 to 3 minutes more. Set aside in a bowl.

Heat the remaining oil in a 5-quart saucepan and add the onion, jalapeño, garlic, and red and green peppers. Sauté over high heat, stirring frequently for 5 minutes, then reduce the heat and cook for 10 minutes more without browning, until the vegetables become soft. Stir in the zucchini and eggplant, and continue to cook for 5 minutes over medium-high heat, allowing the vegetables to release their water.

Add the tomatoes, tomato paste, and spices, stirring well to combine. Bring to a boil, then reduce the heat and simmer for 40 to 45 minutes; all the vegetables should be very tender. Five minutes before serving, add the black beans, corn, and cilantro, and season to taste with salt.

---

- One serving provides more than 130% of the DV for vitamin C, 35% of the DV for folate, and 30% of the DV for vitamin A.
- Mushrooms not only add an earthy taste and meaty texture to this chili, but also are a potentially good source of selenium as well as other minerals.
- High in fiber—more than 45% of the DV per serving.

**Per serving (based on yield of 6 servings):**

| calories | protein | carbohydrates | fat | cholesterol | dietary fiber | saturated fat |
|---|---|---|---|---|---|---|
| 253 | 10 Gm | 41 Gm | 6 Gm | 0 mg | 12 Gm | 1 Gm |

**% of Calories**: 65% carbohydrate, 15% protein, 20% fat

**Major Sources of Potential Cancer Fighters**
**Phytochemicals**: capsaicin, phytic acids, plant polyphenols (flavonoids, phenolic acids), plant sterols, protease inhibitors, terpenes (carotenoids, monoterpenes, triterpenes)

# ❧ *Herbed Vegetable and Parmesan Frittata* ❧

Maria Helm, PlumpJack Cafe, San Francisco, California

6 SERVINGS

•   *Makes a great vegetarian entrée, menu item for brunch, or first course to a dinner menu.*

4   teaspoons olive oil
1   small red onion (about
      4 ounces), thinly sliced
1   large leek, white part only
      (about 2 ounces), washed
      thoroughly, halved,
      and thinly sliced
3   garlic cloves, peeled and
      thinly sliced
1   large bunch Swiss chard
      (about 1 pound), leaves thinly
      sliced (reserve stems for
      another use)
2   cups shiitake mushrooms
      (about 10 ounces), sliced

1   large red bell pepper (about
      7 ounces), seeded and diced
      pinch red pepper flakes
1   medium zucchini (about 7 ounces),
      halved and thinly sliced
1/2   teaspoon dried rosemary
1/2   teaspoon dried thyme leaves
1/4   cup fresh basil, julienned
      salt and pepper
1   cup unseasoned bread crumbs
2   cups egg whites, nonfat egg
      product, or egg substitute
2   medium beefsteak tomatoes
      (about 12 ounces), sliced
1/4   cup Parmesan cheese, grated

Preheat the oven to 375 degrees F.

In an oven-safe, nonstick skillet, heat 1 teaspoon of olive oil over medium-high heat and sauté the onion, leek, and garlic until tender, about 15 minutes. Reserve in a small bowl.

Meanwhile, blanch the Swiss chard in boiling salted water for 3 minutes. Drain and place in a large bowl filled with ice water until it is completely chilled (this refreshing process helps keep the color a vibrant green). Drain and squeeze out as much water as possible. Reserve in a bowl.

Heat 2 teaspoons of olive oil in a nonstick skillet over high heat until almost smoking and add the mushrooms. After the mushrooms become slightly browned, turn down the heat to medium and add the red bell pepper and red pepper flakes. Continue to sauté for another 2 to 3 minutes, tossing to cook evenly and combine the ingredients. Add the zucchini and cook until all water from the vegetables has evaporated and the vegetables are tender but slightly firm, about 5 minutes. Add the Swiss chard and continue cooking for another minute, then add the leek mixture and herbs. Season with salt and pepper. Mix in 3/4 cup bread crumbs and the egg whites and pat down firmly. Top with the sliced tomatoes.

Combine the remaining 1 teaspoon olive oil, the Parmesan, and the remaining bread crumbs and sprinkle on top of the tomatoes.

Bake for 35 minutes or until the egg whites are set.

---

- Swiss chard is a good source of vitamin C (provides more than 45% of the DV), carotenoids, folate (provides 20% of the DV), and calcium (provides more than 10% of the DV).
- A good source of fiber.

---

**Per serving:**

| calories | protein | carbohydrates | fat | cholesterol | dietary fiber | saturated fat |
|----------|---------|---------------|-----|-------------|---------------|---------------|
| 189 | 12 Gm | 25 Gm | 5 Gm | 1 mg | 3 Gm | 1 Gm |

**% of Calories**: 50% carbohydrate, 25% protein, 25% fat

### Major Sources of Potential Cancer Fighters

**Phytochemicals**: allium compounds, capsaicin, plant polyphenols (flavonoids, phenolic acids), terpenes ( carnosol, carotenoids, monoterpenes)

# ✢ Scrambled Egg Burrito ✢

1 SERVING

- *A quick, nutritious weekday dinner or weekend breakfast. Substitute whatever vegetables you have on hand for those listed below.*

3 egg whites
2 tablespoons skim milk
  salt and pepper
1 teaspoon olive oil
1/2 small red onion (about
    1 1/2 ounces), diced
1/3 cup diced green bell pepper
    (about 2 ounces)
1/3 cup diced red bell pepper
    (about 2 ounces)

2 cups spinach, rinsed
  and stemmed
1 10-inch whole wheat tortilla
1/3 cup cooked black beans
  or canned black beans,
  drained and rinsed
1 1/2 ounces soy jalapeño Monterey
  Jack cheese, shredded
2 tablespoons tomato salsa

Whip the egg whites, skim milk, and salt and pepper in a small bowl. Set aside.

Heat the olive oil in an 8-inch nonstick skillet and sauté the red onion over medium heat for 2 to 3 minutes; add the peppers and continue to cook for another 5 minutes.

Meanwhile, heat a small sauté pan brushed with olive oil. Add the spinach, season with salt and pepper, and cook over medium heat until the leaves just wilt, 1 to 2 minutes. When cool enough to handle, squeeze out any excess water. Reserve.

Heat the tortilla in the microwave or on a heated pan (cast iron works well) until just warmed. Place the tortilla on a large plate.

Add the egg mixture to the sautéed onion and peppers and cook, stirring frequently, to desired firmness. Transfer the eggs to the center of the tortilla and add the spinach, black beans, and shredded soy cheese. Roll up the tortilla, folding in both ends. Garnish with a commercial or homemade tomato salsa.

---

- One serving provides 190% of the DV for vitamin C and more than 85% of the DV for vitamin A.
- Both soybeans and black beans contain isoflavones that may lower the risk of breast and other types of cancer. They are also high in fiber and folate, providing 50% and 85% of the DVs, respectively.

---

*Per serving:*

| calories | protein | carbohydrates | fat | cholesterol | dietary fiber | saturated fat |
|---|---|---|---|---|---|---|
| 389 | 30 Gm | 43 Gm | 11 Gm | 1 mg | 13 Gm | 1 Gm |

**% of Calories**: 44% carbohydrate, 30% protein, 26% fat

### Major Sources of Potential Cancer Fighters

**Phytochemicals**: allium compounds, phytic acids, plant polyphenols (flavonoids, isoflavones, phenolic acids), plant sterols protease inhibitors, terpenes (carotenoids, monoterpenes, triterpenes)

# ⚘ Mexican Lasagne ⚘

## 6 SERVINGS

• *This tortilla lasagne is loaded with flavor and nutrients. Vegetables can be added or substituted using leftovers or trimmings that you have on hand.*

• *If you think you do not like tofu, try it in a well-seasoned composition like this. If tofu is not for you, chicken strips can be sautéed and seasoned with chili powder.*

• *You can prepare this lasagne 1 to 2 days before serving. Or freeze and then bake to have a healthy meal at your fingertips on a busy day.*

| | |
|---|---|
| 2 teaspoons olive oil | 6 ounces soy Monterey Jack cheese, shredded (about 1½ cups shredded) |
| 1 medium red onion (about 6 ounces), chopped | |
| 1 small jalapeño, seeded and diced | 1½ cups cooked brown rice (see Notes) |
| 1 large sweet red bell pepper (about 9 ounces), seeded and chopped | 16 ounces cooked or canned black beans, drained |
| 1 large green bell pepper (about 8 ounces), seeded and chopped | 16 ounces salsa or picante sauce |
| | 4 ounces fat-free sour cream (see Notes) |
| 1 pound extra-firm "lite" tofu, drained and cubed | 8 8-inch fat-free, whole wheat tortillas or corn tortillas |
| 1 teaspoon chili powder | |

Preheat the oven to 350 degrees F.

Heat the olive oil in a nonstick skillet and sauté the onion for 5 minutes; add the jalapeño and red and green peppers and sauté for 5 minutes more. Remove from the heat and reserve in a medium bowl.

Add the tofu to the skillet and cook for 2 to 3 minutes on high heat. Add the chili powder, stirring gently to combine. Turn up the heat and cook for 2 minutes more to evaporate most of water from the tofu. Remove from the skillet and add to the bowl containing the onion and peppers.

Arrange all ingredients (tofu-pepper mixture, shredded soy cheese, brown rice, black beans, salsa, sour cream, and tortillas) for easy assembly of the lasagne.

Spread a small amount of salsa on the bottom of an 11 by 7 by 2-inch rectangular baking dish. Next, place a single layer of tortillas (each layer will require 2 tortillas, slightly trimmed to fit the rectangular baking dish). Lightly spread the sour cream on top of the tortilla then layer with a quarter of the rice, followed by the tofu-pepper mixture, beans, salsa, and shredded soy cheese. Place down the next tortilla layer and continue layering as above 3 more times, ending with the tortillas and reserving 1/3 cup of shredded cheese.

Cover the baking dish with aluminum foil and bake for 50 minutes. Remove the foil and cover the top tortilla layer evenly with the reserved cheese. Bake for 10 minutes more. Remove from the oven and let cool for 10 minutes before serving.

*Notes:* If you do not have leftover brown rice, start it before cooking the tofu and peppers. Simply measure out 1 cup of long-grain brown rice and add to 2 1/2 cups of boiling water. Stir in 1/3 teaspoon of salt, reduce to a simmer, and cook, covered, for 25 to 30 minutes.

To make this lasagne completely dairy free and even richer in soy, substitute pureed silken tofu or soy sour cream for the fat-free sour cream.

---

- With only 10% of calories from fat, this entrée can help keep you below the goal of 20% of calories from fat in a day.
- Eighteen of the 21 grams of protein per serving are derived from soy and other legume sources.
- Black beans are high in fiber and like soy contain isoflavones and other phytochemicals that may lower the risk of breast and other types of cancer. They are also rich in folate; one serving of Mexican lasagne provides 35% of the DV.
- Each serving provides more than 175% of the DV for vitamin C and more than 10% of the DV for vitamin A.
- Brown rice is a potentially good source of selenium and is a good source of fiber. One slice of lasagne provides more than half of the DV for fiber.

---

***Per serving:***

| calories | protein | carbohydrates | fat | cholesterol | dietary fiber | saturated fat |
|----------|---------|---------------|-----|-------------|---------------|---------------|
| 377 | 28 Gm | 55 Gm | 5 Gm | 0 mg | 15 Gm | 1 Gm |

**% of Calories**: 58% carbohydrate, 30% protein, 12% fat

### Major Sources of Potential Cancer Fighters

**Phytochemicals**: capsaicin, phytic acids, plant polyphenols (flavonoids, isoflavones, phenolic acids), plant sterols, protease inhibitors, terpenes (carotenoids, monoterpenes, triterpenes)

# ❧ *Root Vegetable Lasagne* ❧

## 6 SERVINGS

• *Serve as a colorful, nutritious vegetarian entrée or a vegetable side dish with meat, fish, or poultry.*

• *Soy cheese melts well and tastes great when cooked in casseroles such as this. Unlike its dairy counterpart, the soy Monterey Jack cheese used in this recipe is cholesterol free, very low in total and saturated fat, and contains all of the protective phytochemicals found in soybeans.*

| | | | |
|---|---|---|---|
| 2 | dried ancho chiles (see Notes) | 3 | medium turnips (about 12 ounces), peeled and sliced into 1/8-inch-thick slices |
| 1 1/2 | cups vegetable stock (page 146) or low-sodium canned broth | | |
| 1/2 | teaspoon olive oil | | salt |
| 2 | large baking potatoes (about 1 pound), peeled and sliced lengthwise into 1/8-inch-thick slices | 2 | medium sweet red bell peppers (about 12 ounces), seeded and diced |
| 2 | medium sweet potatoes (about 14 ounces), peeled and sliced lengthwise into 1/8-inch-thick slices | 8 | ounces soy Monterey Jack cheese (not fat-free), shredded (see Notes) |
| 2 | medium parsnips (about 8 ounces), peeled and sliced lengthwise into 1/8-inch-thick slices | | |

Preheat the oven to 375 degrees F.

In a small saucepan, simmer the ancho chiles in the vegetable broth for 10 minutes. Turn off the heat and let steep while preparing the lasagne.

Rub an 11 by 7 by 3-inch rectangular baking pan with olive oil. Arrange the root vegetable slices, starting with a layer of slightly overlapping potatoes, followed by sweet potato, parsnip, and turnips; repeat the sequence. Season each layer with salt and sprinkle with diced red pepper and shredded cheese; reserve about 1/3 cup of shredded cheese. Layer the vegetables slightly above the rim of the baking dish because they will shrink down when cooked.

Strain the broth and pour evenly over the casserole. Cover with foil wrap and bake for 50 minutes. Remove the foil, sprinkle with the remaining cheese, and bake for 15 more minutes. Let cool for 15 minutes before serving.

*Notes:* Ancho chiles are dried poblano peppers available at some supermarkets and most gourmet specialty stores. When soaked or steeped, they lend a rich smoky flavor to sauces and broths without too much heat.

Soy cheeses are available at some supermarkets and most natural food stores.

Use a mandoline to slice vegetables quickly and easily. Made of stainless steel or plastic, they are usually sold with a variety of blades for thin slicing, julienning, and french-fry cutting. Inexpensive, good-quality plastic mandolines are available at most culinary stores.

---

- One serving provides more than 100% of the DV for vitamin C and vitamin A, and 20% of the DV for calcium.
- Turnips belong to the cruciferous family of vegetables and have protective phytochemicals.
- Moderate consumption of capsaicin, a phytochemical found in chile peppers, may help the body neutralize carcinogens.
- High in fiber—20% of the DV.

---

**Per serving:**

| calories | protein | carbohydrates | fat | cholesterol | dietary fiber | saturated fat |
|---|---|---|---|---|---|---|
| 285 | 13 Gm | 41 Gm | 8 Gm | 0 mg | 5 Gm | 1 Gm |

% of Calories: 57% carbohydrate, 18% protein, 25% fat

### Major Sources of Potential Cancer Fighters

**Phytochemicals:** capsaicin, glucosinolates, phytic acids, plant polyphenols (flavonoids, isoflavones, phenolic acids), plant sterols, terpenes (carotenoids, triterpenes)

# FISH

## ✧ *Tuna with Provençal Crust* ✧ *and Baby Greens with Red Wine Vinaigrette*

Susan Weaver, Fifty Seven, Four Seasons Hotel, New York, New York

### 4 SERVINGS

- *The ingredients of Provence not only taste good but also contain cancer-fighting nutrients and phytochemicals.*
- *Tuna with Provençal Crust can be served with almost any salad, such as a simple tomato salad with grilled or toasted bread, a Niçoise salad, or Francesco Antonucci's Venetian Pepperonata, page 126, served at room temperature.*
- *Garlic Mashed Potatoes, page 258, or Rosemary Roasted Potatoes, page 221, also marry well with the flavors of this dish.*

### *Tuna*

| | | | |
|---|---|---|---|
| 2 | cups fresh bread crumbs, finely ground (about 10 slices white bread, crusts removed; see Note) | 2 | tablespoons finely chopped basil, tarragon, oregano, and parsley |
| 2 | tablespoons finely chopped drained capers | 4 | 6-ounce portions ahi tuna (see Notes) |
| 2 | tablespoons finely chopped anchovies | 1 | cup flour seasoned with salt and freshly ground pepper |
| 1 | tablespoon finely chopped garlic | 2 | eggs, slightly beaten |
| | | 1 | tablespoon olive oil |

### *Vinaigrette*

#### MAKES 1¹/₂ CUPS (1 SERVING = 1 TABLESPOON)

| | | | |
|---|---|---|---|
| ¹/₃ | cup red wine vinegar | | salt and freshly ground pepper |
| 2 | tablespoons finely chopped shallots | 1 | cup extra virgin olive oil |
| 2 | teaspoons finely chopped garlic | | |
| 2 | tablespoons finely chopped basil, tarragon, oregano, and parsley | 4 | cups baby greens or mesclun |

Preheat the oven to 350 degrees.

To make the tuna, combine the bread crumbs, capers, anchovies, garlic, and herbs. Roll each portion of tuna in the flour, shake off any excess, and coat with the egg. Drain off any excess egg and evenly cover with the bread crumb mixture; gently shake off any excess.

Heat the olive oil in a large, oven-safe, nonstick skillet. When almost smoking, place the tuna in the skillet, shake the pan gently, and sauté over medium-high to high heat until a light brown crust forms on one side, about 2 minutes, then turn over and transfer to the oven. Cook until medium-rare, about 3 minutes.

To make the red wine vinaigrette, in a medium bowl, combine the vinegar, shallots, garlic, and herbs and season with salt and pepper. Whisk in the olive oil and adjust the seasoning, if necessary.

Just before serving, toss the baby greens with 4 tablespoons of vinaigrette.

With a sharp knife, slice each tuna steak in 3 slices on the bias. Pile the dressed baby greens in a neat mound at the top of the plate. Fan the tuna slices in front of the greens.

*Notes:* Ahi is the Hawaiian name for yellowfin or bigeye tuna. This type of tuna is available at many supermarkets or fish markets. To help assure freshness, select pieces with firm, red flesh without a distinct odor.

You can substitute commercial unseasoned bread crumbs for the fresh, but grind them in a food processor if they are coarse.

---

- The fat sources in this recipe are predominantly monounsaturated (more than 50%), including potentially protective omega-3 fatty acids.
- Tuna is a potentially good source of selenium.
- Rich in vitamins A, C, and folate, providing more than 20% of the DV for each.
- A good source of fiber.

---

**Per serving of Tuna with Provençal Crust:**

| calories | protein | carbohydrates | fat | cholesterol | dietary fiber | saturated fat |
|----------|---------|---------------|------|-------------|---------------|---------------|
| 418 | 49 Gm | 34 Gm | 9 Gm | 160 mg | 2 Gm | 1 Gm |

**Per 1-tablespoon serving of Red Wine Vinaigrette:**

| calories | protein | carbohydrates | fat | cholesterol | dietary fiber | saturated fat |
|----------|---------|---------------|------|-------------|---------------|---------------|
| 80 | 0 Gm | 0 Gm | 9 Gm | 0 mg | 0 Gm | 1 Gm |

**Per serving of Tuna with Provençal Crust and Baby Greens with Red Wine Vinaigrette:**

| calories | protein | carbohydrates | fat | cholesterol | dietary fiber | saturated fat |
|----------|---------|---------------|------|-------------|---------------|---------------|
| 507 | 50 Gm | 36 Gm | 18 Gm | 160 mg | 3 Gm | 3 Gm |

**% of Calories**: 28% carbohydrate, 29% protein, 33% fat

**Major Sources of Potential Cancer Fighters**
**Phytochemicals**: allium compounds, plant polyphenols (flavonoids, phenolic acids), terpenes (carotenoids, monoterpenes)

# ❧ Herb and Spice Crusted ❧ Mahimahi with Watermelon Salsa

Erasmo "Razz" Kamnitzer, Razz's Restaurant and Bar, Scottsdale, Arizona

4 SERVINGS

• *Use this herb and spice mixture to crust other fish, such as swordfish, tuna, halibut, or wild bass.*

• *Serve the watermelon salsa as a topping for grilled, seared, or roasted salmon, tuna, or swordfish (try it over Coriander, Fennel, and Pepper Crusted Tuna page 217). It also marries well with spicy chicken.*

## Watermelon Salsa

| | | | |
|---|---|---|---|
| 2 | cups watermelon, peeled, seeded, and diced | 1/2 | cup diced sweet yellow pepper |
| 1 | tablespoon sliced onion | 1 | teaspoon chopped garlic |
| 1 | tablespoon diced poblano pepper or 1 teaspoon diced jalapeño pepper | 3 | tablespoons chopped cilantro juice of 2 limes plus |
| | | 1 | teaspoon grated zest salt and pepper |

## Herb and Spice Crusted Mahimahi

| | | | |
|---|---|---|---|
| 1 | tablespoon *each* fresh chopped herbs: basil, tarragon, marjoram, thyme, rosemary, parsley | 1 | tablespoon maple sugar (optional) |
| | | 1/2 | teaspoon cayenne |
| | | 1/2 | teaspoon salt |
| 1 | tablespoon *each* cracked black pepper, ground cumin, curry powder, ground coriander seeds | 1 1/2 | pounds mahimahi (4- to 6-ounce steaks) |
| | | 3 | teaspoons olive oil |

To prepare the salsa, in a mixing bowl, combine all ingredients and season with salt and pepper.

To prepare the herb and spice mixture, combine the herbs and spices and spread them out on a large plate. Place one side of the mahimahi steaks into the herb-spice blend, lift it up, and shake off any excess.

Heat 1½ teaspoons of olive oil in a 10-inch nonstick skillet until almost smoking. Carefully place 2 of the mahimahi steaks, herb and spice–coated side down, into the skillet. A crust should form within 1 minute. Using kitchen tongs, turn over the fish, lower the heat, and continue to cook for 3 to 4 minutes more, until the flesh is firm when touched. Repeat the process with the remaining mahimahi steaks.

---

- Curry powder contains curcumin, a plant polyphenol that lends yellow color and acts as an antioxidant; it may also play a role in blocking cancer at the initiation stage.
- Though watermelon is not often thought of as a nutrient-rich fruit, its red color is provided by the carotenoid lycopene. It is also a good source of vitamin C and potassium.

---

*Per serving of Watermelon Salsa (¹/₃ cup):*

| calories | protein | carbohydrates | fat | cholesterol | dietary fiber | saturated fat |
|---|---|---|---|---|---|---|
| 38 | 1 Gm | 7 Gm | 1 Gm | 0 mg | 1 Gm | 0 Gm |

*Per serving of Herb and Spice Crusted Mahimahi:*

| calories | protein | carbohydrates | fat | cholesterol | dietary fiber | saturated fat |
|---|---|---|---|---|---|---|
| 297 | 38 Gm | 8 Gm | 12 Gm | 86 mg | 1 Gm | 2 Gm |

*Per serving of Herb and Spice Crusted Mahimahi with Watermelon Salsa.*

| calories | protein | carbohydrates | fat | cholesterol | dietary fiber | saturated fat |
|---|---|---|---|---|---|---|
| 335 | 39 Gm | 15 Gm | 13 Gm | 86 mg | 2 Gm | 2 Gm |

**% of Calories**: 20% carbohydrate, 47% protein, 33% fat

### Major Sources of Potential Cancer Fighters

**Phytochemicals**: allium compounds, capsaicin, plant polyphenols (flavonoids), terpenes (carotenoids, monoterpenes, limonenes, triterpenes)

# ❧ *Tandoori Sea Bass with Minted* ❧ *Couscous, Banana Salsa, and* *Fresh Coconut-Mango Chutney*

Adam Busby, Director of Culinary Programs, Dubrulle Culinary School,
Vancouver, British Columbia, Canada

### 4 SERVINGS

•   *This dish has great contrasts: hot and cold temperatures and sweet and savory flavors. All components are easy to prepare and are very versatile.*

•   *The Banana Salsa and Coconut-Mango Chutney also marry well with other well-spiced fish, such as snapper, tuna, or swordfish. Try it with Coriander, Fennel, and Pepper Crusted Tuna, page 217.*

•   *The Minted Couscous is the perfect bed for braised or stewed meat or vegetables. Try it with Indian Spiced Vegetable Stew, page 198, or Curry Roasted Summer Vegetables, page 191.*

## Sea Bass

| | | | |
|---|---|---|---|
| 1 | garlic clove, minced | 3/4 | cup low-fat or fat-free sour cream |
| 1 | shallot, coarsely chopped | 1 1/2 | pounds sea bass, cut into |
| 1/2 | bunch cilantro, chopped | | 4 medallions |
| 1/2-inch gingerroot, | | 2 | teaspoons butter, cut into |
| | peeled and minced | | small pieces |
| 2 | teaspoons ground cumin | | salt and freshly ground pepper |
| 2 | tablespoons paprika | | |

## Banana Salsa

| | | | |
|---|---|---|---|
| 1 | large banana (about 4 ounces), | 1/2 | shallot, finely chopped |
| | peeled and cut into fine dice | 1 | tablespoon chopped cilantro |
| 1 | tablespoon lime juice | | salt and freshly ground black |
| | | | pepper |

## Couscous

| | | | |
|---|---|---|---|
| 1 | cup couscous | | salt |
| 2 | cups boiling chicken stock, | 1/3 | cup chopped mint |
| | vegetable stock, or water | 1 | teaspoon butter |

## Coconut-Mango Chutney

¹/₂  cup shredded coconut                    4  tablespoons mango chutney

To prepare the marinade, in a food processor, puree the garlic, shallot, cilantro, ginger, cumin, and paprika. Transfer to a mixing bowl and mix with the sour cream. Place the sea bass medallions into this marinade, cover, and refrigerate for at least 2 hours (preferably overnight).

To prepare the banana salsa, in a mixing bowl, combine all ingredients being careful not to mash the banana. Cover and refrigerate until ready to use.

To prepare the coconut-mango chutney, toss the coconut and mango chutney together in a small mixing bowl. Cover and refrigerate.

To cook the sea bass, preheat the oven to 400 degrees F. Wipe excess marinade off the sea bass, leaving an even thin coating on the top and sides. Place the medallions on a nonstick baking sheet. Dot with pieces of butter and season with salt and pepper. Bake until a little golden crust forms and the fish is just cooked, 10 to 12 minutes.

To prepare the couscous, in a medium saucepan, add the couscous to the boiling stock. Stir and then simmer for about 2 minutes. Season with salt and add mint and butter. Let sit, covered, for 5 minutes. Fluff with a fork.

Put a portion of couscous into the center of each plate. Place a sea bass medallion on top and spoon the coconut-mango chutney and banana salsa over the fish.

---

- Sea bass is a potentially very good source of selenium and protective omega-3 fatty acids.
- Mint contains monoterpenes that act as antioxidants and blocking agents to interfere with carcinogens.
- Each serving provides more than a third of the DV for vitamin A.
- A good source of fiber.

---

*Per serving of Banana Salsa (¹/₄ cup):*

| calories | protein | carbohydrates | fat | cholesterol | dietary fiber | saturated fat |
|---|---|---|---|---|---|---|
| 28 | 0 Gm | 7 Gm | 0 Gm | 0 mg | 1 Gm | 0 Gm |

*Per serving of Couscous (³/₄ cup):*

| calories | protein | carbohydrates | fat | cholesterol | dietary fiber | saturated fat |
|---|---|---|---|---|---|---|
| 185 | 6 Gm | 36 Gm | 1 Gm | 3 mg | 2 Gm | 1 Gm |

*Per serving of Coconut-Mango Chutney (2 tablespoons):*

| calories | protein | carbohydrates | fat | cholesterol | dietary fiber | saturated fat |
|---|---|---|---|---|---|---|
| 75 | 0 Gm | 11 Gm | 3 Gm | 3 mg | 1 Gm | 3 Gm |

*Per serving of Tandoori Sea Bass with Minted Couscous, Banana Salsa, and Fresh Coconut-Mango Chutney:*

| calories | protein | carbohydrates | fat | cholesterol | dietary fiber | saturated fat |
|----------|---------|---------------|-----|-------------|---------------|---------------|
| 515 | 40 Gm | 63 Gm | 11 Gm | 78 mg | 4 Gm | 6 Gm |

**% of Calories**: 50% carbohydrate, 31% protein, 19% fat

### Major Sources of Potential Cancer Fighters

**Phytochemicals**: allium compounds, plant polyphenols (flavonoids, phenolic acids), terpenes (carotenoids, monoterpenes, triterpenes, gingerol)

# ❧ Shrimp with Garlic and Capers ❧

### 4 SERVINGS

- *Serve as a first course along with some crusty bread or as a main course over rice.*

| | | | |
|---|---|---|---|
| 1½ | pounds large shrimp, peeled and deveined | 2 | tablespoons chopped parsley |
| | salt and pepper | 2 | tablespoons fresh squeezed lemon juice |
| 3 | teaspoons olive oil | | |
| 1 | tablespoon minced garlic | 2 | tablespoons drained capers |
| ¼ | cup dry white wine | 2 | teaspoons butter |

Season the shrimp with salt and pepper.

Heat 2 teaspoons of olive oil in a large nonstick skillet. When almost smoking, add the shrimp and cook at high heat until nicely browned and just cooked, about 2 minutes per side. Transfer the shrimp to 4 plates and cover to keep warm.

Add the remaining 1 teaspoon of olive oil and the garlic to the skillet and cook over medium-high heat while stirring. After about 1 minute, when the garlic is lightly browned, add the white wine and parsley. Using a wooden spoon, stir to dissolve caramelized particles on the bottom of the pan. Simmer for less than 1 minute and add the lemon juice, capers, and 1 tablespoon water to the pan. Cook for another minute, whisk in the butter, and pour over the shrimp. Serve immediately.

- With less than 2 grams of fat per 5-ounce serving, shrimp is a very lean protein source. It can quickly become a high-fat dish, however, if cooked in butter- or cream-based sauces or if served with high-fat condiments. For recipes that include shrimp and other low-fat shellfish, such as scallops, crab, or lobster, try sautéing in a nonstick pan heated with a minimal amount of olive or canola oil or cooking in a flavorful liquid medium, such as in soups, stews, risotto, and paellas.
- Shrimp is a potentially good source of selenium.

*Per serving:*

| calories | protein | carbohydrates | fat | cholesterol | dietary fiber | saturated fat |
|---|---|---|---|---|---|---|
| 228 | 34 Gm | 3 Gm | 7 Gm | 260 mg | 0 Gm | 2 Gm |

**% of Calories**: 5% carbohydrate, 63% protein, 40% fat, 2% alcohol

**Major Sources of Potential Cancer Fighters**

**Phytochemicals**: allium compounds, plant polyphenols (flavonoids), terpenes (monoterpenes)

# ❧ Chimayo Chile Crusted Ahi ❧ Tuna with Soba Noodle–Cucumber Salad and Cilantro-Honey Vinaigrette

Ming Tsai, Santacafé, Santa Fe, New Mexico

4 SERVINGS

- *This Asian-Southwestern salad is a terrific light meal or first course. It characterizes the type of modern fusion cuisine created by Ming Tsai.*
- *The Soba Noodle–Cucumber Salad with Cilantro-Honey Vinaigrette can be served alone as a vegetarian course.*

## Chile Oil

MAKES 1 CUP (1 SERVING = ½ TABLESPOON)

2 tablespoons chili powder
1 teaspoon ground cumin

1 cup canola oil

## Tuna

<sup></sup>

| | |
|---|---|
| 1/3 cup chili powder (preferably chimayo or ancho) | 12 ounces center-cut ahi tuna loin (must be block shaped) |
| 1/3 cup freshly ground cumin seeds | salt |
| 1/3 cup freshly ground fennel seeds | 1 teaspoon canola oil |

## Cilantro-Honey Vinaigrette

MAKES 3/4 CUP (1 SERVING = 1/2 TABLESPOON)

| | |
|---|---|
| 2 small serrano chiles, seeded and minced | 1 tablespoon Dijon mustard |
| 1 1/2 tablespoons honey | 1/4 cup ice water |
| 1/2 cup cilantro leaves | 3/4 cup canola oil |
| | salt and pepper |

## Soba Noodle–Cucumber Salad

| | |
|---|---|
| 8 ounces dried soba noodles | salt and pepper |
| 1 seedless cucumber, peeled and julienned | 1 cup daikon sprouts (optional) |
| 2 scallions, green part only, thinly sliced | |

To prepare the chile oil, heat the chili powder and cumin together in a sauté pan until barely smoking. Whisk in the oil. Carefully transfer to a glass jar and let stand overnight for proper separation.

To prepare the ahi tuna, grind the spices in a spice grinder or small food processor. Spread the spice mixture out evenly on a large flat plate. Season the tuna with salt and roll in the spice mixture. Heat the oil in a nonstick skillet; when almost smoking, add the tuna and sear for 10 seconds on each side. (It is best to keep high-quality tuna very rare, but if you prefer it more cooked, you can place the skillet with the seared tuna in an oven preheated to 400 degrees F for 2 to 5 minutes depending on desired doneness. Refrigerate for easy slicing.

To prepare the vinaigrette, in a blender or food processor, combine the serrano chiles, honey, cilantro, mustard, and ice water and puree until smooth. With the motor running, slowly drizzle in the oil. Season to taste with salt and pepper. Store excess vinaigrette in a sealed container in the refrigerator for up to 1 week.

To cook the soba noodles, bring 5 quarts of salted water to a boil. Cook the noodles according to package instructions, drain, rinse thoroughly under cold water, and drain again.

Toss the soba noodles, cucumber, and scallions with 1/4 cup of the vinaigrette. Adjust seasoning with salt and pepper, if necessary. Place a mound of salad in the center of

4 plates. Surround with thin slices of the tuna. Drizzle with 2 tablespoons of vinaigrette and the chile oil. Garnish with daikon sprouts, if desired.

---

- The types of fatty acids in this recipe are predominantly cancer-protective monounsaturated fatty acids and linolenic fatty acids. Use a little less vinaigrette and/or chile oil if you wish to further reduce fat.
- Chiles contain capsaicin, which may help to neutralize carcinogens.

---

**Per serving of seared Ahi Tuna with Chile Oil:**

| calories | protein | carbohydrates | fat | cholesterol | dietary fiber | saturated fat |
|---|---|---|---|---|---|---|
| 164 | 19 Gm | 0 Gm | 9 Gm | 38 mg | 0 Gm | 1 Gm |

**Per serving of Soba Noodle–Cucumber Salad with Cilantro-Honey Vinaigrette:**

| calories | protein | carbohydrates | fat | cholesterol | dietary fiber | saturated fat |
|---|---|---|---|---|---|---|
| 183 | 7 Gm | 28 Gm | 6 Gm | 0 mg | 1 Gm | 1 Gm |

**Per serving of Chimayo Chile Crusted Ahi Tuna with Soba Noodle–Cucumber Salad and Cilantro-Honey Vinaigrette:**

| calories | protein | carbohydrates | fat | cholesterol | dietary fiber | saturated fat |
|---|---|---|---|---|---|---|
| 347 | 26 Gm | 28 Gm | 15 Gm | 38 mg | 1 Gm | 2 Gm |

**% of Calories**: 32% carbohydrate, 30% protein, 38% fat

**Major Sources of Potential Cancer Fighters**

**Phytochemicals**: allium compounds, capsaicin, plant polyphenols (flavonoids, phenolic acids)

# ✧ Coriander, Fennel, and ✧ Pepper Crusted Tuna

## 4 SERVINGS

- *The spice blend lends this recipe some heat. A nice cool fruit salsa such as Razz Kamnitzer's Watermelon Salsa, page 210, helps put out the fire and balance the flavor.*
- *With a salad and Minted Couscous, page 212, preparation time is less than 30 minutes—a quick weekday meal.*
- *Double or triple the amount of spice blend and store in a sealed container.*

## Spice Blend

1    tablespoon coriander seeds    2    teaspoons black peppercorns
1    tablespoon fennel seeds

## Tuna

24    ounces tuna (4 pieces    salt
      1½ inches thick)    2    teaspoons olive oil

To prepare the spice blend, grind all spices in a mini food processor or spice grinder until they are powdery. Spread the spice mixture evenly on a large plate.

Rinse the tuna fillets and pat dry. Place one side of each piece of tuna into the spice mixture. Shake off any excess.

In a 10-inch nonstick skillet, heat 1 teaspoon of olive oil over high heat until almost smoking. Carefully place two of the tuna fillets, spiced side down, into the skillet. A spice crust should form within 1 minute. Using kitchen tongs, turn over the tuna, lower the heat to medium, and cook for 2 to 5 minutes to desired doneness. Repeat the process with the remaining tuna fillets.

---

Tuna is a potentially good source of omega-3 fatty acids.

---

**Per serving:**

| calories | protein | carbohydrates | fat | cholesterol | dietary fiber | saturated fat |
|----------|---------|---------------|-----|-------------|---------------|---------------|
| 198 | 40 Gm | 0 Gm | 4 Gm | 74 mg | 0 Gm | 1 Gm |

**% of Calories**: 1% carbohydrate, 81% protein, 18% fat

**Major Sources of Potential Cancer Fighters**

**Phytochemicals**: omega-3 fatty acids

# ✧ *Fillet of John Dory* ✧ in Lettuce and Fennel Broth

Cesare Casella, Il Cantinori, New York, New York

6 SERVINGS

- *Other lean whitefish, such as sole, flounder, cod, or halibut, can be substituted for John Dory. The more firm and thick the fish fillet, the longer the poaching time.*
- *The addition of cooked beans, such as chickpeas or white beans, during the poaching of the fillets adds texture and increases the fiber and phytochemical content of this recipe.*

| | |
|---|---|
| 2 heads Boston lettuce (about 7 ounces) | 1 medium lemon |
| | 4 quarts cold water |
| 2 medium carrots (about 4 ounces) | salt |
| 2 small red onions (about 5 ounces) | 2½ pounds San Pietro |
| 2 celery stalks (about 4 ounces) | (John Dory) fillets, cleaned |
| 1 large fennel bulb (about 1 pound), halved; reserve feathery leaves for garnish | freshly ground pepper |
| | 10 to 15 fresh basil leaves |
| | pinch red pepper flakes |

To prepare the broth, using a chef's knife, shred the lettuce into long thin strips and add to a large saucepan. Put 1 carrot, 1 onion cut into 2 halves, 1 celery stalk, and half of the fennel bulb in a large saucepan, cover with water, and season with salt. Bring to a rolling boil, then reduce the heat so that the mixture remains at a low boil for 1 hour. Drain the liquid into a large bowl and discard the vegetables.

Trim the remaining vegetables. Peel the carrot and run a fork or vegetable channeler down the lengthwise side at even increments (this will give it an attractive flower shape when sliced). Set the blade of a mandoline on its smallest setting (for very thin slices), and slice the carrot, lemon, fennel, celery, and onion crosswise.

Combine the vegetables in a sauté pan that is large enough to hold the fish fillets in a single layer. Toss to evenly distribute, and season with salt and pepper. Add 4 cups of the fennel-lettuce broth and bring to a boil. Reduce the heat and simmer for 10 minutes.

Place the fish fillets over the vegetables, season with salt and pepper, and sprinkle with the basil leaves and red pepper flakes. Cook over moderate heat, covered, for approximately 3 minutes (time will depend on the thickness of the fillets).

Using a large slotted spatula, carefully transfer the fish to a wide bowl. Adjust the seasoning of the broth, then spoon the vegetables and broth over the top of the fish. Garnish with the reserved fennel leaves.

*Note*: Cesare provides a tomato salsa recipe as an alternate garnish:

| | | | |
|---|---|---|---|
| 3 | tomatoes, seeded, peeled, and chopped | 1 | small jalapeño pepper (or peperoncini), diced |
| 1/4 | cup extra virgin olive oil | | salt and pepper |
| 2 | tablespoons white wine vinegar | | |

In a medium bowl, combine all ingredients.

---

- One serving provides 50% of the DV for vitamin A.
- With more than 40 grams of protein and less than 5 grams of fat, this recipe makes an excellent lean protein choice.

---

**Per serving:**

| calories | protein | carbohydrates | fat | cholesterol | dietary fiber | saturated fat |
|---|---|---|---|---|---|---|
| 233 | 40 Gm | 7 Gm | 4 Gm | 60 mg | 2 Gm | 1 Gm |

**% of Calories**: 12% carbohydrate, 71% protein, 17% fat

**Major Sources of Potential Cancer Fighters**

**Phytochemicals**: allium compounds, capsaicin, plant polyphenols (flavonoids, phenolic acids), terpenes (carotenoids, monoterpenes, triterpenes)

---

# ⩔ *Slow-roasted Salmon* ⩔
# *with a Warm Salad of Arugula, Rosemary Roasted Potatoes, Shiitake Mushrooms, and Balsamic Essence*

Michael Otsuka, Chasen's, Beverly Hills, California

4 SERVINGS

- *Slow-roasting the salmon is easy and it concentrates the flavor and retains the moisture. Serve the salmon with this salad or on its own.*
- *Prepare the Rosemary Roasted Potatoes (with or without the mushrooms) to accompany other entrées, such as roasted or grilled chicken, fish, or game.*

## Rosemary Roasted Potatoes

1½  pounds red skin potatoes,
    scrubbed and halved or quartered
    if they are medium size
3 to 4  fresh rosemary sprigs
    left on stem
4 to 5  garlic cloves, crushed
    and peeled (do not chop)

1½  tablespoons extra virgin olive oil
    salt and freshly ground
    white pepper
¼  pound shiitake mushrooms
    (about 2½ cups), stems removed
    and caps sliced into long strips

## Salad

¾  cup plus 2 tablespoons
    balsamic vinegar
    Rosemary Potatoes (recipe above)

4  cups baby arugula (about 2 small
    bunches), rinsed and spun dry

2  tablespoons extra virgin olive oil
    salt and freshly ground pepper

## Salmon

4  5-ounce salmon fillets
2  teaspoons coarse sea salt

2  teaspoons cracked black pepper

To roast the potatoes, preheat the oven to 425 degrees F. In a large bowl, toss the potatoes with the rosemary, garlic, and 1 tablespoon of the olive oil and season with salt and pepper. Spread the potatoes out in a single layer on a nonstick baking sheet and roast for 10 minutes. In a medium bowl, toss the mushrooms with the remaining ½ tablespoon olive oil and add them to the potatoes, stirring to combine. Continue roasting until the potatoes and mushrooms are tender and golden brown, about 10 minutes. Remove from the oven and cool. Discard the rosemary sprigs and garlic. Set the potatoes aside and lower the oven heat to 275 degrees F.

To prepare the salad, place ¾ cup of the balsamic vinegar into a small stainless-steel saucepan, bring to a boil, then reduce the heat to keep the vinegar at a low boil until it reduces to a syruplike consistency. Set aside.

In a large bowl, combine the potatoes and mushrooms. Set aside. Dress and season the salad when the salmon is cooked.

To cook the salmon, place a small roasting pan filled with water in the oven to increase the humidity. Place a piece of foil paper that has been lightly rubbed with olive oil (less than ½ teaspoon) on top of a baking sheet pan. Place the salmon fillets on top of the foil, skin side up, and season with salt and pepper. Put in the oven and bake at 275 degrees F for 8 minutes, then remove and let rest for about 5 minutes. Gently inspect the center of the largest fillet for doneness; if it is still translucent in the center it will require a little more cooking, 2 to 3 minutes. When done, peel off the skin and gently scrape off the gray areas under the skin with a small spoon or knife until the fish is all pink.

In a large bowl, combine the arugula with the remaining 2 tablespoons balsamic vinegar and 2 tablespoons olive oil and season with salt and pepper. Gently toss to combine. Divide the arugula among 4 salad plates and place the potato-mushroom mixture on top. Place the cooked salmon over the potatoes and mushrooms and drizzle with a little balsamic syrup.

---

- Salmon is a potentially very good source of omega-3 fatty acids and selenium.
- Rosemary contains the phytochemical carnosol, which is a potent antioxidant and may increase enzymes that help neutralize and dispose of carcinogens.
- Dark, leafy greens like arugula contain substantial amounts of folate; combined with other sources in this recipe (salmon, potatoes, and mushrooms) they provide more than 20% of the DV per serving.
- Arugula and potatoes provide more than 40% of the DV for vitamin C.
- High in fiber—20% of the DV per serving.

---

*Per serving of Rosemary Roasted Potatoes:*

| calories | protein | carbohydrates | fat | cholesterol | dietary fiber | saturated fat |
|---|---|---|---|---|---|---|
| 164 | 6 Gm | 25 Gm | 5 Gm | 0 mg | 6 Gm | 1 Gm |

*Per serving of Warm Salad of Arugula, Rosemary Roasted Potatoes, Shiitake Mushrooms, and Balsamic Essence:*

| calories | protein | carbohydrates | fat | cholesterol | dietary fiber | saturated fat |
|---|---|---|---|---|---|---|
| 248 | 6 Gm | 32 Gm | 11 Gm | 0 mg | 6 Gm | 2 Gm |

*Per serving of Slow-roasted Salmon:*

| calories | protein | carbohydrates | fat | cholesterol | dietary fiber | saturated fat |
|---|---|---|---|---|---|---|
| 194 | 28 Gm | 0 Gm | 9 Gm | 75 mg | 0 Gm | 1 Gm |

*Per serving of Slow-roasted Salmon with a Warm Salad of Arugula, Rosemary Roasted Potatoes, Shiitake Mushrooms, and Balsamic Essence:*

| calories | protein | carbohydrates | fat | cholesterol | dietary fiber | saturated fat |
|---|---|---|---|---|---|---|
| 442 | 34 Gm | 32 Gm | 20 Gm | 75 mg | 6 Gm | 3 Gm |

**% of Calories**: 29% carbohydrate, 31% protein, 40% fat

### Major Sources of Potential Cancer Fighters

**Phytochemicals**: allium compounds, omega-3 fatty acids, plant polyphenols (flavonoids, phenolic acids), terpenes (carotenoids, carnosol, monoterpenes)

# ❦ *Seared Salmon with Fresh Corn Relish* ❦

Jimmy Sneed, The Frog and the Redneck, Richmond, Virginia

4 SERVINGS

• *This sweet and sour relish is also wonderful over other seared or grilled fish, such as tuna and swordfish.*

### Relish

| | | | | |
|---|---|---|---|---|
| 3/4 | cup sherry vinegar | | 1 | tablespoon olive oil |
| 1/2 | cup sugar | | 1/2 | small red onion (about |
| 1 1/2 | teaspoons celery seed | | | 2 1/2 ounces), diced |
| | sea salt | | 1 | red bell pepper (about 8 ounces), |
| | cracked black pepper | | | seeded and finely diced |
| 4 | ears corn or 10 ounces frozen | | | |
| | corn, thawed and drained | | | |

### Salmon

| | | | |
|---|---|---|---|
| 1 | teaspoon olive oil | sea salt and freshly ground pepper |
| 4 | 6-ounce salmon fillets | |

Prepare the relish 1 day in advance. In a 2-quart saucepan, bring the vinegar, sugar, 2 cups water, the celery seed, 1 teaspoon sea salt, and 2 teaspoons cracked black pepper to a boil. Reduce to a simmer for 5 minutes. Set aside.

Cook the corn cobs in boiling salted water for 2 minutes. Remove and place in cold water for 5 minutes. Slice the kernels off the cob, being careful not to slice too deeply into the cob. Puree 1/4 of the corn in a food processor or blender using just enough water to liquefy (1 to 2 tablespoons). Season the puree with salt and pepper and refrigerate. Put the remaining corn in a large mixing bowl.

Heat the olive oil in a small nonstick skillet. Sauté the onion for 2 to 3 minutes and add the red bell pepper. Season with salt and pepper and sauté for 5 minutes more without browning. Transfer to the mixing bowl with the corn. Add the marinade and refrigerate for at least 12 hours.

To cook the salmon, preheat the oven to 375 degrees F.

Heat the olive oil in a large cast-iron pan (or oven-safe nonstick skillet). Season both sides of the salmon fillets with sea salt and pepper. Place the fillets, skin side up, into the heated pan and sear until golden brown. Flip the fillets over and finish in the oven for 3 to 5 minutes, depending on the thickness of the fillets.

Strain the relish, discarding the liquid, and place the corn-vegetable mixture in a small bowl. Add the corn puree and mix well. Serve atop the salmon fillets.

- Salmon is a potentially good source of protective omega-3 fatty acids.
- Although corn is not substantially high in vitamin A or beta-carotene, it does contain other carotenes, such as lutein, that may protect against certain types of cancer.
- This recipe provides more than 30% of the DV for vitamin C per serving.

*Per serving of Fresh Corn Relish:*

| calories | protein | carbohydrates | fat | cholesterol | dietary fiber | saturated fat |
|---|---|---|---|---|---|---|
| 202 | 3 Gm | 44 Gm | 4 Gm | 0 mg | 2 Gm | 0 Gm |

*Per serving of Seared Salmon with Fresh Corn Relish:*

| calories | protein | carbohydrates | fat | cholesterol | dietary fiber | saturated fat |
|---|---|---|---|---|---|---|
| 453 | 36 Gm | 44 Gm | 15 Gm | 93 mg | 2 Gm | 2 Gm |

**% of Calories**: 40% carbohydrate, 30% protein, 30% fat

**Major Sources of Potential Cancer Fighters**
**Phytochemicals**: allium compounds, plant polyphenols (flavonoids), terpenes (carotenoids)

# ✤ *Seared Sea Scallops,* ✤ *Enoki Mushrooms, and Grilled Asparagus*

Janos Wilder, Janos, Tucson, Arizona

4 SERVINGS

- *The perfect spring or summer lunch or light dinner.*
- *Use the minted vinaigrette to dress other salads.*

## Scallop and Mushroom Salad

| | |
|---|---|
| 2 tablespoons balsamic vinegar | 1 pound very large sea scallops (8 to 10 each) |
| 1/4 cup fresh squeezed orange juice | |
| 1 tablespoon olive oil | 3/4 pound Enoki mushrooms, brushed clean |
| 3/4 pound fresh pencil-thin asparagus (about 1 bunch), ends trimmed | salt and pepper |

## Minted Vinaigrette

MAKES 1¹/₄ CUPS

| | |
|---|---|
| ¹/₄  cup chopped mint | 1  teaspoon minced gingerroot |
| ³/₄  teaspoon minced garlic | 1  tablespoon soy sauce |
|     (2 small cloves) | 2  tablespoons sesame oil |
| 1  tablespoon honey | ¹/₄  cup peanut oil |
| ¹/₃  cup rice wine vinegar | ¹/₄  cup boiling water |
| ¹/₄  cup lime juice |     salt and pepper |

Prepare the marinade and vinaigrette in advance. To make the marinade, in a small bowl, combine the balsamic vinegar and orange juice and then whisk in the olive oil. Set aside.

Blanch the asparagus in 3 quarts of boiling, salted water until al dente. Drain and chill immediately in ice water. Drain again and place in a rectangular container or baking dish. Pour the balsamic marinade over the top, cover, and refrigerate overnight.

To make the vinaigrette, in a stainless-steel bowl, combine the mint, garlic, and honey. Whisk until well combined and then whisk in all the remaining ingredients. Let steep for 6 hours at room temperature, strain, and adjust the seasoning with salt and pepper. Pour into a squirt bottle. Shake before each use.

Preheat the oven to 400 degrees F and preheat the grill.

Brush a nonstick oven-safe skillet (with a metal handle for oven transfer) with olive oil and heat until almost smoking. Season the scallops with salt and pepper and place in the skillet. Sear them on both sides, until the outside rims are well browned, then lower the heat and continue cooking until they are opaque and spring back when gently probed for about 2 minutes. When cool enough to handle, slice the scallops horizontally into 3 "coins" each. Set aside.

Remove the asparagus from the marinade and drain; grill for 1 to 2 minutes. When the asparagus brown slightly they are done. The asparagus may also be sautéed in a nonstick pan. Heat 1 teaspoon olive oil until almost smoking and add the asparagus.

In a bowl, toss the scallop slices with 3 tablespoons of the vinaigrette. Arrange the scallop slices in a semicircle about 3 inches in diameter in the center of each plate.

Place the asparagus spears in the center of the semicircle, with the stems in the center and the tips pointed toward the rim of the plate.

Remove any "noody" parts from the mushrooms and separate them if they are attached. Gently toss the mushrooms with 4 tablespoons of the vinaigrette. Place them in a neat mound on top of the asparagus. Lightly drizzle the vinaigrette over the salads.

- Scallops and mushrooms are potentially good sources of selenium.
- Sesame, peanut and olive oils provide vitamin E and contain protective plant sterols (but use these fats moderately). In this recipe, more than 10% of the DV for vitamin E is provided per serving.
- Mint contains monoterpenes that act as antioxidants and blocking agents to interfere with carcinogens.
- Asparagus is a good source of vitamin C and folate, providing more than 75% and 40% of the DVs, respectively, per serving.

*Per serving of Minted Vinaigrette (2 tablespoons):*

| calories | protein | carbohydrates | fat | cholesterol | dietary fiber | saturated fat |
|---|---|---|---|---|---|---|
| 89 | 0 Gm | 5 Gm | 8 Gm | 0 mg | 0 Gm | 1 Gm |

*Per serving of Seared Sea Scallops, Enoki Mushrooms, and Grilled Asparagus:*

| calories | protein | carbohydrates | fat | cholesterol | dietary fiber | saturated fat |
|---|---|---|---|---|---|---|
| 290 | 25 Gm | 19 Gm | 13 Gm | 40 mg | 1 Gm | 2 Gm |

**% of Calories**: 26% carbohydrate, 34% protein, 40% fat

### Major Sources of Potential Cancer Fighters

**Phytochemicals**: plant polyphenols (flavonoids), plant sterols, terpenes (carotenoids, gingerol, monoterpenes)

# ✦ Fresh Rockfish with Mussel, ✦ Basil, and Tomato Sauce on Redneck Caviar

Jimmy Sneed, The Frog and the Redneck, Richmond, Virginia

4 SERVINGS

- *This Mussel, Basil, and Tomato Sauce is also terrific over pasta.*

## Rockfish

| | |
|---|---|
| 4   6-ounce fillets of rockfish (striped bass) | 1/4   cup flour |
| sea salt and freshly ground pepper | 1   tablespoon extra virgin olive oil |

## Mussel, Basil, and Tomato Sauce

| | |
|---|---|
| 1/2   cup shallots, chopped | 20   mussels in shell, brushed clean |
| 1/2   cup dry white wine | and beards removed |

1/2   cup tomatoes, diced                    2   garlic cloves, finely chopped
2     tablespoons chopped fresh basil


## Redneck Caviar

2     cups chicken stock                         salt and pepper
3/4   cup coarse stone-ground grits          1   tablespoon squid ink (optional)
      (see Note)


To make the Redneck Caviar, in a heavy 2-quart saucepan, bring the chicken stock to a boil. While stirring with a wooden spoon, add the grits. Simmer over low heat, stirring frequently, for about 30 minutes, until the grits thicken. Season to taste with salt and pepper and add the squid ink.

To make the tomato sauce, in a large sauté pan, simmer the shallots in white wine for 2 minutes. Add the mussels and cover until they open. Reserve the cooking liquid in the sauté pan and set aside. Pick the meat out of the shell, adding any mussel juice to the reserved cooking liquid. Heat the liquid in the sauté pan to a simmer and add the mussel meat, tomatoes, basil, and garlic and season with salt and pepper. After 1 minute, remove from the heat.

To prepare the rockfish, preheat the oven to 400 degrees F. Season the rockfish fillets with salt and pepper. Dredge in flour, shaking off any excess. Heat the olive oil in a large nonstick or cast iron sauté pan until almost smoking. Lay the rockfish fillets in the pan and brown on one side over high heat, 1 to 2 minutes. Turn the fillets and transfer to the oven. Roast for 4 to 6 minutes.

Put some of the redneck caviar into 4 bowls, and place a rockfish fillet over it. Pour the sauce over the fillet.

*Note:* Grits or hominy grits are available at supermarkets and specialty stores in a choice of grinds: coarse, medium, and fine. The amount of cooking liquid and cooking time is directly related to the size of the grind—the more coarse, the more liquid and longer cooking required.

---

- Striped bass is a good source of protective omega-3 fatty acids.
- Both striped bass and mussels are potentially good sources of selenium.

---

**Per serving of Mussel, Basil, and Tomato Sauce (1/3 cup):**

| calories | protein | carbohydrates | fat | cholesterol | dietary fiber | saturated fat |
|----------|---------|---------------|-----|-------------|---------------|---------------|
| 70 | 7 Gm | 4 Gm | 1 Gm | 24 mg | 0 Gm | 0 Gm |

**Per serving of Striped Bass:**

| calories | protein | carbohydrates | fat | cholesterol | dietary fiber | saturated fat |
|----------|---------|---------------|-----|-------------|---------------|---------------|
| 195 | 30 Gm | 0 Gm | 7 Gm | 136 mg | 0 Gm | 1 Gm |

**Per serving of Redneck Caviar:**

| calories | protein | carbohydrates | fat | cholesterol | dietary fiber | saturated fat |
|----------|---------|---------------|-----|-------------|---------------|---------------|
| 128 | 5 Gm | 24 Gm | 1 Gm | 0 mg | 1 Gm | 2 Gm |

**Per serving of Fresh Rockfish with Mussel, Basil, and Tomato Sauce on Redneck Caviar:**

| calories | protein | carbohydrates | fat | cholesterol | dietary fiber | saturated fat |
|----------|---------|---------------|-----|-------------|---------------|---------------|
| 393 | 42 Gm | 28 Gm | 9 Gm | 160 mg | 1 Gm | 3 Gm |

**% of Calories**: 29% carbohydrate, 44% protein, 22% fat, Alcohol 5%

**Major Sources of Potential Cancer Fighters**

**Phytochemicals**: allium compounds, plant polyphenols (flavonoids), terpenes (carotenoids)

# ❧ Grilled Salmon with Yellow ❧ Pepper Coulis and Beet Oil Vinaigrette

Anthony Bourdain, Ed Sullivan Restaurant, New York, New York

4 SERVINGS

- *Serve as a light lunch entrée or with roasted potatoes for dinner.*
- *Use the Beet Vinaigrette with other salads and the Yellow Pepper Coulis as a bed for other grilled or seared fish, such as tuna, swordfish, and snapper.*

## Yellow Pepper Coulis

MAKES 3/4 CUP

| | |
|---|---|
| 2  medium yellow bell peppers (about 14 ounces) | (see Note) |
| 1  garlic clove | 1  tablespoon olive oil |
| 1  tablespoon rice wine vinegar | salt and freshly ground pepper |

## Beet Vinaigrette

MAKES 3/4 CUP

| | |
|---|---|
| 1  medium beet (about 6 ounces) | 1  tablespoon olive oil |
| 1  tablespoon rice wine vinegar | salt and pepper |

*Salmon*

| | | | |
|---|---|---|---|
| 1¹/₂ | pounds salmon (4 6-ounce fillets) | | salt and pepper |
| | | 1 | teaspoon olive oil |
| 4 | cups mesclun, rinsed and well drained | | |

Preheat the oven to 375 degrees F.

To roast the peppers, rub them with a small amount of olive oil (less than ¹/₂ teaspoon) and place in an oven-safe skillet under the broiler. Using kitchen tongs, rotate the peppers to assure even cooking (browning) on all sides. Remove the peppers from the oven, place in a bowl, and cover with foil or plastic wrap so that steam helps to loosen the skins. When cool, remove the skins, seeds, and stems.

Puree the peppers in a blender or food processor with the garlic, rice wine vinegar, and ¹/₄ cup cold water until very smooth. With the motor running, drizzle in the olive oil. If necessary, slowly add a bit more water to achieve a thick liquid consistency. Season with salt and pepper.

To prepare the beet vinaigrette, trim the beet, but leave the root stem and do not puncture the skin to prevent "bleeding" when cooking. Place the beet in foil wrap and roast for approximately 1 hour and 15 minutes, until tender. Let cool. Peel, roughly chop, and puree in a blender with the rice wine vinegar and ¹/₂ cup cold water. With the motor running, drizzle in the olive oil. Strain through a fine sieve. Season with salt and pepper.

To cook the salmon, season the salmon with salt and pepper, lightly brush with oil, and place on a preheated grill. Cook until medium rare and moist in the center. If you do not have a grill, salmon can be seared in a heated nonstick pan which has been brushed with olive oil. After a crispy golden brown has formed on one side, flip over the salmon fillets and transfer to the oven for 4 to 5 minutes, depending on the thickness of the fillets.

While the salmon cooks, mask the bottom of 4 plates with the yellow pepper coulis. Toss the mesclun in the beet vinaigrette and then divide evenly onto the center of the 4 plates, leaving a border of yellow pepper coulis. Place the cooked salmon fillets on top of the salad and serve.

*Note:* Rice wine vinegar is found at some supermarkets and most gourmet specialty shops and health food stores.

---

- Salmon is a potentially good source of protective omega-3 fatty acids.
- Beets, yellow peppers, and mesclun add up to more than 200% of the DV for vitamin C per serving; it's a good source of vitamin A as well: 20% of the DV per serving.
- Both beets and mesclun are rich in folate, providing more than 50% of the DV per serving.

*Per serving of Yellow Pepper Coulis (3 tablespoons):*

| calories | protein | carbohydrates | fat | cholesterol | dietary fiber | saturated fat |
|---|---|---|---|---|---|---|
| 60 | 1 Gm | 7 Gm | 4 Gm | 0 mg | 1 Gm | 0 Gm |

*Per serving of Beet Vinaigrette (2 tablespoons):*

| calories | protein | carbohydrates | fat | cholesterol | dietary fiber | saturated fat |
|---|---|---|---|---|---|---|
| 33 | 1 Gm | 4 Gm | 2 Gm | 0 mg | 1 Gm | 0 Gm |

*Per serving of Grilled Salmon with Yellow Pepper Coulis and Beet Oil:*

| calories | protein | carbohydrates | fat | cholesterol | dietary fiber | saturated fat |
|---|---|---|---|---|---|---|
| 336 | 37 Gm | 11 Gm | 16 Gm | 93 mg | 2 Gm | 1 Gm |

**% of Calories**: 13% carbohydrate, 44% protein, 43% fat

**Major Sources of Potential Cancer Fighters**
**Phytochemicals**: allium compounds, plant polyphenols (flavonoids, phenolic acids), plant sterols, terpenes (carotenoids)

# ❧ *Linguine with Soft-Shell Crab Sauce* ❧

Roberto Donna, Galileo, Washington, D.C.

4 SERVINGS (6 SERVINGS FIRST COURSE)

•  *Roberto Donna first visualized this dish when visiting a friend in the beautiful Italian Riviera. After seeing the abundance of soft-shell crab, he thought, "If crab meat goes so well with linguine, why not use this beautiful, juicy soft-shell crab?"*

| | | | |
|---|---|---|---|
| 3/4 | pound dried linguine | 5 | basil leaves |
| 4 | soft-shell crabs (see Note) | 1 | tablespoon chopped fresh parsley |
| 2 | tablespoons olive oil | 1/2 | cup tomato sauce (see Note) |
| 2 | garlic cloves, crushed | | salt |
| pinch red pepper flakes | | | |

Bring 5 quarts of salted water to a boil and cook the linguine until al dente. Drain thoroughly. Rinse the soft-shell crabs and cut each crab into 6 pieces.

Heat the olive oil in a large, nonstick sauté pan. Sauté the garlic until it begins to turn golden brown, then remove from the pan. Add the soft-shell crab pieces to the pan and sauté for 1 minute. Add the red pepper flakes, basil, parsley, and tomato sauce and sauté 4 minutes more. Remove from the heat and season to taste with salt.

Drain the pasta and transfer to the sauté pan. Toss with the sauce and serve immediately.

*Note:* In the United States soft-shell crabs are found along the Atlantic and Gulf coasts. They are available throughout the country from May to September at some supermarkets and fish markets.

Chef Donna provides the option of omitting the tomato sauce and adding 3/4 cup of white wine (before adding the herbs), reducing it almost completely, and then proceeding with the recipe.

---

- This quick, easy dish contains less than 20% of calories from fat.
- Vegetables such as blanched asparagus tips can be added to help boost your daily fruit and vegetable servings.
- Crab is a potentially good source of selenium.
- A good source of fiber.

---

**Per serving:**

| calories | protein | carbohydrates | fat | cholesterol | dietary fiber | saturated fat |
|----------|---------|---------------|------|-------------|---------------|---------------|
| 442 | 23 Gm | 67 Gm | 9 Gm | 56 mg | 3 Gm | 1 Gm |

**% of Calories:** 61% carbohydrate, 21% protein, 18% fat

**Major Sources of Potential Cancer Fighters**

**Phytochemicals:** capsaicin, phytic acids, plant polyphenols (flavonoids, phenolic acids), plant sterols, terpenes (carotenoids, monoterpenes)

# ❧ Grilled Swordfish Steaks ❧ with Roasted Pepper Marinara

Tom Pustizzi, The Dilworthtown Inn, West Chester, Pennsylvania

4 SERVINGS

- *This marinara sauce is slightly picante and very flavorful. It is also versatile, marrying well with a variety of whitefish and white meats, such as chicken, pork, or veal. It goes well over pasta. This recipe prepares 2 extra cups of sauce; freeze the extra for another use.*

- *Serve with rice, boiled potatoes tossed with fresh herbs, or Rosemary Roasted Potatoes, page 221.*

*Swordfish*

| | | | | |
|---|---|---|---|---|
| 2 | fresh rosemary sprigs | | 2 | garlic cloves, crushed |
| 3 | teaspoons olive oil | | 1¹/₂ | pounds swordfish |
| 2 | tablespoons fresh lemon juice | | | (4 6-ounce steaks) |
| | freshly ground black pepper | | | salt |

*Marinara Sauce*

MAKES 4 CUPS (1 SERVING = ¹/₄ CUP)

| | | | | |
|---|---|---|---|---|
| 1 | tablespoon olive oil | | 3 | small red bell peppers (about |
| 1 | medium onion (about 6 ounces), | | | 12 ounces), roasted, peeled, |
| | chopped | | | seeded, and chopped |
| 1 | small jalapeño pepper, | | 2 | garlic cloves, minced |
| | seeded and diced | | ¹/₄ | cup chopped fresh basil |
| | pinch crushed red pepper flakes | | 2 | tablespoons chopped fresh oregano |
| 2 | small green bell peppers | | ¹/₂ | cup red wine |
| | (about 8 ounces), roasted, | | 1 | can tomato puree (28 ounces) |
| | peeled, seeded, and chopped | | | salt and pepper |
| | (see roasting procedure, below) | | | |

To roast the peppers, rub them with a small amount of olive oil (less than ¹/₂ teaspoon) and place in an oven-safe skillet under the broiler. Using kitchen tongs, rotate the peppers to assure even cooking (browning) on all sides. Remove the peppers from the oven, place in a bowl, and cover with foil or plastic wrap so that steam helps to loosen the skins. When cool, remove the skins, seeds, and stems.

To prepare the marinara sauce, heat ¹/₂ tablespoon of the olive oil in a large nonstick skillet and sauté the onion and jalapeño over medium heat until tender, about 5 minutes. Add the red pepper flakes, roasted bell peppers, garlic, basil, and oregano and sauté over medium-high heat for 2 to 3 minutes, then add the red wine. Let the wine reduce to about 1 tablespoon and add the tomato puree; bring to a boil. Reduce the heat, simmer for 30 minutes, remove from the heat, and let cool slightly. Puree in batches in a food processor or blender until smooth. Return the puree to the sauté pan, bring to a boil, reduce the heat, and simmer for another 15 to 20 minutes. Season with salt and pepper to taste.

While the marinara sauce cooks, marinate the swordfish. In a rectangular baking dish, combine the rosemary (leave on stem), 2 teaspoons of the olive oil, the lemon juice, black pepper, and garlic. Place the swordfish in the marinade, cover, and refrigerate. After 30 minutes turn the steaks over and marinate for another 30 minutes.

Preheat the grill. Season the swordfish with salt. Place the steaks on the grill and cook for 3 to 4 minutes per side. They should be grill-marked, but not charred, on the outside, and just cooked through. Swordfish fillets can be seared instead of grilled.

To sear, heat the remaining 1 teaspoon olive oil in a large nonstick skillet until almost smoking. Wipe the marinade from the swordfish, season with salt, and place in the skillet. Sear over high heat until golden brown on one side, about 1 to 2 minutes. Turn over and cook on medium-low heat until cooked through, about 4 minutes.

Spoon the marinara sauce over the grilled swordfish.

---

- The pepper varieties load this recipe with vitamin C: one serving provides more than 200% of the DV! It also provides 30% of the DV for vitamin A per serving.
- Swordfish is a good source of protective omega-3 fatty acids and a potentially good source of selenium.
- Rosemary contains carnosol, a potent anitoxidant and blocking agent against cancer-causing substances.
- High in fiber—20% of the DV per serving.

---

*Per ½ cup serving of Marinara Sauce (1/2 cup):*

| calories | protein | carbohydrates | fat | cholesterol | dietary fiber | saturated fat |
|---|---|---|---|---|---|---|
| 103 | 3 Gm | 19 Gm | 2 Gm | 0 mg | 4 Gm | 0 Gm |

*Per serving of Grilled Swordfish Steaks with Roasted Pepper Marinara:*

| calories | protein | carbohydrates | fat | cholesterol | dietary fiber | saturated fat |
|---|---|---|---|---|---|---|
| 292 | 35 Gm | 11 Gm | 11 Gm | 66 mg | 2 Gm | 2 Gm |

**% of Calories**: 15% carbohydrate, 49% protein, 35% fat, 1% alcohol

### Major Sources of Potential Cancer Fighters

**Phytochemicals**: allium compounds, capsaicin, plant polyphenols (flavonoids, phenolic acids), plant sterols, terpenes (carotenoids, monoterpenes)

## ❧ *Lobster and Squash Risotto* ❧

Gianni Scappin, Bigoli, Inc., New York, New York; Trattoria alla Pesa, Mason Vicentino, Veneto, Italy

4 SERVINGS (6 FIRST COURSE SERVINGS)

- *Gianni remarks that the combination of lobster, butternut squash, and sage with tortellini, ravioli, or, as in this case, risotto, is "la fine del mondo (the best in the world)."*

2 tablespoons extra virgin olive oil
1 small onion (3 ounces),
    finely diced
2½ cups butternut squash (about
    10 ounces), peeled, seeded, and
    chopped into small cubes
3 fresh sage leaves
10 ounces Italian rice (1½ cups;
    preferably Carnaroli or Superfino
    Arborio or Semifino
    Vialone Nano)

7 cups light fish stock (page 149),
    vegetable stock (page 146), or
    low-sodium canned broth, or
    water, simmering
3 tablespoons canned
    pumpkin puree
    salt and pepper
8 to 10 ounces lobster meat
    or shrimp, cooked
1 tablespoon chopped parsley

Heat 1 tablespoon of the olive oil in a large, heavy saucepan. Sauté the onion over medium heat until limp, 2 to 3 minutes; do not brown. Add the butternut squash and sage leaves and cook for another minute, then add the rice.

Stir in 4 cups of the fish stock and the pumpkin puree; season with salt, and bring to a boil. Cook at a low simmer, stirring frequently. After 10 minutes, add half of the lobster and continue to cook for about 8 minutes, adding stock ½ cup at a time as rice absorbs the liquid. The rice should be tender but firm and should have movement when pan is shaken, but no excess liquid. Add the remaining lobster, remove from the heat, and adjust the seasoning, if necessary, with salt and pepper. Stir in the parsley and the remaining olive oil and serve immediately.

---

- Butternut squash is among the richest sources of beta-carotene. It helps provides most of the vitamin A in this recipe—more than 80% of the DV per serving. It also provides the majority of the vitamin C—more than 20% of the DV per serving.
- The natural oils found in sage have potent antioxidant properties.
- Lobster is a potentially excellent source of selenium.

---

*Per serving (based on 4 servings):*

| calories | protein | carbohydrates | fat | cholesterol | dietary fiber | saturated fat |
|----------|---------|---------------|-----|-------------|---------------|---------------|
| 475 | 26 Gm | 73 Gm | 9 Gm | 46 mg | 2 Gm | 2 Gm |

**% of Calories**: 62% carbohydrate, 22% protein, 16% fat

### Major Sources of Potential Cancer Fighters
**Phytochemicals**: allium compounds, plant polyphenols (flavonoids), plant sterols, terpenes (carotenoids, monoterpenes)

# ❧ Cod Brodetto Venetian Style ❧

Gianni Scappin, Maximillian, New York, New York; Trattoria alla Pesa, Mason Vicentino, Veneto, Italy

4 SERVINGS

- *Gianni provides the option of substituting snapper, grouper, tilefish, halibut, or monk-fish for the cod to make this a versatile "one-pot" meal.*
- *Total preparation time is less than 30 minutes.*
- *Vegetables such as snow peas, haricot verts, asparagus tips, and/or thinly sliced carrots can be added.*

| | |
|---|---|
| 3 medium tomatoes (about 14 ounces) | 2 tablespoons chopped fresh parsley |
| 1 tablespoon olive oil | 10 fresh basil leaves, sliced into long strips |
| 8 small shallots (about 7 ounces), thinly sliced, or 2 small onions, thinly sliced | salt and pepper |
| 2 bay leaves | 3/4 cup white wine |
| 4 medium Yukon Gold potatoes (about 1 pound) sliced 1/4 to 1/2 inch thick | 4 skinless, boneless cod fillets (about 6 ounces each), 1 1/2 inches thick |

Preheat the oven to 375 degrees F.

To peel and seed the tomatoes, bring 2 quarts of water to a boil in a large pot. Cut the core from the tomatoes with a paring knife and plunge them into boiling water for 30 seconds. Remove with a slotted spoon and immediately immerse in ice water until cool. Use a knife to gently peel the skin, which should be discarded. Slice the tomatoes in half and gently squeeze to force out the seeds. Use your fingers to remove any remaining seeds. Discard the seeds, dice the tomatoes, and reserve.

Heat the olive oil in a braising pan or large nonstick oven-safe skillet and sauté the shallots and bay leaves over medium heat for 5 minutes without browning. Transfer to a small bowl.

Spread the potato slices in a single layer in the pan. Place half of the sautéed shallots with bay leaves and half of the parsley and basil on top. Season with salt and pepper, add the wine and 1/2 cup water, and bring to a boil. Reduce the heat to medium-low and simmer for 3 to 4 minutes.

Season the cod fillets with salt and pepper and place on top of the potatoes in a single even layer. Sprinkle with the remaining parsley, basil, shallot-bay leaf mixture, and the tomatoes. Return the mixture to a low simmer, cover, and transfer to the oven for

7 minutes. (You can also leave the fish on the stovetop to cook at a low simmer.) Be sure that the pan is well sealed to keep in flavor and moisture.

Remove the cod carefully from the pan with a spatula. Remove the bay leaves. Using a slotted spoon, divide the potatoes between 4 large soup or pasta bowls. Place a cod fillet on top of the potatoes. Bring the remaining juices and vegetables to a boil. Season to taste with salt and pepper and pour on top of each cod fillet. Serve with a grilled piece of crusty bread rubbed with crushed garlic.

Use a mandoline for uniform potato slices and uniform cooking. Made of stainless steel or plastic, they are usually sold with a variety of blades for thin slicing, julienning, and French fry cutting. Inexpensive, good-quality plastic mandolines are available at most culinary stores.

- Cod is a potentially very good source of selenium and omega-3 fatty acids.
- One serving provides more than 50% of the DV for vitamin C and 40% for vitamin A.
- A good source of fiber.

*Per serving:*

| calories | protein | carbohydrates | fat | cholesterol | dietary fiber | saturated fat |
|---|---|---|---|---|---|---|
| 345 | 30 Gm | 35 Gm | 5 Gm | 65 mg | 4 Gm | 1 Gm |

**% of Calories**: 37% carbohydrate, 40% protein, 14% fat, 9% alcohol

### Major Sources of Potential Cancer Fighters
**Phytochemicals**: allium compounds, plant polyphenols (phenolic acids, flavonoids), plant sterols, terpenes (carotenoids, monoterpenes)

# ❧ *Poached Maine Halibut with* ❧ *Texas Sweet Onions, Boiled Potatoes, and Carrot-Lemongrass Broth*

Scott Cohen, Ocean Grill, New York, New York

4 SERVINGS

- *This beautiful and fragrant dish can be made in less than 30 minutes.*
- *Other fish, such as sea bass, red snapper, and salmon, can be substituted for halibut.*

| | |
|---|---|
| 2 stalks lemongrass, sliced | 2 cups fish stock (page 149) or bouillon |
| 2 medium carrots (about 5 ounces), juiced or 1/2 cup bottled or canned carrot juice | salt and pepper |
| | 1 1/2 pounds boneless halibut (4-6 ounce fillets) |
| 1 1/2 tablespoons sugar | 1/2 bunch fresh coriander (cilantro), stems trimmed and whole leaves reserved |
| 1 teaspoon olive oil | |
| 2 small Texas Sweet or Vidalia onions, sliced (about 2 ounces) | |
| 1/2 cup white wine | |
| 4 to 5 small red potatoes (about 1 pound), sliced 1/4 inch thick | |

*Garnish*

| | |
|---|---|
| 1 large carrot (about 3 ounces), peeled | 16 snow peas, cut into diamond shapes |
| 1 medium parsnip (about 3 ounces), peeled | 1 bunch sunflower sprouts (optional) |

Put the lemongrass, carrot juice, and sugar into a small saucepan and bring to a boil. Reduce the heat to low and simmer slowly until it becomes syrupy, about 20 minutes. Strain and reserve. Meanwhile, proceed with the recipe.

To make the garnish, using a vegetable channeler or the back of a fork, create lengthwise grooves down the carrot and parsnip (this will give a flower shape when sliced). Cut into even, very thin slices (preferably with a mandoline), and set aside.

In a 4-quart saucepan, heat the olive oil and sauté the onions over medium heat until soft, 3 to 4 minutes. Add the white wine and cook for 3 minutes, until the wine reduces by three-quarters, then add the potatoes and fish stock. Season with salt and pepper and simmer until the potatoes are half cooked. Season the fish with the coriander. Add the snow peas and carrot and parsnip slices, and simmer for 5 minutes; lower the seasoned fish fillets into the saucepan. Sprinkle with the coriander and gently simmer, covered, until the fish just begins to flake, 7 to 9 minutes depending on thickness.

Using a slotted spoon, carefully transfer the fish fillets to serving bowls. Scatter the vegetable garnish around the fish and spoon the carrot syrup over the top. Top the fish with a small handful of sunflower sprouts, if desired.

- Each serving provides more than 150% of the DV for vitamin A, 40% for vitamin C, and 15% for folate.
- Halibut is a potentially good source of selenium.
- A good source of fiber.

*Per serving:*

| calories | protein | carbohydrates | fat | cholesterol | dietary fiber | saturated fat |
|----------|---------|---------------|-----|-------------|---------------|---------------|
| 359 | 40 Gm | 30 Gm | 6 Gm | 53 mg | 4 Gm | 1 Gm |

**% of Calories**: 34% carbohydrates, 45% protein, 16% fat, 5% alcohol

### Major Sources of Potential Cancer Fighters
**Phytochemicals**: allium compounds, plant polyphenols (flavonoids, phenolic acids), terpenes (carotenoids, monoterpenes)

# POULTRY AND MEAT

## ✦ *Free-Range,* ✦
## *Full-Flavor Roasted Chicken*

### 4 SERVINGS

• *Roasting chicken creates a dilemma: if you remove the skin before roasting the meat is unpalatably dry when cooked, but if you season and cook the chicken with the skin it makes it difficult to remove and dispose of this crispy, seasoned part later. The ideal solution is to season the chicken underneath the skin so the meat has the flavor, not the skin. In this recipe the natural oils and essences from the garlic, rosemary, and lemon peel seep into the meat, providing nutrients and great flavor. Other possibilities include orange, lime, or grapefruit peel, herbes de Provence, fresh thyme or tarragon—the combinations are limitless.*

• *Try these accompaniments: Robert McGrath's Garlic Mashed Potatoes, page 257, Gianni Scappin's Crispy Oven-roasted Vegetables, page 171, and Sautéed Spinach with Garlic, page 179.*

1  4 to 5 pound free-range roasting chicken, giblets removed
    salt and pepper
    6 to 7 strips of peel from
1  large lemon

4  fresh rosemary sprigs
4  garlic cloves, crushed

Preheat the oven to 400 degrees F.

Rinse the whole chicken and pat dry with paper towels or a clean cloth. Trim off any excess skin. Running your fingers underneath the skin, separate the thin lining that holds the skin to the meat without removing or tearing the skin. Sprinkle some salt and pepper under the skin then place the strips of lemon peel, yellow side touching the meat, whole rosemary sprigs, and crushed garlic cloves underneath the skin of the breasts and legs.

Place the chicken on its back in a roasting pan and place in preheated oven for approximately 50 minutes, or until the juices run clear. Remove from the oven and let rest for 5 minutes before carving.

Remove the breasts and legs from the carcass. Remove the skin, cut the breasts in half diagonally, and separate the thighs from the drumsticks. Dispose of the seasonings. Serve a piece of breast and leg meat on each plate.

Limonene, found in citrus peels, and carnosol, a phytochemical in rosemary, are potent antioxidants and help increase cancer-fighting enzymes in the body.

**Per serving (skin removed):**

| calories | protein | carbohydrates | fat | cholesterol | dietary fiber | saturated fat |
|---|---|---|---|---|---|---|
| 220 | 35 Gm | 3 Gm | 8 Gm | 105 mg | 0 Gm | 2 Gm |

**% of Calories**: 5% carbohydrate, 64% protein, 31% fat

**Major Sources of Potential Cancer Fighters**
**Phytochemicals,** allium compounds, terpenes (monoterpenes, limonenes, carnosol)

## ❧ *Roast Baby Chicken* ❧

Andre Soltner, The French Culinary Institute, New York, New York

2 SERVINGS

• *Andre Soltner served his simple and very popular dish at Lutece every day for the thirty years he was the chef-proprietor.*

• *Almost any vegetable is the perfect accompaniment to this classic dish.*

2  baby chickens (about
    1 pound each), washed inside
    and out and dried with
    paper towels
   salt and freshly ground
   black pepper
5  fresh tarragon sprigs with leaves
4  thyme sprigs
4  parsley sprigs

2  small onions (about 5 ounces)
2  teaspoons peanut oil
1/4  cup white wine
1/4  cup chicken stock (page 147
    or 148), or low-sodium
    canned broth
2  tablespoons minced
    Italian parsley
1  tablespoon unsalted butter

Sprinkle the chickens with salt and pepper, inside and out. Put 2 whole tarragon sprigs, 2 thyme sprigs, 2 parsley sprigs, and 1 onion in the cavity of each chicken. Cross the legs of the chickens and truss with string.

Remove the leaves from the remaining sprig of tarragon, and set them aside.

Preheat the oven to 450 degrees F.

On the stove, over high heat, heat the oil in a roasting pan or a cast-iron pan, and brown the chickens on all sides.

Transfer the pan, with the chickens, to the oven and roast, basting often, about every 5 minutes, until the chickens are crisp and golden brown, 20 to 25 minutes. (To baste means to coat with pan juices. This can be done by simply spooning the juices over the chickens or using a baster, which is available at many supermarkets and most culinary stores.) Remove the chickens from the oven, put them on a serving platter, and keep them warm.

Pour off the fat from the pan, and put the pan over medium heat on the stove. Add the wine and scrape the pan thoroughly with a wooden spoon. Add the veal or chicken stock, the reserved tarragon leaves, and the Italian parsley. Simmer for 2 minutes. Remove the pan from the heat and stir in the butter. Pour this sauce around the chickens and serve immediately.

---

Rosemary and thyme contain phytochemicals that are antioxidants.

---

**Per serving:**

| calories | protein | carbohydrates | fat | cholesterol | dietary fiber | saturated fat |
|----------|---------|---------------|-----|-------------|---------------|---------------|
| 264 | 29 Gm | 3 Gm | 15 Gm | 93 mg | 1 Gm | 5 Gm |

**% of Calories**: 4% carbohydrate, 44% protein, 51% fat, 1% alcohol

**Major Sources of Potential Cancer Fighters**
**Phytochemicals**: allium compounds, terpenes (monoterpenes)

# ✲ *Poached Chicken Breast* ✲
# *with Ratatouille Orzo Ragout*

David Burke, Park Avenue Cafe, New York, New York
Adapted from *Cooking with David Burke*, Alfred A. Knopf, 1995.

### 4 SERVINGS

- *The chicken becomes very moist and flavorful when poached in the ratatouille.*
- *Ratatouille by itself is an excellent low-fat, high-nutrient topping for starches such as rice, potatoes, or pasta.*

2   cups cooked orzo pasta
1½   cups chicken stock (page 147 or 148) or low-sodium canned broth

1½   cups tomato sauce, homemade (page 125), or canned

1½  pounds boneless, skinless chicken
     breasts (4 6-ounce split breasts)
     coarse or kosher salt and
     freshly ground pepper
1    large red bell pepper
     (about 8 ounces), diced
1    yellow bell pepper
     (about 5 ounces), diced
1    medium zucchini (about
     8 ounces), diced
1    medium yellow squash
     (about 10 ounces), diced

1    small eggplant (14 ounces),
     unpeeled, pulp scooped out
     leaving outer 1½ inches close
     to the skin, diced
½    small onion (about 2 ounces),
     diced
3    garlic cloves, minced
1    cup chopped fresh basil
¼    cup mascarpone or grated
     Parmesan cheese (see Note)
4    basil or parsley leaves

To cook the orzo, bring 4 quarts of salted water to a boil. Add the orzo and cook for 7 to 9 minutes (check package directions). Drain, rinse with cold water, and reserve.

Combine the chicken stock and tomato sauce in a soup pot. Bring to a simmer.

Season the chicken with salt and pepper and add to the pot. Cover and simmer for 10 minutes, or until the chicken is cooked. Add the peppers, zucchini, yellow squash, eggplant, onion, and garlic. Stir to combine and simmer for an additional 2 minutes. Remove the chicken breasts and keep warm.

Continue to cook the vegetable mixture, covered, until the vegetables are tender. Add the cooked orzo just before serving. Adjust the seasoning with salt and pepper and add the chopped basil.

Spoon the ragout into 4 large bowls. Cut each chicken breast horizontally into 2 pieces and place over the ragout. Top with 1 tablespoon of mascarpone or grated Parmesan and garnish with the basil or parsley leaves.

*Note:* Mascarpone cheese has about 13 grams of fat per ounce; Parmesan varieties average about 8 grams of fat per ounce. Due to the intense flavor of parmesan, one can generally use less and still get the full effect.

---

- One serving provides three times the DV for vitamin C, 25% of the DV for folate, and enough carotenoids to supply 20% of the DV for vitamin A.
- A good source of dietary fiber.

---

**Per serving:**

| calories | protein | carbohydrates | fat | cholesterol | dietary fiber | saturated fat |
|----------|---------|---------------|-----|-------------|---------------|---------------|
| 478 | 64 Gm | 35 Gm | 9 Gm | 150 mg | 4 Gm | 3 Gm |

**% of Calories**: 29% carbohydrate, 53% protein, 18% fat

**Major Sources of Potential Cancer Fighters**
**Phytochemicals**: allium compounds, plant polyphenols (flavonoids, phenolic acids), plant sterols, terpenes (carotenoids, monoterpenes)

# ❧ Middle Eastern Chicken ❧ Breasts with Smoky Lentils

Katy Keck, New World Grill, New York, New York

4 SERVINGS

• *Prepare the marinade for this great weeknight meal in under 10 minutes in the morning and let the chicken breasts marinate all day—they will become incredibly tender and flavorful. They will only require transfer to a preheated oven and will cook in less than 30 minutes. Serve the chicken with or without the lentils.*

• *Use Smoky Lentils as a bed for other well-seasoned meats or poultry.*

## Middle Eastern Chicken Breasts with Marinade

| | |
|---|---|
| ²/₃ cup nonfat plain yogurt | 2 teaspoons paprika |
| 1 bunch scallions, white part and a little green, thinly sliced | 1 teaspoon ground coriander |
| | 1 teaspoon ground cumin |
| ¹/₄ cup chopped parsley | ¹/₂ teaspoon salt |
| 2 garlic cloves, minced | ¹/₂ teaspoon cayenne |
| juice of 1 lime | 4 boneless, skinless chicken |
| 1 tablespoon olive oil | breasts (4 to 6 ounces each) |

## Smoky Lentils

| | |
|---|---|
| 2 teaspoons olive oil | 4 cups chicken stock (page 147 or 148), or vegetable stock (page 146), or low-sodium canned broth |
| ¹/₂ small onion, minced | |
| 2 garlic cloves, minced | |
| 2 medium carrots (about 7 ounces), peeled and diced | 4 teaspoons pureed chipotle pepper (see Note) |
| 2 celery stalks (about 4 ounces), chopped | 1 teaspoon ground coriander |
| | ¹/₂ teaspoon salt |
| 1¹/₂ cups tiny lentils, such as Massor Dal or DePuy | ¹/₄ cup chopped parsley |

To prepare the chicken marinade, combine all ingredients, except the chicken, in a small mixing bowl and stir to mix well. Place the chicken in a small rectangular baking dish lightly rubbed with olive oil. Pour the marinade over the chicken, turning to coat both sides. Cover and refrigerate for 2 to 4 hours.

One hour before cooking the chicken, begin to prepare the lentils. Heat the olive oil in a medium (3-quart) saucepan. Add the onion and garlic and sauté over medium-high heat for 2 to 3 minutes, stirring constantly. Add the carrots and celery and sauté for 5 minutes more, or until slightly softened.

Add the lentils and stir to coat with oil, then add the chicken broth, chipotle puree, coriander, and salt. Bring to a boil, then reduce the heat and simmer for 45 to 50 minutes, or until the lentils are tender and most of the liquid has been absorbed. Add water if additional liquid is needed. Remove from the heat and stir in the parsley.

To cook the chicken breasts, preheat the oven to 350 degrees F. Bake the chicken, uncovered, for 25 to 30 minutes, or until the juices run clear. Remove from the oven and let rest for 5 minutes.

Divide the lentils among 4 dinner plates. Slice each chicken breast into 4 slices and fan out over the lentils.

*Note:* Pureed chipotle pepper is available at gourmet specialty stores and some supermarkets.

---

- Chicken is potentially a very good source of selenium.
- Each serving provides more than 150% of the DV for vitamin A and 50% of the DV for vitamin C.
- Lentils are a very good source of folate, providing more than 90% of the DV per serving.
- Very high in fiber—each serving provides more than 80% of the DV.

---

*Per serving of Middle Eastern Chicken Breasts:*

| calories | protein | carbohydrates | fat | cholesterol | dietary fiber | saturated fat |
|---|---|---|---|---|---|---|
| 344 | 55 Gm | 6 Gm | 10 Gm | 143 mg | 1 Gm | 2 Gm |

*Per serving of Smoky Lentils:*

| calories | protein | carbohydrates | fat | cholesterol | dietary fiber | saturated fat |
|---|---|---|---|---|---|---|
| 303 | 22 Gm | 50 Gm | 3 Gm | 0 mg | 20 Gm | 0 Gm |

*Per serving of Middle Eastern Chicken Breasts with Smoky Lentils:*

| calories | protein | carbohydrates | fat | cholesterol | dietary fiber | saturated fat |
|---|---|---|---|---|---|---|
| 647 | 77 Gm | 56 Gm | 13 Gm | 143 mg | 21 Gm | 2 Gm |

**% of Calories**: 35% carbohydrate, 47% protein, 18% fat

### Major Sources of Potential Cancer Fighters

**Phytochemicals**: allium compounds, capsaicin, phytic acids, plant polyphenols (flavonoids), protease inhibitors, terpenes (carotenoids, monoterpenes)

# ❧ Chicken Cacciatore ❧

### 4 SERVINGS

• *In this quick and healthful "one-pot meal," the chicken becomes very tender when braised in the flavorful vegetable stew.*

| | | | |
|---|---|---|---|
| 4 | split boneless, skinless chicken breasts (1½ pounds), all visible fat removed | 1 | garlic clove, minced |
| | salt and pepper | 1 | tablespoon flour |
| 1 | tablespoon olive oil | ¼ | cup white wine or 2 tablespoons white wine vinegar plus 2 tablespoons water |
| 1 | medium onion (about 6 ounces), halved and sliced | 14½ | ounces canned stewed tomatoes |
| 1 | large green pepper (about 8 ounces), seeded and cut into long, thin strips | 1 | cup domestic mushrooms (about 2½ ounces), sliced |
| 2 | medium celery stalks (about 3 ounces), chopped | 1 | teaspoon grated lemon zest |
| 2 | medium carrots (about 5 ounces), peeled and sliced ¼ inch thick | 2 | tablespoons chopped fresh Italian parsley |

Season the chicken with salt and pepper. Heat the olive oil in a medium nonstick saucepan or casserole and sauté the chicken over medium-high heat until nicely browned on both sides. Remove and reserve.

In the same pan, sauté the onion, pepper, celery, carrots, and garlic over medium heat for 10 minutes; stir frequently. Sprinkle the flour over the vegetables and stir to evenly incorporate the flour into the vegetables—there should be no lumps or large particles.

Add the white wine and stir to dissolve all particles on the bottom of the pan. Add the tomatoes, mushrooms, lemon zest, and salt and pepper to taste; stir the mixture well. Bring to a boil, then reduce the heat, so that the mixture simmers.

Return the chicken breasts to the pan and braise, covered, until the chicken is done, about 15 minutes.

Place the chicken breasts into large shallow soup bowls and spoon the sauce and vegetables over the top. Garnish with parsley.

- Both chicken and mushrooms are potentially good sources of selenium.
- Using grated citrus zest (or peel) in cooking is recommended. Limonene, a phytochemical that may help your body eliminate carcinogens, is found in the peel.
- One serving provides more than 110% of the DV for vitamin A, 100% of the DV for vitamin C, and 10% of the DV for folate.
- A good source of fiber.

*Per serving:*

| calories | protein | carbohydrates | fat | cholesterol | dietary fiber | saturated fat |
|----------|---------|---------------|-----|-------------|---------------|---------------|
| 404 | 55 Gm | 20 Gm | 10 Gm | 143 mg | 4 Gm | 2 Gm |

**% of Calories**: 20% carbohydrate, 55% protein, 22% fat, 3% alcohol

**Major Sources of Potential Cancer Fighters**
**Phytochemicals**: allium compounds, plant polyphenols (flavonoids, phenolic acids), plant sterols, terpenes (carotenoids, monoterpenes)

# ❧ *Veggie-packed Chicken Pot Pie* ❧

## 4 SERVINGS

- *This version is rich and creamy, but contains almost half the fat of traditional chicken pot pie.*
- *A great way to introduce new vegetables to kids.*
- *Use the Olive Oil Pastry for other savory recipes that call for a crust.*

### Olive Oil Pastry

| | | | |
|---|---|---|---|
| 1 | cup flour | 2 | tablespoons olive oil |
| 1/4 | teaspoon salt | 1 | large egg, beaten |

### Filling

1 tablespoon olive oil

1 small onion (about 4 ounces), chopped

1 large celery stalk (about 2 ounces), sliced

2 small carrots (about 5 ounces), peeled and cut into small cubes

3 cups chicken stock (page 147 or 148) or low-sodium canned broth

1 medium potato (about 6 ounces), peeled and cut into medium-size cubes

1   small sweet potato (about       4   teaspoons cornstarch
    6 ounces), peeled and cut into    1/2   cup plus 1 tablespoon evaporated
    medium-size cubes                     skim milk
1   medium turnip (about 5 ounces),   2   tablespoons chopped parsley
    peeled and cut into small cubes   3/4   cup frozen peas, thawed, or
12   ounces boneless, skinless            fresh, removed from pod
    chicken breast, trimmed of all    salt and pepper
    visible fat and cut into
    small strips

Preheat the oven to 400 degrees F.

To make the pastry, in the bowl of a food processor, combine the flour and salt. Pulse quickly to evenly combine. Add the olive oil and pulse again for 2 to 3 seconds. Add 1 tablespoon water and the egg and turn on the processor for about 10 seconds. At this point the pastry dough should be crumbly but moist. Remove the dough from the food processor bowl and compact it to form a disk (do not knead). Wrap in plastic wrap or wax paper and let the dough rest in the refrigerator for at least 30 minutes. (Resting is especially important for low-fat doughs; it relaxes the gluten that can make the dough tough and chewy.)

Cut the pastry dough into quarters. Place the quarters of pastry dough between two sheets of plastic wrap or in the center of 4 large plastic bags. Flatten the dough, then, making circular motions with the palm of your hand, spread out the dough evenly to form 1/8- to 1/4-inch-thick circles large enough to cover the tops of ramekins (an individual baking dish usually made of porcelain or earthenware). Put the dough in the refrigerator for at least 5 minutes—this will make it easier to peel the plastic wrap from the dough.

To make the filling, in a large nonstick (or heavy-bottomed) saucepan, heat the olive oil and sauté the onion on medium heat until limp but not browned. Add the celery and carrots and sauté for 5 minutes more. Pour the chicken stock into the pan and bring to a boil, then reduce the heat so that the mixture simmers. Add the potatoes, sweet potato, and turnip and cook, covered, until the vegetables are just cooked but still slightly firm, about 15 minutes, depending on the size of the cut vegetables. Strain the broth from the vegetables, placing the broth back into the saucepan and dividing the vegetables between 4 8-ounce ramekins or oven-proof casseroles. Add the chicken to the broth and simmer until the chicken is just barely cooked through. Dilute the cornstarch in 1/2 cup evaporated skim milk and stir until well combined; add to the saucepan. While stirring, bring to a full boil for 4 minutes to cook the starch and thicken the sauce. Remove from the heat; stir in the parsley and peas, and season to taste with salt and pepper.

Divide the chicken and thickened broth among the ramekins with vegetables. Place circles of dough over the filled ramekins and press to form a tight seal. Place the ramekins on a baking sheet and brush the surface with the remaining evaporated milk. Bake at 400 degrees F until the crust becomes golden brown, about 15 minutes.

- These pot pies are rich in cancer-protective vitamins; one serving provides more than 125% of the DV for vitamin A and 40% of the DV for vitamin C. They also contain cancer-protective cruciferous vegetables (turnips) and onions, and are rich in beta-carotene and other carotenoids.
- Olive oil, rich in protective monounsaturated fatty acids, provides more than 75% of the fat in this recipe.
- A potentially good source of selenium.
- High in fiber—21% of the DV per serving.

*Per serving:*

| calories | protein | carbohydrates | fat | cholesterol | dietary fiber | saturated fat |
|---|---|---|---|---|---|---|
| 508 | 38 Gm | 53 Gm | 16 Gm | 128 mg | 5 Gm | 3 Gm |

**% of Calories**: 42% carbohydrate, 30% protein, 28% fat

### Major Sources of Potential Cancer Fighters

**Phytochemicals**: allium compounds, glucosinolates, plant polyphenols (flavonoids, phenolic acids), terpenes (carotenoids, monoterpenes)

# ❧ Turkey Steaks with ❧ Grape and Currant Sauce

Jacques Pépin, Dean of Special Studies, The French Culinary Institute, New York, New York
Reprinted from *Jacques Pépin's Simple and Healthy Cooking*, copyright 1994 by Jacques Pépin. Permission granted by Rodale Press, Inc., Emmaus, PA 18098. For ordering information, please call 1-800-848-4735.

6 SERVINGS

- *Jacques recommends serving this as a dinner party entrée. He suggests either buying a whole turkey breast and cutting it into 1/2-inch steaks or asking your butcher to do it for you.*

6 turkey breast steaks (6 ounces each and about $^1/_2$ inch thick)

2 tablespoons extra virgin olive oil

1 small leek (3 to 4 ounces), trimmed, chopped, and washed

1 medium onion (4 ounces), peeled and chopped

$^1/_4$ cup balsamic vinegar

$^1/_4$ cup red wine vinegar

$1^1/_2$ cups brown chicken stock (page 148)

$2^1/_2$ cups seedless grapes

$^1/_4$ cup dried currants

$^1/_2$ teaspoon sea salt

$^1/_4$ teaspoon freshly ground black pepper

2 tablespoons chopped fresh chives

Preheat the oven to 180 degrees F.

Season the turkey steaks with salt and pepper. Heat the olive oil in a very large, heavy skillet set over high heat. When the oil is hot, add the turkey steaks and cook them for 2 to 3 minutes on each side. They will be slightly undercooked at this point; transfer them to a gratin dish and place them in the oven while you make the sauce. (They can wait there up to 30 minutes.)

Add the leek and onion to the skillet and sauté them for 2 minutes. Add the balsamic vinegar and red wine vinegar; cook until they have almost evaporated.

Add the chicken stock, grapes, currants, salt, pepper, and any juices that have accumulated around the turkey steaks in the oven. Boil for 2 to 3 minutes, until the sauce thickens slightly.

Arrange the turkey steaks on a platter, cover them with the sauce, and sprinkle the chives on top. Serve.

---

- Turkey breast is very low in fat, and with the flavorful Grape and Currant Sauce, very moist. Turkey is also a potentially very good source of selenium.
- The skins of currants and grapes contain flavonoids, which act as potent antioxidants and may boost enzymes that help rid the body of carcinogens.
- Each serving provides 10% of the DV for vitamin C.

---

*Per serving:*

| calories | protein | carbohydrates | fat | cholesterol | dietary fiber | saturated fat |
|----------|---------|---------------|------|-------------|---------------|---------------|
| 288 | 44 Gm | 18 Gm | 4 Gm | 108 mg | 2 Gm | 1 Gm |

**% of Calories**: 25% carbohydrate, 62% protein, 13% fat

### Major Sources of Potential Cancer Fighters

**Phytochemicals**: allium compounds, plant polyphenols (flavonoids, phenolic acids)

# ❧ Smothered Boneless Pork ❧ Chops with Lentils

Frank Brigtsen, Brigtsen's, New Orleans, Louisiana

4 SERVINGS

• *Frank explains that the term "smothered" is a method of cooking whereby food is braised with moist heat. After browning meat in its own fat or a small amount of added fat, liquid and seasonings are added. Long, slow cooking softens the meat and develops flavor.*

| | |
|---|---|
| 1/2 cup dried lentils (3 ounces) | 1/2 teaspoon salt |
| 4 teaspoons olive oil | 1/8 teaspoon freshly ground white pepper |
| 1/2 cup plus 2 tablespoons carrots, peeled and cut into 1/4-inch dice | 1/8 teaspoon freshly ground black pepper |
| 1/2 cup plus 2 tablespoons celery, cut into 1/4-inch dice | 3 cups chicken stock (page 147 or 148), low-sodium canned broth, or water |
| 2/3 cup plus 2 tablespoons onions, cut into 1/4-inch dice | 4 4-ounce lean center-cut pork chops, trimmed of all visible fat |
| 1 1/2 teaspoons minced garlic | |
| 1 bay leaf | salt and freshly ground black pepper |
| 1/8 teaspoon dried whole leaf thyme | |
| 1/8 teaspoon dried whole leaf oregano | 1/4 teaspoon Tabasco |
| 1/4 teaspoon dried whole leaf summer savory | |

Soak the lentils in water to cover for 1 hour; drain.

Heat 2 teaspoons of the olive oil in a 2-quart saucepan and add 1/2 cup carrots, 1/2 cup celery, and 2/3 cup onions. Cook the vegetables, stirring often, over moderate heat until they begin to brown, 12 to 15 minutes. Add another teaspoon of olive oil, the garlic, bay leaf, thyme, oregano, and summer savory and season with 1/2 teaspoon salt, 1/8 teaspoon white pepper, and 1/8 teaspoon black pepper. Continue cooking, stirring constantly, until the mixture is well browned but not burnt.

Add the stock or water and bring the mixture to a boil. Add the lentils and reduce to a simmer for 15 minutes. Add the remaining 2 tablespoons of carrot, celery, and onion, and continue to cook.

Meanwhile, season the pork chops with salt and black pepper. Heat a 12-inch cast-iron skillet with the remaining teaspoon of oil over medium-high heat. When hot, add the pork chops and brown on both sides. Reduce the heat to medium-low and add the lentils and Tabasco. Simmer, uncovered, for 10 to 15 minutes, or until the pork is cooked and the lentils are tender.

Place 1 pork chop on each plate and top with the lentils.

---

- Lean cuts of pork, such as center cut loin chops, can contain less than 1.5 Gm fat per ounce.
- Both pork and lentils are potentially good sources of selenium.
- This recipe is rich in the cancer-protective vitamins A, C, and folate, providing more than 90%, 15%, and 30% of the DVs, respectively.
- High in fiber—37% of the DV per serving.

---

**Per serving:**

| calories | protein | carbohydrates | fat | cholesterol | dietary fiber | saturated fat |
|----------|---------|---------------|-----|-------------|---------------|---------------|
| 353 | 36 Gm | 22 Gm | 13 Gm | 60 mg | 9 Gm | 3 Gm |

**% of Calories:** 25% carbohydrate, 41% protein, 34% fat

### Major Sources of Potential Cancer Fighters
**Phytochemicals**: allium compounds, phytic acids, plant polyphenols (flavonoids), protease inhibitors, terpenes (carotenoids, monoterpenes)

---

# ❧ Marinated Pork Tenderloin with ❧ Smashed Orange-scented Sweet Potatoes

Gianni Scappin, Maximillian, New York, New York; Trattoria alla Pesa, Mason Vicentino, Veneto, Italy

8 SERVINGS

- *The tenderloin of pork has less than 1.5 grams of fat per cooked ounce (less than a chicken breast), so take a break from chicken and incorporate some variety into your protein selections.*
- *Marinade combinations for pork tenderloin are limitless, making it a very versatile lean meat selection. (See Note for Chef Scappin's marinade suggestions.)*
- *Serve with Sweet and Sour Cabbage, page 181.*

*Pork*

| | | | |
|---|---|---|---|
| 2 | large shallots (about 2 ounces), sliced | 1/2 | teaspoon cracked or coarsely ground black peppercorns |
| 5 | garlic cloves, crushed | 2 | fresh rosemary sprigs |
| 2 | tablespoons tamari (Japanese soy sauce) | 1 | fresh thyme sprig |
| 1 | tablespoon Dijon mustard | 2 | pork tenderloins (about 2 1/2 pounds), trimmed of all visible fat |
| 1 | tablespoon sherry vinegar | | salt and pepper |
| 1 | tablespoon canola olive oil | | |
| 1/2 | tablespoon honey | | |

*Smashed Orange-scented Sweet Potatoes*

| | | | |
|---|---|---|---|
| 8 | medium sweet potatoes (about 3 1/2 pounds) | | grated zest of 2 oranges (orange part only) |
| | salt | 1 | tablespoon olive oil |
| | pinch cinnamon | | |

To prepare the marinade, in a rectangular dish, combine the shallots, garlic, tamari, mustard, sherry vinegar, canola oil, honey, 2 tablespoons water, and the cracked pepper. Stir to combine, then add the rosemary and thyme sprigs.

Place the pork tenderloins into the marinade, rolling to make sure they are well coated. Cover with plastic wrap and refrigerate for at least 1 hour. (You can marinate the pork a day in advance.)

Preheat the oven to 350 degrees F. Prick the potatoes with a fork and place on top of a sheet of foil in the oven for 60 to 70 minutes, or until very tender. Remove and set aside to cool slightly. Turn the oven temperature up to 375 degrees F.

When the potatoes are almost cooked, begin cooking the pork tenderloin. Wipe the marinade off the pork loin and season with salt and pepper. Heat a large cast-iron or non-stick oven-safe skillet (with a metal handle for transfer into the oven). When hot, sear the pork, browning all sides evenly. Transfer the pan to the oven and cook until pork is only slightly pink in the center, about 12 to 15 minutes. Remove the tenderloin from the pan and place on a plate to rest for 5 minutes. Loosely cover with a piece of foil paper to keep hot.

Remove any fat from the bottom of the sauté pan. Place the sauté pan over medium heat and add 1/3 cup water (or white wine or veal or chicken stock) while stirring with a wooden spoon to dissolve all particles on the bottom of the pan. Set aside.

Peel the sweet potatoes and put the flesh in a medium bowl. Add the salt, cinnamon, orange zest, and olive oil. Whip with an electric mixer or wooden spoon until well combined. Season to taste with salt.

Spoon the sweet potatoes slightly above the center of each plate. Slice the pork tenderloins into 3/4-inch slices on the bias and fan out four slices in front of the sweet potatoes on each plate (about 5 ounces cooked pork). Top the pork slices with the reserved juices from the sauté pan.

*Note:* Gianni Scappin suggests other marinade combinations:

- 1 tablespoon tamari or teriyaki, 1 teaspoon sesame oil, 2 teaspoons canola oil, grated zest of 1/2 orange or 1 whole lemon or lime, pinch coriander, 1 tablespoon of rice wine vinegar, 2 tablespoons water, and a sprinkle of brown sugar
- grated zest from 1 lemon, 1 tablespoon olive oil, 2 teaspoons herbes de Provence, 3 tablespoons orange juice.

These marinade combinations may also be used for lean pork loin chops.

---

- Fresh rosemary not only adds a wonderful flavor dimension to roasted meat, fish, and vegetables, but also contains carnosol, a potent antioxidant.
- Pork is a potentially good source of selenium.
- Sweet potatoes are rich in both beta-carotene and flavor. To maximize sweetness, roast the potatoes at a lower temperature for a longer time and let them cool slightly in their skins before serving.
- Provides almost 250% of the DV for vitamin A and more than 50% for vitamin C.
- A good source of fiber.

---

*Per serving of 5 ounces Marinated Pork Tenderloin with natural juices:*

| calories | protein | carbohydrates | fat | cholesterol | dietary fiber | saturated fat |
|---|---|---|---|---|---|---|
| 261 | 40 Gm | 2 Gm | 9 Gm | 112 mg | 0 Gm | 3 Gm |

*Per serving of Smashed Orange-scented Sweet Potatoes:*

| calories | protein | carbohydrates | fat | cholesterol | dietary fiber | saturated fat |
|---|---|---|---|---|---|---|
| 133 | 2 Gm | 28 Gm | 2 Gm | 0 mg | 3 Gm | 0 Gm |

*Per serving of Marinated Pork Tenderloin with Smashed Orange-scented Sweet Potatoes:*

| calories | protein | carbohydrates | fat | cholesterol | dietary fiber | saturated fat |
|---|---|---|---|---|---|---|
| 394 | 42 Gm | 30 Gm | 11 Gm | 112 mg | 3 Gm | 3 Gm |

**% of Calories**: 31% carbohydrate, 44% protein, 25% fat

**Major Sources of Potential Cancer Fighters**
**Phytochemicals**: allium compounds, plant polyphenols (flavonoids), terpenes (carnosol, carotenoids, limonene)

# ❧ *Venison Medallions in Tamarind* ❧ *with Creamy Horseradish Mashed Potatoes*

Adam Busby, Director of Culinary Programs, Dubrulle Culinary School,
Vancouver, British Columbia, Canada

4 SERVINGS

• *Venison is a very lean red meat alternative. It cooks quickly and easily and stands up to intense flavors, such as the tamarind and horseradish in this recipe.*

• *The creamy low-fat mashed potatoes can be made with or without horseradish and served with many other dishes.*

### Creamy Horseradish Mashed Potatoes

| | | | | |
|---|---|---|---|---|
| 4 | medium potatoes (about 1 pound) | | 1 | tablespoon creamed horseradish |
| 1/2 | cup 2% milk | | 1 | tablespoon extra virgin olive oil |
| | | | | salt and pepper |

### Venison

| | | | | |
|---|---|---|---|---|
| 2 | tablespoons tamarind concentrate (see Note) | | 2 | teaspoons peanut oil |
| | | | | salt |
| 2 | venison tenderloins (about 20 ounces), cut into 8 equal-size medallions | | 1 | tablespoon crushed black peppercorns |
| | | | 1 | teaspoon aged balsamic vinegar |

To make the mashed potatoes, boil the potatoes in salted water until tender, about 20 minutes. Drain, peel, and pass through a food mill into a medium bowl (if you do not have a food mill, mash the potatoes with a fork or potato masher).

Heat the milk in a small saucepan until very warm. Add to the potatoes with the horseradish. Whip rapidly with an electric mixer (or wooden spoon), and slowly add the olive oil.

Season to taste with salt and pepper. If the potatoes are done before the venison, place wax paper directly on the surface of the potatoes to keep heat in and prevent a skin from forming.

To make the venison, whisk the tamarind concentrate and 1/4 cup hot water together until smooth. Set aside.

Press the pieces of venison down with the palm of your hand to form 2-inch-thick round medallions. Brush the medallions with the peanut oil and season with salt and crushed peppercorns. Heat a large nonstick or cast-iron pan; when hot, sear the medallions over medium heat until nicely browned on each side, then turn down the heat to medium and cook until medium-rare, about 5 minutes.

Transfer the venison to a plate and add the tamarind mixture to the sauté pan. Turn off the heat and stir with a wooden spoon to remove all flavorful particles from the bottom of the pan. Add any juices released from the venison to the sauté pan.

Place a mound of horseradish mashed potatoes in the center of each plate. Rest 2 medallions against the mashed potatoes with tops slightly crossing. Spoon the tamarind sauce over the venison and then drizzle with aged balsamic vinegar.

*Note:* Tamarind is a large bean pod native to Asia, India, and North Africa. The pulp, which is concentrated into a paste, is sweet and sour and is used in full-flavored foods, such as chutneys, relishes, and marinades. It is available at Indian and Asian markets and some gourmet specialty stores. If you cannot find tamarind, substitute hoisin sauce, a spicy-sweet sauce made from Asian spices and ground soybeans.

---

- Mashed potatoes provide more than 10% of the DV of vitamin C per serving.
- Horseradish contains cancer protective glucosinolates and kaempferol, a flavonoid.

---

*Per serving of Creamy Horseradish Mashed Potatoes:*

| calories | protein | carbohydrates | fat | cholesterol | dietary fiber | saturated fat |
|---|---|---|---|---|---|---|
| 142 | 3 Gm | 22 Gm | 5 Gm | 4 mg | 0 Gm | 1 Gm |

*Per serving of Venison Medallions with Tamarind Sauce:*

| calories | protein | carbohydrates | fat | cholesterol | dietary fiber | saturated fat |
|---|---|---|---|---|---|---|
| 203 | 32 Gm | 3 Gm | 6 Gm | 118 mg | 0 Gm | 1 Gm |

*Per serving of Venison Medallions in Tamarind with Creamy Horseradish Mashed Potatoes:*

| calories | protein | carbohydrates | fat | cholesterol | dietary fiber | saturated fat |
|---|---|---|---|---|---|---|
| 345 | 35 Gm | 26 Gm | 11 Gm | 122 mg | 0 Gm | 2 Gm |

**% of Calories**: 30% carbohydrate, 42% protein, 28% fat

### Major Sources of Potential Cancer Fighters

**Phytochemicals**: allium compounds, glucosinolates, plant polyphenols (flavonoids, phenolic acids)

# ❧ Roasted Boned Quail ❧ with Dungeness Crab

Adam Busby, Director of Culinary Programs, Dubrulle Culinary School,
Vancouver, British Columbia, Canada

4 SERVINGS

• *Quail are game birds with a fairly low fat content. If bought already boned they are very easy to prepare.*

• *This crab filling is also perfect for crab cakes: simply form patties and sauté them in 1 teaspoon of oil heated in a nonstick sauté pan.*

## Crab Filling

| | | | |
|---|---|---|---|
| 10 | ounces Dungeness or other lump crabmeat, cooked | 1/2 | cup fine bread crumbs, unseasoned |
| 1/4 | cup chopped cilantro | 2 | tablespoons lemon juice |
| 2 | teaspoons Dijon mustard | 1 | egg, beaten |
| 1/4 | cup low-fat mayonnaise | | salt and white pepper |
| 1/4 | cup fat-free sour cream | | |

## Quail

| | | | |
|---|---|---|---|
| 4 | quail, whole, boned but not split | 1 | teaspoon melted butter |
| | | | salt and freshly ground pepper |
| 1 | tablespoon honey | 2 | tablespoons white wine |
| 1 | teaspoon Dijon mustard | 1 | teaspoon butter |

Preheat the oven to 400 degrees F.

To prepare the crab filling, in a mixing bowl, combine all ingredients and season with salt and white pepper. Set aside.

To stuff the quail, place the neck side down in the palm of your hand. With your other hand, open the legs and fill the cavity with the crab. Cross the legs and fit the stuffed quail neatly into an 8-inch oven-safe, nonstick skillet.

In a small bowl, combine the honey, mustard, and melted butter. Brush the quail with the honey-mustard mixture and season with salt and pepper. Roast for 18 to 20 minutes. Remove the skillet from the oven, transfer the quail to a clean plate, cover loosely with foil wrap, and let rest for 2 to 3 minutes.

Over medium heat, add the white wine to the skillet used for roasting quail. Stir with a wooden spoon, scraping to dissolve any particles from the bottom. Add 2 table-spoons water and any juice released from the quail, and simmer for less than 1 minute. Turn off the heat and stir in the butter. Place the quail in the center of 4 plates and pour pan juices over the top.

---

- The natural gums and pectins found in most fat-free sour creams are useful to help bind ingredients in cooking while also adding creaminess without fat.
- Crab is a potentially good source of selenium.
- One serving provides 10% of the DV for vitamins A and folate.

---

*Per serving of Crab Filling (4 ounces):*

| calories | protein | carbohydrates | fat | cholesterol | dietary fiber | saturated fat |
|----------|---------|---------------|-----|-------------|---------------|---------------|
| 179 | 17 Gm | 18 Gm | 4 Gm | 95 mg | 1 Gm | 1 Gm |

*Per serving of Roasted Boned Quail with Dungeness Crab:*

| calories | protein | carbohydrates | fat | cholesterol | dietary fiber | saturated fat |
|----------|---------|---------------|-----|-------------|---------------|---------------|
| 268 | 30 Gm | 23Gm | 6 Gm | 130 mg | 1 Gm | 2 Gm |

**% of Calories**: 34% carbohydrate, 45% protein, 21% fat

**Major Sources of Potential Cancer Fighters**
**Phytochemicals**: plant sterols, terpenes (monoterpenes)

---

# ❧ Grilled Ostrich Fillet ❧
## with Blueberry Barbecue Sauce
## and Garlic Mashed Potatoes

Robert McGrath, Windows on the Green, Phoenix, Arizona

4 SERVINGS

- *Ostrich is a very lean red meat alternative to beef. Although its flavor is full, it is not "gamey."*
- *The Blueberry Barbecue Sauce is lower in fat and higher in nutrients than traditional barbecue sauce. Use it in place of standard barbecue sauce for other grilled or seared meats or chicken.*
- *Serve these vegetable-fortified mashed potatoes with other full-flavored entrées.*

*Blueberry Barbecue Sauce*

| | | | |
|---|---|---|---|
| 1 | teaspoon olive oil | 1½ | tablespoons brown sugar |
| ¼ | cup onions, finely diced | 1 | tablespoon Dijon mustard |
| 1 | tablespoon jalapeño pepper, seeded and diced | ¼ | cup water |
| 1 | pint fresh blueberries | 1 | teaspoon butter |
| 2 | tablespoons rice wine vinegar | | salt and pepper |

*Garlic Mashed Potatoes*

| | | | |
|---|---|---|---|
| 2 | large potatoes (about 1 pound), peeled, cut into cubes | ¼ | cup fresh sweet corn or frozen, thawed and drained |
| ¼ | cup roasted garlic, (page 178) | 2 | tablespoons diced red bell pepper |
| ¼ | cup 2% milk | 2 | tablespoons diced green bell pepper |
| ¼ | cup fat-free sour cream | 2 | tablespoons diced red onion |
| 1 | tablespoon butter | | salt and pepper |

*Ostrich*

| | | | |
|---|---|---|---|
| 4 | 6-ounce ostrich fillets | | salt and pepper |
| 1 | teaspoon canola oil | ¼ | cup blueberries (for garnish) |

To prepare the sauce, in a medium nonstick skillet, sauté the onions and jalapeño in olive oil over medium-high heat until limp, 2 to 3 minutes. Add the remaining ingredients, except the butter, and cook at a low boil for 15 minutes, stirring often. Puree the sauce in a blender or food processor until smooth. Strain through a fine mesh strainer, using a rubber spatula to push as much sauce as possible through the mesh. Return the sauce to clean sauté pan, reheat, adjust seasoning with salt and pepper and stir in the butter just before serving.

To prepare the potatoes, preheat the oven to 400 degrees F. Bring 3 quarts of salted water to a boil, add the potatoes, and cook until tender when pierced with a knife, 15 to 20 minutes. Drain thoroughly. Spread the potatoes in a single layer on a nonstick baking pan and roast for 8 minutes. Remove the potatoes from the oven and place in a medium bowl. Using a kitchen mixer or handheld mixer, begin whipping the potatoes while gradually adding the milk, sour cream, butter, and roasted garlic. Stop mixing when all ingredients have been well incorporated and the potatoes are creamy. Fold in the vegetables and season with salt and pepper. Place a piece of waxpaper directly on the surface of the potatoes to keep heat in and prevent a skin from forming. Set aside.

To grill or sear the ostrich fillets, preheat the grill to medium heat, about 10 minutes.

Brush the fillets with canola oil and season with salt and pepper. Grill to desired doneness, about 2 to 3 minutes on each side for medium-rare, depending on the thickness of the fillets. To sear the fillets, instead of grilling, heat the canola oil in a medium nonstick skillet, and when almost smoking add the fillets. Brown on all sides, lower the heat, and cook to desired doneness.

Spoon a mound of mashed potatoes onto the center of the plate. Slice each fillet into 4 slices and fan out in front of the mashed potatoes. Spoon the blueberry barbecue sauce over the ostrich. Sprinkle blueberries around the perimeter.

---

- Blueberries and potatoes are rich in vitamin C, providing 70% of the DV per serving. Blueberries also contain ellagic acid, a phytochemical, that may help boost enzymes that rid the body of cancer-causing substances.
- Each serving provides more than 110% of the DV for vitamin A
- A good source of fiber.

---

*Per serving of Blueberry Barbecue Sauce (1/4 cup):*

| calories | protein | carbohydrates | fat | cholesterol | dietary fiber | saturated fat |
|---|---|---|---|---|---|---|
| 115 | 1 Gm | 18 Gm | 5 Gm | 3 mg | 4 Gm | 1 Gm |

*Per serving of Garlic Mashed Potatoes:*

| calories | protein | carbohydrates | fat | cholesterol | dietary fiber | saturated fat |
|---|---|---|---|---|---|---|
| 161 | 5 Gm | 29 Gm | 4 Gm | 9 mg | 2 Gm | 2 Gm |

*Per serving of Grilled Ostrich Fillet with Blueberry Barbecue Sauce and Garlic Mashed Potatoes:*

| calories | protein | carbohydrates | fat | cholesterol | dietary fiber | saturated fat |
|---|---|---|---|---|---|---|
| 513 | 41 Gm | 47 Gm | 18 Gm | 162 mg | 5 Gm | 6 Gm |

**% of Calories**: 34% carbohydrate, 34% protein, 32% fat

### Major Sources of Potential Cancer Fighters

**Phytochemicals:** allium compounds, plant polyphenols (flavonoids, phenolic acids), terpenes (carotenoids)

# ❦ *Medallions of Antelope* ❦ *with Wild Blueberry Sauce*

Roberto Donna, Galileo, Washington, D.C.

4 SERVINGS

- *As this low-fat red meat becomes more popular on restaurant menus, it has become available at specialty stores and by mail-order.*
- *Lean game such as venison, buffalo, ostrich, or quail also works nicely with this blueberry sauce.*
- *Serve with mashed potatoes or Smashed Orange-scented Sweet Potatoes, page 251.*

| | |
|---|---|
| 1 pint wild blueberries | 1 tablespoon cognac (optional; see Note) |
| 1/4 cup sugar | |
| 1 1/2 pounds antelope loin, cut into 8 2 1/2-inch-thick medallions | 2 tablespoons gin (optional; see Note) |
| salt and pepper | 1 cup brown stock, such as chicken, veal, or beef |
| 2 teaspoons olive oil | |

In a medium sauté pan, cook the blueberries with 2 tablespoons water for 10 minutes over medium-high heat, until they reduce to a syrupy consistency. Add the sugar and cook on low heat for 10 minutes more. Set aside to cool.

While the blueberry sauce is cooking, cook the antelope. Season the medallions on both sides with salt and pepper. In a nonstick pan, heat the olive oil over high heat. When almost smoking, add the medallions and cook until both sides are a rich brown color. Turn down the heat to medium, and cook to medium-rare, another 2 minutes per side, and transfer to a large plate. (Because antelope is a very lean meat it will become tough if overcooked.)

Pour any excess fat out of the sauté pan. Away from the stove, carefully pour the cognac and gin into the pan, stirring with a wooden spoon to "deglaze" or remove the flavorful particles from the bottom. Return the pan to medium heat and reduce until most of the alcohol has cooked off, then add the stock and bring to a simmer. Reduce the volume by half. Stir in any juice released from the cooked medallions and the reserved wild blueberry syrup. Adjust the seasoning with salt and pepper.

Place the medallions, slightly overlapping, in the center of each plate and sprinkle with a few wild blueberries. Top with the blueberry sauce.

*Note:* If you omit the cognac and gin, add stock to the sauté pan after you pour off the excess fat.

---

- Blueberries are a good source of vitamin C and also contain ellagic acid, a phytochemical that may help boost enzymes that may rid the body of cancer-causing substances.
- Antelope has only 0.5 Gm of fat per ounce; skinless, roasted chicken breast has 1 Gm of fat per ounce.

---

*Per serving:*

| calories | protein | carbohydrates | fat | cholesterol | dietary fiber | saturated fat |
|----------|---------|---------------|-----|-------------|---------------|---------------|
| 315 | 35 Gm | 24 Gm | 7 Gm | 146 mg | 2 Gm | 2 Gm |

**% of Calories:** 30% carbohydrate, 46% protein, 19% fat, 5% alcohol

**Major Sources of Potential Cancer Fighters**

**Phytochemicals:** plant polyphenols (flavonoids, phenolic acids), terpenes (carotenoids)

# BREADS

## ❧ *Whole Wheat Rosemary Rolls* ❧

### 24 ROLLS

• *These fragrant rolls can be served with lamb, lean beef, hearty stews, and spicy grilled or roasted chicken. They also make a great bread for a small sandwich, such as smoked turkey with a fruit chutney.*

| | | | | |
|---|---|---|---|---|
| 1 1/2 | packages active dry yeast | | 5 | cups whole wheat flour |
| 3 | cups lukewarm water | | 2 1/2 | cups all-purpose flour |
| 1/4 | cup olive oil | | 1 | tablespoon plus 1 teaspoon salt |
| 1/4 | cup honey | | | |
| 3 | tablespoons chopped fresh rosemary or 1 tablespoon dried | | | |

In a large mixing bowl, stir the yeast into 1/2 cup of the warm water; let stand until frothy and creamy, about 8 minutes. Stir in the remaining water, oil, honey, and rosemary. Add the flours and salt gradually to the yeast mixture. Work the flour into the dough, then remove the dough from the bowl and place on a work surface lightly dusted with flour. Knead for 10 minutes, until the dough is smooth and springs back when gently pressed.

Place the dough in a lightly greased bowl, cover tightly with plastic wrap, and let rise in a warm (but not hot) place until doubled in size, about 1 hour and 10 minutes.

Punch down the dough and shape into 24 rolls, placing them under a clean cloth as they are made to prevent them from drying out. Place the rolls about 1/2 inch apart on a lightly oiled or sprayed baking pan. Place a towel over the rolls and let them rise again until almost doubled in size, 20 to 30 minutes.

Preheat the oven to 400 degrees F. Bake the rolls for 20 to 25 minutes on the middle rack of the oven. They should be lightly browned. Let cool slightly on a wire rack. Break the rolls apart and serve warm or at room temperature.

> • Carnosol, a phytochemical in rosemary, is a potent antioxidant and may also help increase cancer-fighting enzymes in the body.
> • Whole grains, as well as some types of beans and seeds, contain phytic acids, phytochemicals that may help reduce oxidative damage to the body.
> • A good source of fiber.

Per roll:

| calories | protein | carbohydrates | fat | cholesterol | dietary fiber | saturated fat |
|----------|---------|---------------|-----|-------------|---------------|---------------|
| 155 | 5 Gm | 28 Gm | 3 Gm | 0 mg | 4 Gm | 1 Gm |

**% of Calories**: 72% carbohydrate, 12% protein, 16% fat

**Major Sources of Potential Cancer Fighters**
**Phytochemicals:** phytic acids, plant polyphenols (flavonoids), protease inhibitors, terpenes (carnosol)

# ✧ Sunflower and Flaxseed Bread ✧

## 2 LARGE LOAVES

- *The combination of flax and sunflower seeds gives this whole wheat bread a rich, nutty flavor.*

- *Flaxseed has been part of the human diet for more than 5,000 years, and it has numerous nutritional benefits. It can be used whole in breads, muffins, and cookies or ground in yeast or quick breads, cereals, waffles, cookies, and crackers.*

| | | | | |
|---|---|---|---|---|
| 2 | packages active dry yeast | | 1 | tablespoon salt |
| 3 | cups lukewarm water | | 1/4 | cup honey |
| 1 | cup ground flaxseed (see Note) | | 1/2 | cup sesame seeds |
| 2 | tablespoons flaxseed oil, olive oil, or canola oil | | 4 | cups whole wheat flour |
| | | | 3 1/2 to 4 | cups all-purpose flour |

Dissolve the yeast in 1/2 cup warm water and let stand until frothy, about 10 minutes.

In a large bowl, combine the yeast, remaining water, ground flaxseed, oil, salt, and honey and beat until smooth. Add the sesame seeds and whole wheat flour and beat again, then gradually work in the all-purpose flour. Turn the dough out onto a flat surface dusted with flour and knead for 8 to 10 minutes, until it springs back when gently pressed.

Place the dough in a large, lightly greased bowl, cover tightly with plastic wrap, and let rise in a warm (but not hot) place until doubled in size, 30 to 40 minutes. Preheat the oven to 375 degrees F.

Punch down the dough. Divide in half, shape into 2 long, wide loaves, and place on a lightly greased baking sheet or into 2 lightly sprayed 9 by 5-inch loaf pans. Cover with a clean towel and let rise for about 30 minutes.

Bake for about 40 minutes, until lightly browned. The loaves should sound hollow when tapped on the bottom.

*Note:* Flaxseed can be ground in a coffee grinder or small food processor.

---

- Flaxseed is a terrific source of protective omega-3 fatty acids. It is also high in protein and fiber.
- Sunflower seeds are a potentially good source of selenium.
- Both sunflower seeds and flaxseeds contain isoflavones, phytoestrogens that may lower the risk of certain types of cancer.
- Whole grains, as well as some types of beans and seeds, contain phytic acids, phytochemicals that may help reduce oxidative damage to the body.

---

**Per serving (1-inch slice):**

| calories | protein | carbohydrates | fat | cholesterol | dietary fiber | saturated fat |
|---|---|---|---|---|---|---|
| 167 | 5 Gm | 28 Gm | 4 Gm | 0 mg | 4 Gm | <1 Gm |

**% of Calories**: 66% carbohydrate, 13% protein, 21% fat

**Major Sources of Potential Cancer Fighters**

**Phytochemicals**: phytic acids, plant polyphenols (isoflavones), plant sterols, protease inhibitors

---

# ❧ *Skillet Jalapeño Corn Bread* ❧

## 10 SERVINGS

- *This great-tasting quick bread can be made in less than 30 minutes and is the perfect side for Shiitake Vegetable Chili, page 199, or any other zesty entrée.*
- *Use small nonstick loaf pans or a nonstick muffin pan to make individual corn breads.*

| | |
|---|---|
| 1 cup all-purpose flour | 1/4 cup olive oil |
| 1 cup yellow cornmeal | 2 tablespoons sugar |
| 3/4 teaspoon salt | 3/4 cup canned creamed corn |
| 1/4 teaspoon cayenne | 2 medium jalapeño peppers, |
| 1 tablespoon baking powder | seeded and sliced |
| 1 cup 1% milk or soy milk | 1/2 teaspoon olive oil or cooking spray |
| 1 large egg | |

Preheat the oven to 425 degrees F.

In a large bowl, sift together the flour, cornmeal, salt, cayenne, and baking powder.

In a separate bowl, beat together the milk, egg, olive oil, and the sugar, then stir in the creamed corn and jalapeño pepper. Add to the dry ingredients and mix until just combined.

On the stove, heat a well-seasoned cast-iron or nonstick skillet that has been sprayed with cooking spray. When moderately hot, add the batter and spread out evenly. Transfer to the oven and bake for 20 to 25 minutes. When a toothpick placed in the center comes out clean, the corn bread is done. Let cool slightly, then cut into 10 wedges.

---

- Although corn does not contain substantial amounts of vitamins, it derives its color from the carotenoid lutein, a potent antioxidant.
- Chile peppers contain capsaicin, a phytochemical that may help neutralize carcinogens.

---

*Per serving (1-inch slice):*

| calories | protein | carbohydrates | fat | cholesterol | dietary fiber | saturated fat |
|----------|---------|---------------|-----|-------------|---------------|---------------|
| 169 | 4 Gm | 26 Gm | 5 Gm | 22 mg | 2 Gm | 1 Gm |

**% of Calories:** 61% carbohydrate, 10% protein, 29% fat

**Major Sources of Potential Cancer Fighters**
**Phytochemicals:** capsaicin, terpenes (carotenoids, monoterpenes)

# ❧ *Banana-Bran Muffins* ❧

### 8 MEDIUM MUFFINS

- *These tasty muffins are great for a healthy breakfast on the run.*
- *Prepare extra batter and refrigerate it for up to 3 days, so you can bake muffins when you want them. Freeze the batter or baked muffins and defrost as needed.*

| | |
|---|---|
| 2 tablespoons low-fat cream cheese or tofu cream cheese, softened | 1 teaspoon vanilla extract |
| 2 tablespoons canola oil | 2 medium bananas (about 10 ounces), peeled and sliced |
| 3/4 cup granulated sugar | 3/4 cup orange juice |
| 1/4 cup packed dark brown sugar | 3/4 cup sifted, defatted or low-fat soy flour (see Note) |
| 1 large egg | |

| | |
|---|---|
| 1 cup sifted all-purpose flour | 1/2 teaspoon baking soda |
| 1 cup 100% bran cereal, such as Bran Buds or All Bran | 1/4 teaspoon ground ginger |
| | 1/2 teaspoon ground cinnamon |
| 2 teaspoons baking powder | 1/4 teaspoon salt |

Preheat the oven to 375 degrees F.

In a food processor or mixer, pulse or beat together the cream cheese, canola oil, granulated sugar, brown sugar, egg, vanilla, and banana. When the mixture becomes creamy, add the orange juice.

Combine the remaining ingredients in a large bowl, stirring to incorporate. Add the banana mixture and beat until just combined.

Spray medium nonstick muffin tins with a canola-based cooking spray or rub lightly with canola oil. Portion the batter into the cups and bake for about 12 minutes, until the muffins are lightly browned and spring back when touched.

*Note:* Defatted and regular soy flours can be found at some supermarkets and most natural food stores.

---

- Baking with soy flour adds a nutty taste to baked goods, as well as protein (it is 50% protein by weight) and protective isoflavones. For other uses of soy flour, see pages 43–44.
- These moist muffins are low in fat—about the equivalent of 1 teaspoon of butter or margarine, but from potentially protective monounsaturated sources, including linolenic and omega-3 fatty acids.
- Each muffin provides more than 20% of the DV for folate; the highest source is soy flour.
- The combination of orange juice, cereal, and banana provide 30% of the DV for vitamin C.
- Whole grains, as well as some types of beans and seeds, contain phytic acids, phytochemicals that may help reduce oxidative damage to the body.
- High in fiber—20% of the DV per serving.

---

*Per serving (1 muffin):*

| calories | protein | carbohydrates | fat | cholesterol | dietary fiber | saturated fat |
|---|---|---|---|---|---|---|
| 308 | 9 Gm | 57 Gm | 5 Gm | 27 mg | 5 Gm | 1 Gm |

**% of Calories**: 74% carbohydrate, 12% protein, 14% fat

### Major Sources of Potential Cancer Fighters

**Phytochemicals**: phytic acids, plant polyphenols (flavonoids, isoflavones), plant sterols, protease inhibitors, terpenes (triterpenes)

# ❧ *Carrot and Zucchini Bread* ❧

## 2 LOAVES

- *This tasty quick bread is easy to prepare and helps contribute to your daily vegetable intake.*
- *Serve with breakfast or brunch or with tea or coffee for an afternoon snack.*

| | | | |
|---|---|---|---|
| 1 | large egg | 1 | cup grated zucchini |
| 1 | large egg white | | (1 small zucchini, 5 ounces) |
| 3/4 | cup granulated sugar | 2 | cups all-purpose flour |
| 1/2 | cup packed dark brown sugar | 1/2 | teaspoon salt |
| 1/4 | cup canola oil | 1 | teaspoon baking soda |
| 3/4 | cup orange juice | 1/2 | teaspoon baking powder |
| | zest of 1 orange | 1/2 | teaspoon ground cinnamon |
| 1 | cup canned pumpkin puree | 2 | teaspoons grated gingerroot |
| 1 | cup grated carrot | | pinch ground cloves |
| | (1 medium-large carrot) | | pinch nutmeg |

Preheat the oven to 350 degrees F.

In a medium bowl, combine the egg, egg white, granulated sugar, brown sugar, canola oil, orange juice, orange zest, and pumpkin puree. Beat by hand with a wooden spoon or with an electric mixer until well combined, then fold in the carrot and zucchini.

In a large bowl, combine the flour, salt, baking soda, baking powder, cinnamon, ginger, cloves, and nutmeg, stirring to mix well. Pour into the carrot-zucchini batter and mix until just combined.

Spray 2 8 by 3 3/4 by 2 1/2 inch loaf pans with a canola-based cooking spray. Dust with flour, coating the pan, then shake out the excess. Divide the batter between the 2 pans and bake for 50 to 55 minutes. Let cool for 10 minutes.

---

- The combination of pumpkin and carrots provides almost 75% of the DV for vitamin A per serving. Each slice also provides 20% of the DV for vitamin C.
- Gingerroot contains 6-gingerol, which may suppress enzymes and hormones related to cancer.
- Using citrus zest in baking is encouraged; it not only lends aroma and flavor, but also contains limonene, a phytochemical that may help your body dispose of carcinogens.

*Per serving (1-inch slice):*

| calories | protein | carbohydrates | fat | cholesterol | dietary fiber | saturated fat |
|----------|---------|---------------|-----|-------------|---------------|---------------|
| 215 | 4 Gm | 38 Gm | 5 Gm | 18 mg | 2 Gm | 1 Gm |

**% of Calories**: 70% carbohydrate, 9% protein, 21% fat

### Major Sources of Potential Cancer Fighters

**Phytochemicals**: plant polyphenols (flavonoids, phenolic acids), terpenes (carotenoids, monoterpenes, triterpenes)

# ✹ *Walnut-Raisin Bread* ✹

## 2 LOAVES

• *This bread has a crisp crust and a tender center. Its nutty flavor marries well with cheese or can stand alone as a breakfast bread. Also, try using it for a sandwich of fresh roast turkey, fresh watercress, and a small amount of a soft cheese, such as brie.*

| | | | |
|---|---|---|---|
| 3 | cups warm water | 1/4 | cup walnut oil |
| 1 | package active dry yeast | 2 | tablespoons olive oil |
| 4 | cups whole wheat flour | 1 | cup crushed walnuts |
| 1 | tablespoon plus 1 teaspoon salt | 3/4 | cup seedless raisins |
| 1/4 | cup honey | 2 1/2 | cups all-purpose flour |

In a small bowl, combine 1/2 cup of water with the yeast. Lightly stir to combine and let sit for 5 minutes.

In a mixer or mixing bowl, combine the whole wheat flour and salt and stir to combine. Make a small well in the center by pushing the flour to the sides. Pour the remaining water, yeast, honey, and walnut and olive oils into the center; mix. Add the walnuts, raisins, and 1 cup of all-purpose flour and mix. Add the remaining all-purpose flour, 1/3 cup at a time; the dough should be moist and slightly sticky.

Place the dough on a work surface lightly dusted with flour and knead for 8 minutes, until the dough is soft and elastic (add more flour only if the dough is very sticky).

Place the dough in a large, lightly greased bowl, cover tightly with plastic wrap, and let rise until doubled in size, in a warm (but not hot) place 1 hour and 30 minutes.

Punch down the dough and shape into 2 oval loaves. Line a baking sheet with parchment paper sprayed lightly with cooking spray. Place the loaves on the baking sheet and let rise until almost doubled in size, about 40 minutes.

Preheat the oven to 375 degrees F. Bake the loaves on the middle oven rack for 40 to

45 minutes, rotating the pan midway through baking; the bread should be lightly browned. Lift off the baking sheet; the loaves should sound hollow when tapped on the bottom.

---

- Walnuts and raisins contain phenolic acids that may act as antioxidants and blocking agents against cancer-causing substances. Walnuts and their extracted oil are also a terrific source of protective omega-3 fatty acids and plant sterols.
- Whole grains, as well as some types of beans and seeds, contain phytic acids, phytochemicals that may help reduce oxidative damage to the body.

---

*Per serving (1/2-inch slice):*

| calories | protein | carbohydrates | fat | cholesterol | dietary fiber | saturated fat |
|----------|---------|---------------|-----|-------------|---------------|---------------|
| 161 | 5 Gm | 25 Gm | 5 Gm | 0 mg | 3 Gm | 1 Gm |

**% of Calories**: 60% carbohydrate, 11% protein, 29% fat

### Major Sources of Potential Cancer Fighters

**Phytochemicals:** phytic acids, plant polyphenols (phenolic acids), plant sterols, protease inhibitors

# DESSERTS

## ❧ *Cocoa Fudge Brownies* ❧

The International Olive Oil Council

25 SERVINGS

• *The International Olive Oil Council's brownie recipe is made moist and low in saturated fat by use of olive oil instead of butter or shortening.*

| | | | |
|---|---|---|---|
| 3/4 | cup plus 1 teaspoon light flavored olive oil | 1 3/4 | cups granulated sugar |
| 3/4 | cup unsweetened cocoa | 4 | large eggs |
| 1/2 | cup all-purpose flour | 1 | teaspoon instant coffee |
| 1/2 | teaspoon salt | 1 | tablespoon hot water |
| | | 1 | cup coarsely chopped walnuts |

Grease and flour a 9-inch-square baking pan with 1 teaspoon of olive oil. Preheat the oven to 350 degrees F.

In a small bowl, sift together the cocoa, flour, and salt.

In a large bowl, beat the sugar and the remaining olive oil with an electric mixer on high speed for 3 minutes. Add the eggs, one at a time, beating after each addition.

Dissolve the coffee in the hot water, and add it to the sugar mixture. Stir in the dry ingredients. Fold in the nuts. Pour into a prepared pan. Bake 30 to 35 minutes, until the center is slightly soft. Cool the brownies in the pan. Chill completely in the refrigerator before cutting them into squares.

---

• Of the total amount of fat, 60% is protective monounsaturated fat.
• Walnuts contain phenolic acids that act as antioxidants, and help rid the body of carcinogens.

---

*Per serving:*

| calories | protein | carbohydrates | fat | cholesterol | dietary fiber | saturated fat |
|---|---|---|---|---|---|---|
| 173 | 3 Gm | 18 Gm | 10 Gm | 34 mg | 1 Gm | 1 Gm |

**% of Calories**: 40% carbohydrate, 7% protein, 53% fat

**Major Sources of Potential Cancer Fighters**
**Phytochemicals**: plant polyphenols (phenolic acids), plant sterols

# ✙ *Gâteau au Chocolat* ✙

The International Olive Oil Council

10 SERVINGS

• *This chocolate cake recipe was developed for the International Olive Oil Council by Carmen Jones, master chef and a member of the International Association of Cooking School. The low-fat Crème Anglaise sauce is from Strang.*

• *This cake can also be served with Strang's Raspberry Sauce—see Creamy Mocha Chocolate and Raspberry "Parfait." (page 290)*

## Crème Anglaise

### MAKES 1⁷/₈ CUPS

| | | | | |
|---|---|---|---|---|
| 2 | tablespoons all-purpose flour | | 2 | large egg yolks |
| 1³/₄ | cups 1% milk | | 1/₃ | cup granulated sugar |
| 1¹/₂ | teaspoons vanilla extract | | | |

## Gâteau au Chocolat

| | | | | |
|---|---|---|---|---|
| 1 | cup plus 1 teaspoon olive oil | | 1/₂ | teaspoon baking powder |
| 3 | cups plus 3 tablespoons all-purpose flour | | 2 | teaspoons baking soda |
| 1 | cup cocoa | | 2¹/₂ | cups granulated sugar |
| 2 | cups hot water | | 4 | large eggs |
| 1¹/₂ | teaspoons salt | | 2 | teaspoons vanilla extract |

To make the Crème Anglaise, in a small bowl, whisk the flour with ¹/₂ cup of the milk. Place it in a medium saucepan with the remaining milk and vanilla. Over low-medium heat, slowly warm the milk, stirring frequently.

In a small bowl, whisk together the egg yolks and sugar until the mixture is a pale yellow color.

When the milk is hot, temper the egg mixture by adding a small amount of the hot milk while whisking. Add all of the egg mixture to the saucepan with the remaining milk, and continue heating until the mixture boils. Lower the heat and allow the mixture to gently simmer and thicken, stirring constantly. Strain the liquid into a medium bowl; let cool. Refrigerate, covered with plastic wrap, for at least 2 hours.

To make the Gâteau au Chocolat, preheat the oven to 350 degrees F. Lightly grease a tube or Bundt pan with 1 teaspoon of olive oil then coat with 3 tablespoons of flour, shaking out the excess. In a medium bowl, mix together the cocoa and water until well combined. Set aside.

In a mixer, combine flour, salt, baking powder, baking soda, and sugar. Turn the mixer on to incorporate the dry ingredients. Pour in the olive oil, eggs, and vanilla and beat at medium speed for 2 to 3 minutes. Add the cocoa mixture and continue beating until well blended, about 3 minutes. Pour into prepared pan and bake for 50 to 60 minutes. A cake tester inserted in the center should emerge clean. Cool for 5 minutes before turning out. Cool thoroughly on a wire rack. Serve in slices with Crème Anglaise sauce.

---

Of the total amount of fat, more than 65% is protective monounsaturated fat.

---

*Per serving of Crème Anglaise (3 tablespoons):*

| calories | protein | carbohydrates | fat | cholesterol | dietary fiber | saturated fat |
|---|---|---|---|---|---|---|
| 62 | 3 Gm | 9 Gm | 1 Gm | 44 mg | 0 Gm | <1 Gm |

*Per serving of Gâteau au Chocolat:*

| calories | protein | carbohydrates | fat | cholesterol | dietary fiber | saturated fat |
|---|---|---|---|---|---|---|
| 461 | 5 Gm | 66 Gm | 20 Gm | 71 Gm | 1 Gm | 3 Gm |

*Per serving of Gâteau au Chocolat with Crème Anglaise:*

| calories | protein | carbohydrates | fat | cholesterol | dietary fiber | saturated fat |
|---|---|---|---|---|---|---|
| 523 | 8 Gm | 75 Gm | 21 Gm | 115 mg | 1 Gm | 3 Gm |

**% of Calories**: 57% carbohydrate, 6% protein, 36% fat

**Major Sources of Potential Cancer Fighters**
**Phytochemicals**: plant polyphenols (phenolic acids), plant sterols

---

# ❧ *Hazelnut Plum Tart* ❧

The International Olive Oil Council

8 SERVINGS

• *This tart is the perfect ending for a summer cookout or picnic.*

| | | | |
|---|---|---|---|
| 1 | cup hazelnuts | 1/3 | cup olive oil |
| 1/4 | cup light brown sugar | 1 | large egg, separated |
| 1 | cup all-purpose flour | 3 | tablespoons granulated sugar |
| | pinch salt | 2 | teaspoons cornstarch |

1/2   teaspoon grated lime rind
pinch nutmeg
pinch cloves

1 1/4   pounds plums (about 5 large),
          halved, pitted
3   tablespoons currant jelly, melted

Preheat the oven to 375 degrees F. Spray a 9-inch removable bottom tart pan with nonstick cooking spray.

Chop the hazelnuts in a food processor with the metal blade until coarsely chopped. Remove 1/4 cup for garnish and set aside. Add the brown sugar and process until the nuts are finely ground, about 15 seconds. Add the flour, salt, olive oil, and egg yolk and process until combined. The mixture will be crumbly.

Spoon the mixture into the prepared pan. Press firmly in an even layer on the bottom and up the sides. Brush the inside of the tart shell with the egg white. Chill in the freezer for 10 minutes.

Blend together the sugar, cornstarch, rind, nutmeg, and cloves in a medium bowl with a large spoon. Cut each plum half into 4 wedges, add to the bowl, and toss until combined. Arrange the plums in the pastry shell and scrape any remaining sugar mixture over the plums. Place the tart on a baking sheet.

Bake in the preheated oven for 45 to 50 minutes, or until the fruit is tender and the juices are thickened. Remove and cool 30 minutes on a rack. Remove the tart ring. Brush the fruit with currant jelly and sprinkle on reserved hazelnuts. Serve warm or at room temperature.

---

- Of the total amount of fat, more than 75% is protective monounsaturated fat.
- Plums provide flavonoids, cancer-fighting phytochemicals, and are a good source of fiber.
- The peel of citrus (or zest) contains limonene, a phytochemical that may help your body to dispose of carcinogens.

---

**Per serving (1 1/2-inch slice):**

| calories | protein | carbohydrates | fat | cholesterol | dietary fiber | saturated fat |
|----------|---------|---------------|-----|-------------|---------------|---------------|
| 380 | 4 Gm | 47 Gm | 22 Gm | 27 mg | 3 Gm | 2 Gm |

**% of Calories:** 47% carbohydrate, 4% protein, 49% fat

### Major Sources of Potential Cancer Fighters
**Phytochemicals:** plant polyphenols (flavonoids), terpenes (monoterpenes, limonene)

# ❧ *Cranberry Pecan Bundt Cake* ❧

The International Olive Oil Council

14 SERVINGS

• *Typically, a Bundt cake is made with two sticks of butter and 4 eggs, making it a high-cholesterol, high–saturated fat pleasure. This olive oil version has only 20% of the cholesterol, and less than 1/3 of the saturated fat.*

| | | | |
|---|---|---|---|
| 2 1/2 | cups unsifted cake flour | 1 | teaspoon vanilla extract |
| 1 | tablespoon baking powder | 1 | cup chopped pecans |
| 1 | teaspoon salt | 3/4 | cup dried cranberries (if not available, substitute other dried fruit such as chopped figs, prunes, or apricots) |
| 1 | teaspoon ground cinnamon | | |
| 1/4 | teaspoon ground cloves | | |
| 2 | large eggs | | |
| 4 | large egg whites | 1 | tablespoon grated orange zest |
| 1 3/4 | cups granulated sugar | 2 | tablespoons confectioner's sugar |
| 1 1/4 | cups light olive oil | | |

Preheat the oven to 325 degrees F. Spray a 10-inch tube or Bundt pan with nonstick cooking spray, then dust with flour. Set aside. In a medium bowl, sift together the flour, baking powder, cinnamon, and ground clove. Set aside. In a large bowl, with an electric mixer on medium speed, beat together the whole eggs, 2 egg whites, and sugar until thick and well blended, about 3 minutes. Reduce speed to low and add the olive oil gradually. Add the vanilla extract, and beat mixture on high for 2 minutes.

Clean and dry the beater of the electric mixer. In a medium bowl, beat the remaining 2 egg whites until soft peaks form. Set aside.

Stir the pecans, dried cranberries, and orange zest into the sugar mixture. Fold the flour mixture into the sugar mixture until just combined. Gently fold beaten egg whites into the batter. Spoon the batter into the prepared pan. Bake for 30 minutes at 325 degrees F, then reduce heat to 300 degrees F and bake an additional 40 to 45 minutes, or until a cake tester inserted in the center comes out clean.

Cool the cake in the pan for 15 minutes. Turn the cake out and cool completely on a wire rack. Transfer the cake to a serving plate and dust with confectioner's sugar.

---

- Of the total amount of fat, more than 85% is protective monounsaturated fat.
- Cranberries contain ellagic acid, a phytochemical that may help boost enzymes that rid the body of cancer-causing substances.
- The peel of citrus (or zest) contains limonene, a phytochemical that may help your body to dispose of carcinogens.

Per serving:

| calories | protein | carbohydrates | fat | cholesterol | dietary fiber | saturated fat |
|----------|---------|---------------|-----|-------------|---------------|---------------|
| 409 | 4 Gm | 43 Gm | 25 Gm | 30 mg | 1 Gm | 3 Gm |

**% of Calories**: 42% carbohydrate, 4% protein, 54% fat

**Major Sources of Potential Cancer Fighters**
**Phytochemicals**: phytic acids, plant polyphenols (flavonoids, phenolic acids), plant sterols, terpenes (monoterpenes, limonene)

# ❧ Lemon Semolina Cake ❧

The International Olive Oil Council

12 SERVINGS

• *Moist and flavorful, this easy to prepare cake can be served as a breakfast or tea cake or as a dessert topped with fresh berries.*

## Cake

| | |
|---|---|
| 2 cups semolina flour or farina | 1½ teaspoons baking powder |
| 2 cups minus 2 tablespoons granulated sugar | 2 cups plain low-fat yogurt |
| zest of 1 lemon | 6 tablespoons light olive oil |
| | ½ cup walnut halves |

## Syrup

| | |
|---|---|
| 1 cup granulated sugar | 1 teaspoon grated lemon zest |
| 1 cup water | few drops lemon juice |

To make the cake, preheat the oven to 350 degrees F. In a large bowl combine the flour, sugar, zest, baking powder, and yogurt with a wooden spoon or spatula. Do not use a mixer. Add the olive oil and mix well.

Oil a 12-inch springform pan, and pour in the batter. With a table knife, cut about ½ inch into the batter. Make 10 to 12 diamond shapes or squares. (The marks will not remain completely visible before baking, but when removed from the oven the cake will be scored.) Arrange a walnut half in the center of each square or diamond shape.

Bake in the preheated oven for about 45 minutes, until golden. Remove the cake from the oven. Cut through scored portions, constantly cleaning the knife. Pour the hot syrup onto the hot cake in the pan. Serve from the pan.

To make the syrup, in a small saucepan, combine all the ingredients. Bring to a boil, reduce heat, and boil gently until the mixture becomes a fairly thick syrup, about 215 degrees F on a candy thermometer.

---

- Of the total amount of fat, more than 65% is from protective monounsaturated fat.
- Walnuts contain phenolic acids that act as antioxidants, and help rid the body of carcinogens.
- The peel of citrus (or zest) contains limonene, a phytochemical that may help your body to dispose of carcinogens.

---

**Per serving:**

| calories | protein | carbohydrates | fat | cholesterol | dietary fiber | saturated fat |
|----------|---------|---------------|-----|-------------|---------------|---------------|
| 416 | 6 Gm | 74 Gm | 11 Gm | 2 mg | 1 Gm | 2 Gm |

**% of Calories**: 71% carbohydrate, 6% protein, 23% fat

**Major Sources of Potential Cancer Fighters**

**Phytochemicals**: phytic acids, plant polyphenols (phenolic acids), plant sterols, terpenes (monoterpenes, limonene)

# ❧ Olive Oil Cake with ❧ Citrus and Toasted Almonds

The International Olive Oil Council

10 SERVINGS

- *Chef Norman Van Aken of NORMAN'S in Coral Gables, Florida created this succulent cake for the International Olive Oil Council.*

| | | | | |
|---|---|---|---|---|
| 6 | kumquats, cut into halves | | 3 | large egg whites |
| 2/3 | cup olive oil | | 1½ | cups granulated sugar |
| 1 | orange | | 1 | cup all-purpose flour |
| 1 | lemon | | 3 | teaspoons baking powder |
| 6 | ounces blanched almonds, lightly toasted | | 1 | mango, peeled, pitted, and finely diced |
| 2 | large eggs | | | |

Combine the kumquats and olive oil in a sauce pan. Bring to a simmer, cooking gently for 3 minutes. Remove from the heat and let stand for 30 to 60 minutes. Strain, pressing out juices. Discard the fruit. Set aside the citrus-infused oil.

Preheat the oven to 350 degrees F. Put the orange and lemon in a small saucepan with water to cover. Simmer for 30 minutes, drain, and cool. Cut off the stem ends of lemon, cut in half, and scoop out the pulp and seeds and discard. Finely chop the rind. Finely chop the whole orange, and combine with the lemon rind. Set aside.

Chop the almonds in a food processor with a metal blade until they resemble finely ground bread crumbs. With an electric mixer, beat the eggs and egg whites until they are a light lemon color. Continue beating, gradually adding the sugar.

In a medium bowl, sift together the flour and baking powder. Stir in the egg mixture. Gently fold in the reserved rind, nuts, mango, and citrus-infused olive oil. Pour the batter into a lightly oiled 9-inch springform pan, and bake in the preheated oven for 1 hour, or until the tip of a knife gently inserted into the center comes out clean. Cool on a rack, and remove the sides of the pan. Garnish with citrus fruit if desired.

- Of the total amount of fat, 70% is from protective monounsaturated fat.
- Each serving of this citrus-infused cake provides more than 30% of the DV for vitamin C.
- The peel of citrus (or zest) contains limonene, a phytochemical that may help your body to dispose of carcinogens.

**Per serving:**

| calories | protein | carbohydrates | fat | cholesterol | dietary fiber | saturated fat |
|---|---|---|---|---|---|---|
| 399 | 7 Gm | 46 Gm | 21 Gm | 42 mg | 1 Gm | 3 Gm |

**% of Calories**: 46% carbohydrate, 7% protein, 47% fat

### Major Sources of Potential Cancer Fighters
**Phytochemicals:** plant polyphenols (flavonoids, phenolic acids), plant sterols, terpenes (monoterpenes, limonene, triterpenes)

## 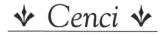 Cenci

The International Olive Oil Council

25 SERVINGS

- *Olive oil can be heated to high temperatures, making it perfect for frying. Achieving a high temperature is essential for the least absorption of oil in the food. Also, olive oil contributes flavor to these crispy cookies.*

3²/₃  cups all-purpose flour
¹/₃  cup granulated sugar
      pinch salt
      grated zest of 1 lemon
2    tablespoons unsalted butter,
      melted

4    large eggs
1    tablespoon brandy or grappa
³/₄  cup olive oil for frying
¹/₄  cup powdered sugar

Place the flour on a clean, flat surface. Add the sugar, salt, and lemon zest. Make a mound with the flour mixture and create a well in the center. Add the melted butter, and work it into the flour with your fingers. Break the eggs into the well. Beat the eggs with a fork and gradually mix in the flour. Bring the flour from the rim into the center and work the mixture to the outside. When most of the flour has been absorbed by the egg and butter mixture, add the brandy or grappa. Knead for approximately 10 minutes.

Place the dough into a bowl, cover it with a napkin, and allow it to rest for 1 hour. Place the dough on a flat, lightly flour-dusted surface and roll into a thin sheet. Use a cookie cutter to cut 2-inch diameter cookies.

Heat the olive oil in a nonstick skillet. When the oil is very hot (it should look loose and have movement, but not smoke), add 12 cookies and fry until they are lightly browned. Remove the cookies from the oil with tongs and place them on a large plate lined with paper towels to drain. Fry and drain the remaining cookies. Dust with the powdered sugar before serving.

---

- Of the total amount of fat, 60% is from protective monounsaturated fat.
- The peel of citrus (or zest) contains limonene, a phytochemical that may help your body to dispose of carcinogens.

---

*Per serving (1 cookie):*

| calories | protein | carbohydrates | fat | cholesterol | dietary fiber | saturated fat |
|----------|---------|---------------|-----|-------------|---------------|---------------|
| 139 | 3 Gm | 18 Gm | 6 Gm | 36 mg | 0 Gm | 1 Gm |

**% of Calories:** 51% carbohydrate, 8% protein, 41% fat

### Major Sources of Potential Cancer Fighters
**Phytochemicals:** plant sterols, terpenes (monoterpenes, limonene)

# ↯ Warm Mango and Yanni ↯ Pear Soup with Fruit Sorbets

Charlie Trotter, Charlie Trotter's, Chicago, Illinois

4 SERVINGS

### Mango-Pear Soup

| | |
|---|---|
| 1 | pound ripe mangoes (about 2 small), peeled and coarsely chopped |
| 1/2 | cup Yanni or any other ripe pear, peeled and diced |

| | |
|---|---|
| 1/4 | cup pineapple, diced |
| 2 | cups water |
| 1/4 | cup sugar |

### Fruit Salad

| | |
|---|---|
| 1/2 | cup pear, diced |
| 1/2 | cup strawberries, diced |
| 2 | tablespoons mango, diced |
| 1/2 | cup melon sorbet (either store-bought or homemade; see Note) |

| | |
|---|---|
| 1/2 | cup banana sorbet (either store-bought or homemade; see Note) |
| 1/2 | cup lemon sorbet (either store-bought or homemade; see Note) |

To make the mango-pear soup, bring the mangoes, pear, pineapple, water, and sugar to a boil. Remove from the heat and let cool for 30 minutes. Puree in a food processor or blender and strain through a fine strainer into a bowl. Warm just before serving.

To make the fruit salad, in a medium bowl, combine the diced pear, strawberries, and mango.

Spoon a small mound of fruit salad into each bowl. Place a small scoop of each sorbet on the mound of fruit. Pour some of the warmed mango-pear soup into each bowl.

*Note:* Chef Trotter's Basic Fruit Sorbet:

| | |
|---|---|
| 1/2 | cup simple syrup equals 1 cup water plus 1/2 cup sugar |
| 2 | cups peeled and diced fruit, such as pear, melon, strawberries, mango, peach, raspberry, passion fruit, and banana |

**Fresh lemon juice, as needed**

Combine the water and sugar in a saucepan. Simmer, stirring occasionally, until the sugar dissolves. Add the fruit and cook for another minute. Let cool slightly, then puree the fruit-syrup mixture. Taste fruit syrup, and add a touch of lemon juice if necessary to balance sweetness. Place in an ice cream maker and follow the manufacturer's instructions.

---

- Strawberries, mango, and pineapple are all terrific sources of vitamin C—one serving of this delicious dessert provides more than 75% of the DV.
- Mangos' orange, sweet, and juicy flesh is rich in beta-carotene.
- A good source of fiber.

---

*Per serving:*

| calories | protein | carbohydrates | fat | cholesterol | dietary fiber | saturated fat |
|----------|---------|---------------|-----|-------------|---------------|---------------|
| 238 | 1 Gm | 60 Gm | <1 Gm | 0 mg | 3 Gm | 0 Gm |

**% of Calories**: 97% carbohydrate, 1% protein, 2% fat

**Major Sources of Potential Cancer Fighters**

**Phytochemicals**: plant polyphenols (flavonoids, phenolic acids), terpenes (carotenoids)

# ✙ *Raspberry Sorbet* ✙

4 SERVINGS

### Simple Syrup

1/2 cup sugar

1/2 cup water

2 cups fresh raspberries
(about 8 ounces)

lemon juice, as needed

To prepare the simple syrup, combine the sugar and water in a small saucepan. Bring to a boil, stirring frequently, until all sugar is dissolved, about 2 to 3 minutes. Let cool slightly.

Puree the raspberries and simple syrup in a blender. Strain and season with lemon juice if the mixture is too sweet. Freeze in an ice cream maker, according to the manufacturer's directions.

*Note:* If you do not have an ice cream maker, try making a granita: Pour the raspberry–simple syrup puree into a shallow, rectangular, stainless-steel pan. Place in the freezer and stir with a whisk every 20 minutes. After 2 hours the granita should be well mixed and slushy. Serve in chilled martini glasses and garnish with fresh berries and mint leaves.

- This sorbet is rich in the antioxidant vitamin C: one serving provides enough vitamin C to supply 30% of the DV.
- Like most berries, raspberries contain ellagic acid, a plant polyphenol that may boost enzymes that help dispose of carcinogens. This phytochemical may reduce the genetic damage caused by cancer-causing substances.
- A good source of fiber.

**Per serving:**

| calories | protein | carbohydrates | fat | cholesterol | dietary fiber | saturated fat |
|---|---|---|---|---|---|---|
| 132 | 1 Gm | 32 Gm | 0 Gm | 0 mg | 3 Gm | 0 Gm |

**% of Calories**: 96% carbohydrate, 4% protein, 0% fat

**Major Sources of Potential Cancer Fighters**
**Phytochemicals:** plant polyphenols (flavonoids, phenolic acids), terpenes (carotenoids, monoterpenes)

# ❧ *Exotic Fruit Soup* ❧
# *with Pineapple Granita*

William Yosses, Pastry Chef, Bouley, New York, New York

6 SERVINGS

- *A tasty way to boost your fruit servings—each portion provides 3 fruit servings.*

1 pineapple, peeled, cored, and cut into small dice (save skins)

1 mango (about 6 ounces), peeled, pitted, and cut into small dice

1 papaya (about 1 pound), peeled, pitted, and cut into small dice

1 star fruit (about 5 ounces), cut into slices (also called carambola; see Note)

3 passion fruits with their seeds (about 4 ounces), peeled and sliced

6 lychees (about 2¹/₂ ounces), shelled (see Note)

1 pint strawberries (about 12 ounces), rinsed and stems removed

1 quart water

6 fresh mint sprigs, reserve tops and stems separately

1 lemongrass stalk
  peel of 1 orange (remove all white pith)
  peel of 1 lime (remove all white pith)

1 vanilla bean, split in half lengthwise

3 tablespoons sugar

Cut the ripe fruit (pineapple, mango, papaya, star fruit, and passion fruit) as indicated. Reserve the fruit in separate small bowls.

Using a hand blender, food processor, or blender, puree the strawberries and then pass them through a strainer. Set aside.

Boil the pineapple skins in 1 quart of water with the mint stems, lemongrass, orange and lime peels, 1/2 vanilla bean, and the sugar. Allow the mixture to boil for 30 minutes, until reduced by half. Strain the liquid into a flat, low-sided container, such as a pie shell or cookie sheet pan, and place in the freezer. With a fork, stir and scrape this mixture every 20 minutes to create ice "flakes" that will be the granita. After 2 hours it should be well mixed and slushy.

Place the diced pineapple, mango, and papaya in the center of a soup plate and place star and passion fruit slices and a lychee on top of them. Spoon the strawberry puree around the edges. When ready to serve, spoon the granita on top. Cut the remaining 1/2 vanilla bean lengthwise into narrow "strings" and tie into circles to decorate the top of the fruit. Add a mint sprig and serve.

*Note:* Star fruit or carambola are juicy, fragrant tropical fruits that can be eaten out of hand, added to desserts or salads, or used as a garnish. When this golden yellow fruit is cut crosswise, a star shape can be noted. They are available at some supermarkets and gourmet specialty stores.

Although lychees are native to Southeast Asia, this small, sweet fruit is also grown in California, Florida, and Hawaii. Available at some supermarkets and gourmet specialty stores.

---

- Provides more than 250% of the DV for vitamin C and 20% for vitamin A per serving.
- The oils of the Asian herb lemongrass contain the protective phytochemical myrcene.
- High in fiber—24% of the DV per serving.

---

**Per serving:**

| calories | protein | carbohydrates | fat | cholesterol | dietary fiber | saturated fat |
|----------|---------|---------------|-----|-------------|---------------|---------------|
| 264 | 2 Gm | 65 Gm | 2 Gm | 0 mg | 6 Gm | 0 Gm |

**% of Calories:** 59% carbohydrate, 36% protein, 5% fat

### Major Sources of Potential Cancer Fighters

**Phytochemicals:** plant polyphenols (flavonoids, phenolic acids), terpenes (carotenoids, limonene, myrcene, triterpenes)

# ❧ *Strawberry Soup* ❧

Dieter Schorner, Pâtisserie Café Didier, Washington, D.C.;
Chairman of Pastry Arts, The French Culinary Institute, New York, New York

6 SERVINGS

- *An easy and light summer dessert.*

| | | |
|---|---|---|
| 3 | cups strawberries (about 1 pound), cleaned and trimmed | 3 tablespoons sugar |
| 2½ | cups fresh orange juice | ½ cup low-fat sour cream |
| ¼ | cup Grand Marnier | sliced strawberries and mint leaves for garnish |

Place 6 bowls in the refrigerator to chill.

Rinse and drain the berries. In a food processor, puree the strawberries with 1 cup of orange juice until smooth. Transfer the puree to a large bowl and whisk in the remaining ingredients, except the garnish. Cover and refrigerate for at least 1 hour.

To serve, divide soup among the chilled bowls and garnish with sliced strawberries and mint leaves.

---

Strawberries contain more vitamin C than any other member of the berry family—½ cup provides 70% of the DV.

---

**Per serving:**

| calories | protein | carbohydrates | fat | cholesterol | dietary fiber | saturated fat |
|---|---|---|---|---|---|---|
| 124 | 2 Gm | 26 Gm | 1 Gm | 0 mg | 2 Gm | 0 Gm |

**% of Calories**: 83% carbohydrate, 6% protein, 3% fat, 8% alcohol

**Major Sources of Potential Cancer Fighters**

**Phytochemicals**: plant polyphenols (flavonoids, phenolic acids), terpenes (carotenoids, monoterpenes)

# ❧ *Chilled Soup of Pineapple* ❧ and Kalamansi with Yogurt-Lime Sorbet

Gray Kunz, Lespinasse, New York, New York

4 SERVINGS

- *A refreshing, almost fat-free dessert full of fruit.*

### Chilled Soup

| | |
|---|---|
| 1 | cup pineapple juice |
| 2 1/2 | ounces juice of kalamansi or lime juice |
| 7 | ounces water |
| 1/2 | cup sugar |

1/2   cup pineapple, peeled, cored, and chopped into small pieces (reserve one small slice for garnish)

### Sorbet

| | |
|---|---|
| 8 | limes, peel grated and reserved, juice strained and reserved |
| 10 | ounces low-fat, plain yogurt (1 1/3 cups) |

1/2   cup sugar

### Garnish

reserved pineapple slice

3   tablespoons grenadine syrup or Campari

To make the soup, in a small saucepan, combine the pineapple juice, lime juice, water, and sugar. Heat to a boil, reduce the heat, and simmer until the sugar dissolves, about 2 minutes. Let cool slightly and combine with the pineapple in the bowl of a food processor or in a blender. Puree until very smooth, then strain. Chill to a very cold temperature.

To make the sorbet, in a bowl, combine the lime juice and zest, yogurt, and sugar. Freeze in an ice cream maker.

To make the garnish, cut the reserved pineapple slice into 1/4-inch diamond shapes. In a small bowl, soak them in grenadine syrup or Campari for 2 to 3 minutes, then drain.

Divide the soup among 4 dessert bowls. Scoop sorbet into each and garnish with the grenadine-soaked pineapple diamonds.

*Note:* Purchase a citrus frozen yogurt if you do not have an ice cream maker.

Both pineapple and lime are rich in vitamin C, providing half of the DV in this recipe. The peel also contains limonenes, a phytochemical that acts as a blocking agent, disarming carcinogens.

---

*Per serving:*

| calories | protein | carbohydrates | fat | cholesterol | dietary fiber | saturated fat |
|----------|---------|---------------|-----|-------------|---------------|---------------|
| 310 | 5 Gm | 71 Gm | 1 Gm | 1 mg | 1 Gm | 0 Gm |

**% of Calories**: 92% carbohydrate, 7% protein, 3% fat

### Major Sources of Potential Cancer Fighters

**Phytochemicals**: plant polyphenols (flavonoids, phenolic acids), plant sterols, terpenes (limonene, triterpenes)

---

# ❧ *Pumpkin–Arborio Rice Pudding* ❧

### 4 TO 6 SERVINGS

• *When stirred during cooking, Italian Arborio rice releases starch, giving it a creamy consistency that is perfect for this low-fat version of rice pudding.*

| | |
|---|---|
| 2¹/₃ cups 1% vanilla soy milk (see Note) | ground cloves |
| ¹/₃ cup packed brown sugar | 1 cup Italian Arborio rice |
| 1 cinnamon stick or ¹/₄ teaspoon ground cinnamon dash | 1 cup canned, unsweetened pumpkin puree |
| | ¹/₃ cup seedless raisins |

Heat the soy milk with the brown sugar, cinnamon stick, and cloves. When the mixture begins to boil, reduce to a simmer and stir in the rice. Cook for 15 minutes, stirring intermittently. Add the pumpkin puree and raisins and continue cooking for about 5 minutes more, stirring constantly until the rice is creamy and the liquid is absorbed. Remove the cinnamon stick. Transfer to dessert bowls and serve warm or chilled.

*Note:* Low-fat soy milk can be purchased at some supermarkets and most natural food stores.

---

- With less than 0.5 Gm of fat per serving, this can be considered a "fat-free" dessert.
- Pumpkin is rich in beta-carotene and provides 100% of the DV for vitamin A per serving.

*Per serving (based on 6 servings):*

| calories | protein | carbohydrates | fat | cholesterol | dietary fiber | saturated fat |
|----------|---------|---------------|-----|-------------|---------------|---------------|
| 270 | 5 Gm | 62 Gm | 0 Gm | 0 mg | 2 Gm | 0 Gm |

**% of Calories**: 92% carbohydrate, 8% protein, 0% fat

### Major Sources of Potential Cancer Fighters

**Phytochemicals**: phytic acids, plant polyphenols (flavonoids, isoflavones), plant sterols, protease inhibitors, terpenes (carotenoids, triterpenes)

# ❧ *Peach and Blueberry Crisp* ❧

## 6 SERVINGS

- *The key to flavor in this easy-to-prepare dessert is using perfectly ripe fruit. Other delicious combinations include strawberry and rhubarb; apple, walnut, and raisin; mango, apple, and grated ginger.*
- *Try it topped with vanilla frozen yogurt.*

| | | | |
|---|---|---|---|
| 6 | medium peaches, peeled, cored, and cut into large chunks | 1/3 | cup granulated sugar<br>juice of 1/2 lemon |
| 2 | cups blueberries, rinsed and drained | 1/2 | cup oatmeal |
| 1/4 | cup plus 2 tablespoons all-purpose flour | 1/4 | cup packed brown sugar |
| | | 1/2 | teaspoon ground cinnamon |
| | | 1 | tablespoon melted butter |

Preheat the oven to 375 degrees F.

Spray an 8 by 8 by 2-inch baking pan with a canola-based cooking spray or lightly rub with canola oil.

In a medium bowl, combine the peaches, blueberries, 2 tablespoons of the flour, the granulated sugar, and lemon juice. Toss with your hands to thoroughly combine. Spread the fruit out in the baking pan.

In a separate bowl, prepare the topping. Mix together the oatmeal, remaining 1/4 cup flour, the brown sugar, and cinnamon. Drizzle with the melted butter, then rub the topping together between your hand until it resembles a coarse meal. Evenly spread the topping over the fruit and bake for 30 to 35 minutes, until the fruit is bubbling and the topping is slightly browned. Remove and let cool slightly. Serve warm or at room temperature.

- Peaches derive their orange color from beta-carotene. They also contain substantial amounts of vitamin C: combined with blueberries, they provide more than 20% of the DV per serving.
- Blueberries contain ellagic acid, a phytochemical that may help boost enzymes that rid the body of cancer-causing substances.
- A good source of fiber.

*Per serving:*

| calories | protein | carbohydrates | fat | cholesterol | dietary fiber | saturated fat |
|----------|---------|---------------|-----|-------------|---------------|---------------|
| 234 | 3 Gm | 49 Gm | 3 Gm | 5 mg | 4 Gm | 1 Gm |

**% of Calories**: 84% carbohydrate, 5% protein, 11% fat

### Major Sources of Potential Cancer Fighters
**Phytochemicals**: plant polyphenols (flavonoids, phenolic acids), terpenes (carotenoids)

# ✦ *Low-Fat Chocolate Soufflé* ✦

## 8 SERVINGS

- *A delicious low-caloric, low-fat "fix" for chocolate lovers.*
- *An impressive low-fat dessert for guests; serve with fresh raspberries, strawberry slices, or Raspberry Sauce, page 290.*

### Soufflé Base

| | |
|---|---|
| 3/4 cup plus 2 tablespoons 1% milk or 1% soy milk | 1 large egg |
| 1 tablespoon plus 1 teaspoon all-purpose flour | 3 tablespoons sugar |
| 1/2 teaspoon vanilla extract | 2 ounces semisweet chocolate, cut into small pieces or grated |

### Soufflé Molds

| | |
|---|---|
| cooking spray or 1/2 teaspoon melted butter | 3 tablespoons sugar |

### Whipped Egg Whites

| | |
|---|---|
| 4 large egg whites | 2 tablespoons sugar |

To prepare the soufflé base, in a small bowl, whisk 1/4 cup of milk with the flour, making sure that no lumps remain. Place in a small, heavy saucepan with the remaining milk and the vanilla and slowly bring to a broil, stirring frequently. Reduce the heat and simmer until it thickens, about 1 minute.

In a small mixing bowl, beat the egg and 3 tablespoons of sugar together until the mixture is pale yellow and the sugar is well incorporated. Add a small amount of hot milk (about 2 to 3 tablespoons) and whisk to combine. Add the egg mixture to the milk in the saucepan. Simmer on medium-low heat, stirring constantly. Cook for 1 to 2 minutes, until thick and creamy. Transfer to a large bowl and stir in the chocolate. Set aside and let cool. (*The soufflés can be made in advance up to this point.*)

Preheat the oven to 400 degrees F.

To prepare the soufflé molds, spray 8 4-ounce soufflé molds (or ramekins) with a canola-based cooking spray or rub lightly with butter. Add 3 tablespoons of sugar to the first mold and tilt the mold to evenly coat the bottom and sides. Pour the remaining sugar into the next mold and repeat the process until all molds are lightly dusted with sugar.

To whip the egg whites, using an electric mixer beat the egg whites to firm peaks and gradually add 2 tablespoons of sugar. Fold the egg whites into the chocolate until just combined. Do not beat.

Fill the soufflé molds three-quarters full and place on a baking pan. Bake for 9 to 10 minutes, until they have risen and spring back when touched. Serve in the mold or invert onto dessert plates and serve immediately.

| *Per serving:* | | | | | | |
|---|---|---|---|---|---|---|
| calories | protein | carbohydrates | fat | cholesterol | dietary fiber | saturated fat |
| 113 | 4 Gm | 19 Gm | 3 Gm | 27 mg | 0 Gm | 2 Gm |

**% of Calories**: 65% carbohydrate, 65% protein, 24% fat

**Major Sources of Potential Cancer Fighters**
**Phytochemicals**: plant polyphenols (phenolic acids)

# ✧ *Low-Fat Cheesecake Brûlée* ✧

### 4 SERVINGS

- *A low-fat creamy cross between cheesecake and crème brûlée.*

| | |
|---|---|
| 4 ounces low-fat cream cheese | 1 tablespoon flour |
| 1 cup low-fat plain yogurt, drained of whey (yogurt cheese; see Note) | grated zest of 1 lemon |
| | 1 teaspoon vanilla extract |
| 1/4 cup plus 2 tablespoons sugar | 1/2 teaspoon butter or butter-flavored baking spray |
| 1 large egg | 2 tablespoons sugar |
| 1 egg white | |

Preheat the oven to 300 degrees F.

Bring 1 quart of water to a boil.

In a large bowl, using an electric mixer, or in a food processor, beat together the cream cheese and yogurt cheese until smooth. Add 1/4 cup plus 2 tablespoons sugar, the egg, egg white, flour, lemon zest, and vanilla and beat until creamy.

Rub 4 4-ounce ramekins with butter. Divide the mixture among the ramekins (see Note) and place them in a shallow baking tray. Pour hot water into the baking tray until it reaches halfway up the ramekins and bake for 50 to 55 minutes, until set. Remove from the oven and let cool to room temperature in the baking tray; refrigerate until ready to serve (at least 2 hours).

Arrange the oven rack so that it is very close to the broiler. Preheat the broiler.

Place the cheesecakes on a baking pan and evenly sprinkle the tops with 2 tablespoons of sugar. Put the baking pan directly under the broiler; let the sugar melt and brown, then immediately remove from the oven. Serve in the mold. (To prevent the cheesecakes from melting, the broiler must be very hot and the molds very close to the heat to limit the time they're exposed to the heat.)

*Note:* Yogurt cheese funnels are available in many culinary stores or kitchen mail-order catalogs. To make yogurt "cheese," place yogurt in a funnel that is resting over a small bowl or container and refrigerate overnight. The part that remains in the funnel is the "cheese" and the liquid in the container is the whey. Whey gives yogurt its distinct taste and, when drained away and discarded, the creamy cheese that remains is a perfect replacement for cream cheese for spreading, cooking, or baking.

Ramekins are individual baking dishes that resemble soufflé molds. They are usually made of porcelain or earthenware and can be used for both sweet and savory dishes.

The peel or zest of citrus fruit contains limonene, which may help boost cancer-fighting enzymes in the body.

*Per serving:*

| calories | protein | carbohydrates | fat | cholesterol | dietary fiber | saturated fat |
|---|---|---|---|---|---|---|
| 218 | 8 Gm | 30 Gm | 7 Gm | 71 mg | 0 Gm | 4 Gm |

**% of Calories**: 55% carbohydrate, 16% protein, 29% fat

**Major Sources of Potential Cancer Fighters**

**Phytochemicals**: terpenes (limonene)

# ❧ Creamy Mocha Chocolate ❧ and Raspberry "Parfait"

## 4 SERVINGS

• *Tofu never tasted so good. The Mocha Chocolate Mousse can be made in less than 5 minutes and served on its own, chilled. It can also be served in elegant dessert glasses with the Raspberry Sauce.*

• *Thin the Raspberry Sauce with a touch more orange juice and use with Low-Fat Chocolate Soufflé, page 287, or the Lemon Tart, page 306.*

### Mocha Chocolate Mousse

2  10 1/2-ounce containers Mori-Nu lite, silken, extra-firm tofu (see Note)
3  tablespoons maple syrup
1/4  cup packed brown sugar
2  tablespoons Tia Maria or another type of coffee liqueur

1/3  cup plus 1 tablespoon good-quality cocoa powder, such as Ghirardelli, Lindt, or Vahlorona
2  teaspoons instant espresso
1/4  teaspoon ground cinnamon

### Raspberry Sauce

2 1/2  cups fresh raspberries, well rinsed, or frozen, thawed
1/3  cup fresh orange juice

juice of 1/2 lemon
2  tablespoons granulated sugar

## Garnish

½ cup raspberries 4 mint leaves

To prepare the mousse, combine all ingredients in the bowl of a food processor and puree until creamy, about 2 minutes. Transfer the mousse to a bowl, cover, and refrigerate.

To prepare the raspberry sauce, combine 1½ cups of raspberries and the remaining ingredients in the bowl of a food processor and puree until smooth. Strain the raspberry sauce through a fine strainer (rubbing with a rubber spatula to work through the mesh) into a small bowl. Mix in the remaining 1 cup of whole raspberries, cover, and refrigerate for about 15 minutes.

Spoon a 1-inch-deep layer of mousse into long, narrow parfait glasses or small glass dessert bowls, spreading out evenly. Top with a layer of raspberry sauce. Repeat, ending with a layer of mousse. Chill for at least 20 minutes. Garnish with some whole raspberries and a mint leaf.

*Note:* Mori-Nu tofu is available at some supermarkets and most natural food stores.

---

- This dessert is rich in the antioxidant vitamin C: each serving provides 40% of the DV.
- Like many other berries, raspberries contain ellagic acid, a phytochemical that may boost enzymes that help rid the body of cancer-causing substances.
- Tofu, the curd of soybean milk, contains numerous cancer-fighting phytochemicals, including protective isoflavones. Each serving provides 8 Gm of soy protein.
- A good source of fiber.

---

*Per serving of Mocha Chocolate Mousse:*

| calories | protein | carbohydrates | fat | cholesterol | dietary fiber | saturated fat |
|----------|---------|---------------|-----|-------------|---------------|---------------|
| 133 | 8 Gm | 20 Gm | 2 Gm | 0 mg | 3 Gm | 0 Gm |

*Per serving of Raspberry Sauce:*

| calories | protein | carbohydrates | fat | cholesterol | dietary fiber | saturated fat |
|----------|---------|---------------|-----|-------------|---------------|---------------|
| 54 | 1 Gm | 13 Gm | 0 Gm | 0 mg | 0 Gm | 0 Gm |

*Per serving of Creamy Mocha Chocolate and Raspberry Parfait:*

| calories | protein | carbohydrates | fat | cholesterol | dietary fiber | saturated fat |
|----------|---------|---------------|-----|-------------|---------------|---------------|
| 187 | 9 Gm | 33 Gm | 2 Gm | 0 mg | 3 Gm | 0 Gm |

**% of Calories**: 66% carbohydrate, 17% protein, 12% fat, 5% alcohol.

**Major Sources of Potential Cancer Fighters**
**Phytochemicals**: phytic acids, plant polyphenols (isoflavones, flavonoids, phenolic acids), plant sterols, protease inhibitors, terpenes (carotenoids, triterpenes)

# ❧ Best Low-Fat Chocolate ❧
# Fondue with Fresh Fruit

### 6 SERVINGS

- *An easy-to-prepare dessert for a weeknight or a nice touch when entertaining.*
- *This chocolate sauce is so rich and creamy you will not believe it is low-fat.*
- *Substitute any fresh seasonal fruit that can be sliced and skewered with a fondue fork.*
- *Try the reduced-fat chocolate sauce over other fruit or frozen yogurt, or as a sauce for cakes or tortes.*

## Chocolate Sauce

### MAKES 2 CUPS (1 SERVING = 1/4 CUP)

| | |
|---|---|
| 1 large egg | 1/4 cup unsweetened cocoa powder |
| 1 large egg white | 2 teaspoons butter |
| 1/3 cup sugar | |
| 1 1/2 cups 1% vanilla soy milk or plain soy milk plus 1/2 teaspoon vanilla extract | |

## Fresh Fruit

| | |
|---|---|
| 12 large strawberries (about 1 pound), stems on, well rinsed, and drained | 3 ripe pears, peeled, cored, rubbed with lemon, and sliced into long strips |
| 2 bananas, peeled and sliced on the bias | |

To prepare the chocolate sauce, in a small bowl, whisk together the egg, egg white, and sugar.

In a small, heavy saucepan, whisk together the soy milk and cocoa powder. Heat slowly over medium heat, stirring frequently, until the mixture almost boils. Pour a small amount of the cocoa mixture into the bowl with the eggs and immediately whisk to combine. Then pour the egg mixture into the saucepan and bring to a boil, stirring constantly. Reduce the heat and simmer the sauce until it thickens, about 2 minutes; remove from the heat. Whisk in the butter and set aside. Pour the sauce into an attractive serving bowl and let cool slightly.

If necessary, heat the sauce on high power in the microwave for about 2 minutes to warm it. Place the bowl in the center of a serving platter and surround with fresh fruit. Use fondue forks to dip the fruit into the warm chocolate.

---

- Strawberries are rich in vitamin C, providing almost 75% of the DV per serving. They also contain ellagic acid, a phytochemical that may help boost enzymes that rid the body of cancer-causing substances.
- The use of soy milk enriches this sauce with all of the protective phytochemicals found in soybeans.
- A good source of fiber.

---

*Per serving of Chocolate Sauce (¹/₄ cup):*

| calories | protein | carbohydrates | fat | cholesterol | dietary fiber | saturated fat |
|----------|---------|---------------|-----|-------------|---------------|---------------|
| 87 | 3 Gm | 13 Gm | 3 Gm | 30 mg | 0 Gm | 1 Gm |

*Per serving of Best Low-Fat Chocolate Fondue with Fresh Fruit:*

| calories | protein | carbohydrates | fat | cholesterol | dietary fiber | saturated fat |
|----------|---------|---------------|-----|-------------|---------------|---------------|
| 169 | 3 Gm | 33 Gm | 3 Gm | 30 mg | 3 Gm | 1 Gm |

**% of Calories**: 77% carbohydrate, 7% protein, 16% fat

**Major Sources of Potential Cancer Fighters**

**Phytochemicals**: phytic acids, plant polyphenols (flavonoids, phenolic acids), plant sterols, protease inhibitors, terpenes (carotenoids, triterpenes)

---

# ✻ Cherry Clafoutis ✻

6 SERVINGS

• *Although cherries are the traditional fruit used for this country French dessert, it can also be made with pears, plums, or peaches.*

| | | | |
|---|---|---|---|
| 1 | cup 1% milk | 2 | large eggs |
| ³/₄ | cup whole milk | 2 | large egg whites |

<sup></sup>

| | |
|---|---|
| ¹/₂ cup granulated sugar | pinch salt |
| 2 tablespoons sifted flour | 3 cups pitted sour cherries |
| 1 tablespoon vanilla extract | 3 tablespoons powdered sugar |
| 1 tablespoon kirsch or cognac (optional) | for sprinkling |

Preheat the oven to 350 degrees F.

Spray a shallow baking dish, such as a pie plate or large, shallow quiche dish, with a canola-based cooking spray or lightly rub with canola oil.

In a small saucepan, stir together the 1% and whole milks. Heat over medium heat until hot but not boiling. Meanwhile, whisk together the eggs, egg whites, vanilla, and sugar in a medium bowl. Add the flour, whisking until no lumps remain. Pour a small amount of the hot milk into the bowl with the egg mixture and whisk together. Add the rest of the milk and the kirsch, if using, and whisk to combine. Pour into the baking dish and arrange the cherries over the batter in a single layer. Bake until it rises and is set, 30 to 35 minutes. Serve the clafoutis warm or at room temperature sprinkled with powdered sugar.

---

Sour cherries have fewer calories and more vitamin C and beta-carotene than sweet cherries. Each serving provides more than 10% and 15% of the DVs, respectively.

---

**Per serving:**

| calories | protein | carbohydrates | fat | cholesterol | dietary fiber | saturated fat |
|---|---|---|---|---|---|---|
| 202 | 7 Gm | 37 Gm | 3 Gm | 76 mg | 1 Gm | 1 Gm |

**% of Calories**: 72% carbohydrate, 14% protein, 14% fat

**Major Sources of Potential Cancer Fighters**
**Phytochemicals**: plant polyphenols (flavonoids, phenolic acids), terpenes (carotenoids)

## ❦ Schaum Torte ❦

RoxSand Scocos, RoxSand's Restaurant & Bar, Phoenix, Arizona

4 SERVINGS

- *This classic Austrian dessert can satisfy one's sweet craving while still providing nutrients and sparing fat.*
- *Both the baked meringue and fruit can be prepared 1 day in advance.*
- *Fresh seasonal berries can replace fruit compote.*

*Meringue*

| | | | |
|---|---|---|---|
| 1/3 | cup almonds | 1/8 | teaspoon cream of tartar |
| 1/2 | cup egg whites (3 large eggs) | 3/4 | cup sugar |

*Fruit Compote (see Note)*

2 tablespoons sugar

10 medium apricots (about 14 ounces), pitted and cut into wedges, or 1/2 pound dried apricots

1/2 cup fragrant white wine, such as Gewürztraminer, Riesling, Sauvignon Blanc

1/2 vanilla bean, split in half lengthwise
zest of 1 lemon, sliced into long, thick strips

1 cup fresh blueberries (about 5 ounces)

1/4 cup raisins

Preheat the broiler. Spread the almonds out on a nonstick baking pan and toast under the broiler until lightly browned. Let cool slightly, then grind in a spice grinder or food processor. Set aside.

Preheat the oven to 250 degrees F.

Line a large baking sheet with a piece of parchment paper. Using a round or heart-shaped cookie cutter, trace 12 separate sketchings of the desired shape onto the paper.

To prepare the meringue, in a dry mixing bowl, beat the egg whites with an electric mixer at low speed. Gradually increase the speed. When the whites are frothy, add the cream of tartar and continue beating. Add the sugar gradually, and continue beating until the meringue stands in stiff, shiny (but not dry) peaks, another 3 to 4 minutes.

Put the meringue into a pastry bag fitted with a 1/2- to 3/4-inch star or plain tip. Fold toasted almonds into the meringue. Pipe the meringue onto the outlines on parchment paper, making the edges slightly higher than the center by adding an extra rotation. (If you do not have a pastry bag, dollop the meringue onto the paper, then use the back of a spoon to push the meringue away from the center toward the perimeter to form a scoop with a rim.) Bake for 1 hour until they are firm and dry, but not browned. Let them dry out in the oven for 4 to 6 hours. Gently peel the meringues from the paper (if they stick, they are not done and should be baked longer).

To prepare the fruit compote, in an 8-inch nonstick skillet, heat the sugar until it dissolves and begins to brown. Add the apricots and cook for 2 to 3 minutes in the bubbling sugar, then add the white wine, vanilla bean, and lemon zest. Bring to a simmer and cook, covered, for 5 minutes, pouring in a little water if it begins to dry out. Add blueberries and raisins and simmer for another 2 to 3 minutes, until the fruit is tender. Remove the zest and let cool slightly.

Spoon a small amount of fruit compote into a meringue shell, cover with another meringue, spoon more fruit over the top, and repeat one more time until you have 3 layers. Dollop with whipped cream, if desired.

*Note:* You can substitute seasonal fresh fruit, such as a mixture of berries, for the Fruit Compote.

---

- Apricots get their orange color from beta-carotene: each serving provides 25% of the DV for vitamin A. Along with blueberries, they also provide more than 25% of the DV for vitamin C.
- A good source of fiber.

---

*Per serving:*

| calories | protein | carbohydrates | fat | cholesterol | dietary fiber | saturated fat |
|----------|---------|---------------|-----|-------------|---------------|---------------|
| 367 | 7 Gm | 70 Gm | 6 Gm | 0 mg | 4 Gm | 1 Gm |

**% of Calories**: 76% carbohydrate, 2% protein, 15% fat, 7% alcohol

**Major Sources of Potential Cancer Fighters**

**Phytochemicals**: plant polyphenols (flavonoids, phenolic acids), terpenes (carotenoids, limonene)

# ❧ *Apple Strudel* ❧

Jacques Torres, Pastry Chef, Le Cirque, New York, New York; Dean of Pastry Arts, The French Culinary Institute, New York, New York

### 3 SERVINGS

- *Crispy and delicious like traditional German strudel, but with less than one-third of the fat and calories.*

| | | | | |
|---|---|---|---|---|
| 2 | tablespoons raisins | | 2 | tablespoons finely ground unseasoned bread crumbs |
| 2 | tablespoons rum | | 2 | teaspoons lemon juice |
| 1 | large apple, peeled, cored, and diced | | | zest of 1/2 lemon |
| 2 | tablespoons chopped walnuts | | 2 | phyllo sheets (see Note) |
| 2 | tablespoons granulated sugar | | 1 | tablespoon melted butter |
| 1/4 | teaspoon ground cinnamon | | 2 1/2 | tablespoons powdered sugar |
| 1/2 | vanilla bean, split lengthwise and beans scraped out, or 1/2 teaspoon vanilla extract | | | |

Preheat the oven to 400 degrees F.

Soak the raisins in the rum for 5 minutes to hydrate them.

Place the apple in a mixing bowl with the nuts. Add the granulated sugar, cinnamon, vanilla bean seeds, bread crumbs, rum-soaked raisins (rum drained), lemon juice, and lemon zest. Mix until well combined.

Spread 1 phyllo sheet onto a parchment-covered baking pan. Using a pastry brush, brush evenly with the butter. With a sifter, sprinkle about 1 tablespoon of powdered sugar over the buttered phyllo sheet. Top with a second phyllo sheet and brush again with butter and sprinkle with about 1 tablespoon of sifted powdered sugar.

Place the apple mixture in a lengthwise row 2 inches from the base of the phyllo rectangle and ending 2 inches from either end. Roll the phyllo dough around the apple mixture (away from you) until you have a long tube. Gently roll the strudel so that the seam end is on the bottom and loosely fold the ends under.

Brush the top of the strudel with butter and sprinkle with the remaining 1/2 tablespoon powdered sugar. Bake for about 12 minutes, until golden brown. Let cool slightly. Slice into 3 even segments and serve.

*Note:* Phyllo dough can be purchased frozen at many supermarkets. Thaw overnight in the refrigerator before unrolling. Phyllo dough can dry out quickly, making it potentially difficult to work with. Do not remove phyllo from its wrapper until the apple filling is prepared and all equipment is ready. Always cover air-exposed phyllo dough with a slightly moistened clean towel.

---

- Both apples and walnuts contain phenolic acids that may act as antioxidants, blocking agents against cancer-causing substances. Walnuts are also good plant sources of protective omega-3 fatty acids.
- Using the peel of citrus in baking is encouraged; it not only lends aroma and flavor, but also contains limonene, a phytochemical that may help your body to dispose of carcinogens.

---

*Per serving:*

| calories | protein | carbohydrates | fat | cholesterol | dietary fiber | saturated fat |
|---|---|---|---|---|---|---|
| 224 | 3 Gm | 34 Gm | 7 Gm | 7 mg | 2 Gm | 2 Gm |

**% of Calories**: 60% carbohydrate, 5% protein, 26% fat, 9% alcohol

**Major Sources of Potential Cancer Fighters**

**Phytochemicals**: phytic acids, plant polyphenols (flavonoids, phenolic acids), plant sterols

# ❧ *Apple Cake (Gâteau aux Pommes)* ❧

Robert Bennett, Le Bec Fin, Philadelphia, Pennsylvania

8 SERVINGS

- *Delicious, easy to prepare, and full of fruit. Serve warm or at room temperature; goes well with vanilla frozen yogurt.*
- *This cake can be made with pears instead of apples.*

| | | | |
|---|---|---|---|
| 1 | teaspoon sweet butter | 1 | teaspoon ground cinnamon |
| 1½ | cups plus 2 tablespoons all-purpose flour | ¼ | cup orange juice grated zest of 1 orange |
| 1 | cup plus 3 tablespoons sugar | 1¼ | teaspoons vanilla extract |
| ½ | teaspoon salt | 2 | large eggs |
| 1½ | teaspoons baking powder | ½ | cup canola oil |
| 3 | apples (about 1 pound), peeled, cored, and cut into cubes | | |

Prepare a 6-cup Bundt pan by rubbing with butter, then sprinkling with 2 tablespoons of flour. Evenly coat, then shake out the excess flour.

Preheat the oven to 350 degrees F.

In a medium bowl, sift together 1½ cups of flour, 1 cup of sugar, the salt, and baking powder and reserve.

In another bowl, combine the apples, 3 tablespoons of sugar, and the cinnamon and reserve.

In a large bowl, beat together the orange juice, orange zest, vanilla, and eggs with an electric mixer, or by hand using a whip, then pour in the oil and beat until well incorporated. Stir in the dry ingredients, mix, then fold in the apple mixture. Pour the batter into the prepared pan and bake for 1 hour and 5 minutes. Cool for 10 minutes, then invert onto a serving plate.

---

- Though apples do not contain substantial amounts of vitamins A or C, they are very good sources of fiber and contain protective plant polyphenols.
- Using the peel or zest of citrus in baking is encouraged; it not only lends aroma and flavor, but also contains limonene, a phytochemical that may help your body to dispose of carcinogens.
- A good source of fiber.

*Per serving:*

| calories | protein | carbohydrates | fat | cholesterol | dietary fiber | saturated fat |
|----------|---------|---------------|-----|-------------|---------------|---------------|
| 296 | 6 Gm | 45 Gm | 10 Gm | 43 mg | 3 Gm | 1 Gm |

**% of Calories**: 61% carbohydrates, 8% protein, 31% fat

### Major Sources of Potential Cancer Fighters

**Phytochemicals**: plant polyphenols (flavonoids, phenolic acids), plant sterols, terpenes (limonene)

# ❧ Raspberry and Chocolate ❧ Soy Protein Shake

### 1 SERVING

- *A high-protein, low-fat shake for breakfast on the run or a snack.*
- *Of particular benefit for people who need to maximize their intake of calories and protein.*

$1/2$ cup soy lite raspberry yogurt (4 ounces; see Note)

1 cup chocolate flavored 1% soy milk or nonfat chocolate soy milk (see Note)

$1/2$ cup fresh or frozen raspberries (about 2 ounces)

2 tablespoon soy protein isolate (protein powder; see Note)

Combine all ingredients in a blender and puree until the shake is very smooth.

*Note:* These soy-based products can be found at most natural food stores.

- Each shake contains as much soy protein as 3 ounces of meat, fish, or poultry—as well as the protective phytochemicals found in soy.
- Raspberries are a good source of ellagic acid, a phytochemical that may help boost enzymes that rid the body of cancer-causing substances.
- High in fiber—20% of the DV.

*Per serving:*

| calories | protein | carbohydrates | fat | cholesterol | dietary fiber | saturated fat |
|----------|---------|---------------|-----|-------------|---------------|---------------|
| 241 | 21 Gm | 36 Gm | 3 Gm | 10 mg | 6 Gm | 0 Gm |

**% of Calories**: 33% carbohydrates, 56% protein, 11% fat

## Major Sources of Potential Cancer Fighters

**Phytochemicals**: phytic acids, plant polyphenols (flavonoids, isoflavones, phenolic acids), plant sterols, protease inhibitors, terpenes (carotenoids, triterpenes).

# HOLIDAY RECIPES

**Easter Menu**

## ❧ Conchiglie with Fresh Asparagus, ❧ Morel Mushrooms, and Tarragon

### 6 SERVINGS

- *This Easter first course incorporates the flavors of spring vegetables and herbs. Best of all, it can be made in less than 20 minutes from start to finish.*
- *Substitute farfalle, orecchiette, or fusilli for the shell pasta.*

| | |
|---|---|
| 1 pound dried conchiglie (small shell pasta) | 14 medium asparagus (about ½ pound), stems peeled and cut on the bias at 2-inch increments, tips reserved |
| 2 tablespoons olive oil | leaves from 2 tarragon sprigs, chopped |
| 5 shallots, peeled and sliced into 6 wedges each | ¾ pound cherry tomatoes (yellow and red), halved |
| 2 tablespoons chopped parsley | salt and pepper |
| ¾ pound fresh morel mushrooms or fresh domestic mushrooms, halved or quartered if large | |

Bring 4 quarts of salted water to a boil.

Cook the pasta according to package directions (usually about 12 minutes for al dente). Meanwhile, heat the olive oil and shallots in a large nonstick sauté pan. Cook over medium-low heat until the shallots are soft, 5 to 7 minutes. Add the parsley and mushrooms and sauté for another minute over medium-high heat. Add the asparagus and continue cooking for another 5 minutes, tossing frequently. Add the tarragon and cherry tomatoes and season with salt and pepper. After 1 to 2 minutes, add to the hot, drained pasta, tossing well to combine. Garnish with asparagus tips.

- Each serving provides approximately 35% of the DV for vitamins A and C, and more than 11% for folate.
- Shallots lend sweetness and protective allium compounds.
- Both pasta and mushrooms are potentially good sources of selenium.
- A good source of fiber.

*Per serving:*

| calories | protein | carbohydrates | fat | cholesterol | dietary fiber | saturated fat |
|----------|---------|---------------|-----|-------------|---------------|---------------|
| 352 | 13 Gm | 67 Gm | 4 Gm | 0 mg | 4 Gm | 1 Gm |

**% of Calories**: 75% carbohydrate, 15% protein, 10% fat

### Major Sources of Potential Cancer Fighters
**Phytochemicals**: allium compounds, plant polyphenols (flavonoids), plant sterols, terpenes (carotenoids, monoterpenes)

# ↓ *Seared Sea Scallops over* ↓ *Wilted Pea Greens with Citrus Vinaigrette*

### 6 SERVINGS

• *Pea greens are tender sprouts that have a flavor that's a cross between peas and spinach. They are delicious added to salads, wilted like spinach, or added to a stir-fry at the last minute.*

### Citrus Vinaigrette

#### MAKES 1/2 CUP

| | |
|---|---|
| 2 tablespoons fresh lemon juice | leaves from 1 fresh tarragon sprig |
| 1 medium orange, peeled | salt |
| 1 tablespoon extra virgin olive oil | |

### Scallops

| | |
|---|---|
| 1/2 teaspoon olive oil | 1 1/2 pounds fresh pea greens |
| 6 very large sea scallops | (or pea sprouts), rinsed |
| (about 10 ounces) | (see Note) |
| salt and pepper | |

To prepare the vinaigrette, combine all ingredients in a blender and puree until smooth and frothy. Pour into a medium bowl. Season with salt. Set aside.

To sear the scallops, brush a nonstick oven-safe skillet (with a metal handle for oven transfer) with olive oil and heat until almost smoking. Season the scallops with salt and pepper and place in the skillet. Sear them on both sides, until the outside rims are well browned, then lower the heat and continue cooking until they are opaque and spring back when gently probed, about 2 minutes. When cool enough to handle, slice the scallops horizontally into 3 "coins" each; place on a large plate and cover loosely with foil to retain heat.

To wilt the pea greens, brush a clean, large, nonstick skillet with olive oil and heat over medium heat. When hot, add the pea greens and cook until just wilted; stir gently to cook evenly. Lift the pea greens out of the skillet, leaving behind any released water, and transfer to the bowl with the vinaigrette. Toss to coat the greens evenly.

Divide the greens among 3 plates and arrange 3 scallop coins on top. Serve immediately.

*Note:* Pea greens are sold at specialty markets and green markets in the spring.

---

- Pea greens are rich in folate, providing more than 25% of the DV per serving. They also supply enough carotenoids to provide 20% of the DV for vitamin A.
- The combination of citrus and pea greens provides more than 50% of the DV for vitamin C.
- Orange zest is a source of limonene, a phytochemical that may help your body to dispose of carcinogens.
- Scallops are very low in fat and are potentially good sources of selenium.

---

*Per serving of Citrus Vinaigrette (1 tablespoon):*

| calories | protein | carbohydrates | fat | cholesterol | dietary fiber | saturated fat |
|---|---|---|---|---|---|---|
| 24 | 0 Gm | 2 Gm | 2 Gm | 0 mg | 0 Gm | 0 Gm |

*Per serving of Seared Sea Scallops over Wilted Pea Greens with Citrus Vinaigrette:*

| calories | protein | carbohydrates | fat | cholesterol | dietary fiber | saturated fat |
|---|---|---|---|---|---|---|
| 74 | 9 Gm | 5 Gm | 2 Gm | 16 mg | 2 Gm | 0 Gm |

**% of Calories**: 27% carbohydrate, 49% protein, 24% fat

### Major Sources of Potential Cancer Fighters

**Phytochemicals**: plant polyphenols (flavonoids, phenolic acids), terpenes (carotenoids, limonene)

# ❦ *Lightly Spiced Lamb Stew* ❦ *with Spring Vegetables*

### 6 SERVINGS

- *The marinade seasoning is exotic but subtle; it makes a flavorful broth that marries well with lamb.*

- *This stew is convenient when entertaining because it can be prepared up to a day in advance and reheated. Substitute seasonal vegetables and make it throughout the winter and spring.*

- *Omit the potatoes, add other vegetables, such as carrots and turnips, and serve over couscous.*

## Marinade

| | | | |
|---|---|---|---|
| 1/2 | teaspoon ground cumin | | grated zest of 1/2 lemon |
| 1/4 | teaspoon ground cinnamon | 1 | teaspoon olive oil |
| | pinch ground cloves | 2 | pounds lamb leg, boned, |
| 1/2 | teaspoon ground turmeric | | trimmed of all visible fat, |
| | pinch nutmeg | | and cut into 2-inch cubes |

## Stew

| | | | |
|---|---|---|---|
| 1 1/2 | tablespoons olive oil | 1 1/2 | pounds small Yukon Gold |
| 2 | celery stalks, cut into | | potatoes, peeled and halved or |
| | 1 1/2-inch cubes | | quartered if large |
| 10 | small shallots, | 1 | small fennel bulb, tough outer |
| | peeled and quartered | | layer discarded, sliced into |
| 1 | tablespoon flour | | 1/4-inch pieces |
| | salt and pepper | 2 | cups fresh, cooked, or frozen |
| 1 | cup orange juice | | artichoke hearts, |
| 4 | cups chicken stock (page 147 or 148), | | thawed and quartered |
| | low-sodium canned broth, | 1 | cup cooked chickpeas or canned, |
| | or water | | drained (see Note) |
| 1 | bay leaf | 2 | tablespoons chopped parsley |

To prepare the marinade and lamb, combine all ingredients in a large bowl; mix well, cover, and refrigerate for at least 1 hour.

To prepare the stew, heat 1 tablespoon of olive oil in a large, heavy pot. Add the celery and shallots, and sauté over medium heat for about 10 minutes, until slightly softened.

Sprinkle the vegetables with the flour and stir to incorporate; no lumps should remain. (See Note)

Season lamb cubes with salt and pepper.

In a large nonstick skillet, heat the remaining $1/2$ tablespoon of oil. When almost smoking, add the lamb cubes. Sear over high heat, browning evenly on all sides. Remove the lamb and add to the pot with the vegetables. Add the orange juice to the skillet, stirring with a wooden spoon to dissolve the flavorful particles on the bottom of the pan. Add this liquid, along with the chicken stock and bay leaf, to the pot with the lamb and vegetables.

Bring the stew to a boil; immediately reduce the heat so that the mixture gently simmers. Cook for 1 hour, then add the potato and continue cooking at a simmer. After another 20 minutes, add the fennel and cook for 10 minutes more. Add the artichokes, chickpeas, and parsley 2 to 3 minutes before serving, and adjust the seasoning with salt and pepper.

*Note:* To cook dried chickpeas, soak them in water to cover for 4 hours; change the water 2 to 3 times. Drain and place in a saucepan, cover with water, and add a bay leaf (1 to 2 celery stalks, a carrot, and half of a large onion may also be added for more flavor). Bring to a boil and then reduce to a gentle simmer. Cook until the beans are tender but firm, 2 to $2^{1}/_{2}$ hours, adding more water as necessary so that the beans are always covered. Drain and use in recipe or as an addition to soups and salads.

The stew will be slightly thickened, but still brothy; if you like a more stewlike consistency, add 1 tablespoon more flour to the vegetables.

---

- Each serving provides more than 90% of the DV for vitamin C, and more than 30% for vitamins A and folate.
- Trimmed leg of lamb contains only 2.5 Gm fat per ounce, and is a good source of protein and B vitamins, and a potentially good source of selenium.
- The peel or zest of citrus fruit contains limonene, which may help boost cancer-fighting enzymes in the body.
- Turmeric contains curcumin, a plant polyphenol that lends yellow color and acts as an antioxidant; it may also play a role in blocking cancer at the initiation stage.
- High in fiber—28% of the DV per serving.

---

**Per serving of Lightly Spiced Lamb Stew with Spring Vegetables:**

| calories | protein | carbohydrates | fat | cholesterol | dietary fiber | saturated fat |
|---|---|---|---|---|---|---|
| 557 | 55 Gm | 45 Gm | 17 Gm | 153 mg | 7 Gm | 5 Gm |

**% of Calories**: 32% carbohydrate, 40% protein, 28% fat

> **Major Sources of Potential Cancer Fighters**
> **Phytochemicals**: allium compounds, phytic acids, plant polyphenols (flavonoids, phenolic acids), protease inhibitors, terpenes (carotenoids, limonene)

# ❧ Lemon Tart ❧

### 8 SERVINGS

- *A refreshing, sweet finish to any meal, this lemon tart has less than three-quarters of the fat of the classic version.*
- *Serve topped with one layer of fresh raspberries or with Raspberry Sauce, page 290.*
- *Use this low-fat pastry shell for other tarts and pies.*

## Pastry Shell

| | | | |
|---|---|---|---|
| 1 1/4 | cups all-purpose flour | 2 | ounces 1% cottage cheese |
| 1/4 | teaspoon baking powder | 1 | large egg white |
| | pinch salt | 2 | tablespoons milk |
| 2 | tablespoons sugar | | |
| 2 | tablespoons cold butter, cut into small cubes | | |

## Lemon Filling

| | | | |
|---|---|---|---|
| | grated zest of 1 lemon | 2 | large eggs |
| 1/2 | cup plus 2 tablespoons sugar | 2 | large egg whites |
| 1/2 | cup fresh lemon juice | 1 | tablespoon butter |
| 3/4 | cup 1% milk | | |

To prepare the pastry shell, place the flour, baking powder, salt, and sugar in the bowl of a food processor; process quickly to just incorporate ingredients.

Add the remaining ingredients and pulse the machine on and off until the dough is well combined, moist, and crumbly. Gather it together and gently press it into a disk shape. Wrap with plastic wrap and refrigerate for at least 30 minutes. (The dough can be made and kept refrigerated up to 2 days in advance.)

Position a rack in the center of the oven and preheat to 350 degrees F.

Roll out the dough to 1/8 to 1/4 inch thick on a work surface lightly dusted with flour. Add a sprinkle of flour if necessary to prevent sticking. Place the dough in a 9-inch tart pan that has been lightly sprayed with cooking spray and center it. Gently mold the pastry dough to the curves of the pan, then trim off the overlapping edges by running a rolling pin flatly across the top.

Bake the shell for about 20 minutes, until the interior is dry and the sides are golden brown. If the bottom of the pastry shell puffs up, tap it down lightly with your fingers as often as necessary. Transfer the shell to a wire rack and let cool completely. Unmold the tart.

To prepare the lemon filling, combine the zest and sugar in a small bowl and rub them together with your hands to coat the sugar with the natural oils and fragrance of the zest.

In a medium bowl, combine the remaining ingredients and whisk in the zest-sugar mixture. Transfer to a medium saucepan and heat over medium heat, stirring constantly, until the mixture just boils. Reduce the heat immediately to a simmer; cook, stirring, for another 1 to 2 minutes. Remove from the heat and strain into a bowl. Let cool slightly, then ladle into the pastry shell. Allow the tart to sit at room temperature until completely cool. Serve at room temperature or refrigerate and serve cool.

---

- Citrus fruits are rich in vitamin C and contain cancer-fighting plant polyphenols.
- The peel or zest of citrus fruit contains limonene that may help boost cancer-fighting enzymes in the body.

---

*Per serving of Pastry Shell (trimmings subtracted):*

| calories | protein | carbohydrates | fat | cholesterol | dietary fiber | saturated fat |
|---|---|---|---|---|---|---|
| 111 | 4 Gm | 17 Gm | 3 Gm | 8 mg | <1 Gm | 2 Gm |

*Per serving of Lemon Tart:*

| calories | protein | carbohydrates | fat | cholesterol | dietary fiber | saturated fat |
|---|---|---|---|---|---|---|
| 209 | 7 Gm | 34 Gm | 5 Gm | 54 mg | <1 Gm | 3 Gm |

**% of Calories**: 65% carbohydrate, 13% protein, 22% fat

### Major Sources of Potential Cancer Fighters

**Phytochemicals**: plant polyphenols (flavonoids, phenolic acids), plant sterols, terpenes (limonene, triterpenes)

**Passover Menu**

# ✤ *Sweet and Sour Braised Brisket* ✤

### 6 SERVINGS

- *This version of the traditional Eastern European dish has a delicious Asian twist.*
- *Feel free to vary your choice of seasonal vegetables (if they cook relatively quickly, such as snow peas, sugar snap peas, or green beans, add them during the last 5 to 10 minutes of cooking).*
- *Serve with White and Sweet Potato Kugel, page 309.*

| | | | |
|---|---|---|---|
| 1 | cup duck sauce | 4 | small turnips (about 1 pound), peeled |
| 1/2 | cup chili sauce | | |
| 3 | pounds brisket, first cut | 2 | medium parsnips (about 10 ounces), peeled |
| | salt and pepper | | |
| 2 | teaspoons olive oil | 4 | medium carrots (about 14 ounces), peeled and stems trimmed |
| 1/4 | cup rice wine vinegar | | |
| 2 | tablespoons brown sugar | | |

Combine the duck sauce and chili sauce in a small baking dish. Coat the brisket with the marinade, cover, and refrigerate overnight.

Preheat the oven to 350 degrees F.

Wipe the marinade from brisket and season with salt and pepper.

Heat the oil in a large, heavy, flameproof casserole. Add the brisket to the pan, and brown on both sides over medium-high heat. Transfer the brisket to a plate and add the vinegar, 1/4 cup water, and the sugar to the casserole, scraping with a wooden spoon to dissolve any particles on the bottom. Remove from the heat and return the brisket, along with any juices that have accumulated, to the casserole. Cover tightly and roast for 1 hour. Remove the casserole from the oven and surround the brisket with the turnips, parsnips, and carrots. Cover and continue roasting for another 2 hours, until fork-tender, basting 2 to 3 times with released juices.

Remove the casserole from the oven and place the brisket on a cutting board. Cut it at an angle into 1/8- to 1/4-inch slices. Place the slices on a serving platter so that they are slightly overlapping and resemble the original shape of the brisket.

Adjust the seasoning of the juices and vegetables in the casserole with salt and pepper. Quarter the turnips and slice the carrots and parsnips. Place them around the brisket. Spoon juices over the meat and vegetables and serve.

- First-cut brisket is very lean, containing less than 2½ Gm of fat per ounce. Cook it slowly, covered, and it will become moist and delicious.
- Beef is a potentially good source of selenium.
- Carrots contribute substantial vitamin A: each serving provides more than 150% of the DV.
- Turnips and parsnips contribute more than 30% of the DV for vitamin C per serving. Like broccoli and cabbage, turnips contain glucosinolates, which may boost enzymes that fight cancer.
- A good source of fiber.

*Per serving:*

| calories | protein | carbohydrates | fat | cholesterol | dietary fiber | saturated fat |
|---|---|---|---|---|---|---|
| 490 | 41 Gm | 47 Gm | 15 Gm | 122 mg | 3 Gm | 5 Gm |

**% of Calories**: 38% carbohydrate, 34% protein, 28% fat

### Major Sources of Potential Cancer Fighters

**Phytochemicals**: glucosinolates, plant polyphenols (flavonoids, phenolic acids), plant sterols, terpenes (carotenoids, monoterpenes)

# ❧ White and Sweet Potato Kugel ❧

## 6 SERVINGS

- *A healthy variation of this traditional holiday menu item features sweet potatoes and a small amount of olive oil.*

| | | | |
|---|---|---|---|
| 2 | small sweet potatoes (about 10 ounces), peeled | 1 | medium onion (about 5 ounces), chopped |
| 3 | medium Idaho potatoes (about 1½ pounds), peeled | | salt and pepper |
| ½ | teaspoon salt | 3 | tablespoons matzo meal |
| 2 | tablespoons olive oil | 2 | large eggs, well beaten |

Preheat the oven to 400 degrees F. Using a grater or a mandoline, grate the sweet potatoes and white potatoes, sprinkle with ½ teaspoon salt, and place in a colander to drain for 15 minutes.

Heat the olive oil in a large nonstick sauté pan, and sauté the onion over medium-high heat until limp, about 5 minutes. Add the potato mixture and continue to sauté for another 5 minutes, stirring frequently, until the potatoes begin to become tender. Season with salt and pepper and remove from the heat. Stir in the matzo meal and eggs and pour into a small, rectangular nonstick baking pan, spreading the mixture out evenly. Bake for 50 minutes or until golden brown.

---

- The addition of sweet potatoes to this traditional Passover dish provides enough carotenoids to supply more than 60% of the DV for vitamin A.
- Both white and sweet potatoes contribute substantial amounts of vitamin C: each serving provides more than 35% of the DV.

---

*Per serving:*

| calories | protein | carbohydrates | fat | cholesterol | dietary fiber | saturated fat |
|---|---|---|---|---|---|---|
| 223 | 6 Gm | 34 Gm | 7 Gm | 71 mg | 2 Gm | 1 Gm |

**% of Calories**: 60% carbohydrate, 10% protein, 30% fat

**Major Sources of Potential Cancer Fighters**

**Phytochemicals:** allium compounds, plant polyphenols (flavonoids, phenolic acids), plant sterols, terpenes (carotenoids, monoterpenes)

# ⬇ Matzo Apple Bread Pudding ⬇

### 8 SERVINGS

- *This delicious version of "bread" pudding was provided by Laurel Reiss, a friend of Strang. She makes this kugel, or pudding, annually as a sweet side dish to her multiple main courses. It makes a terrific dessert for Passover or anytime.*

| | | | | |
|---|---|---|---|---|
| 4 | matzo sheets | | 3/4 | teaspoon salt |
| 2 | large eggs | | 2 | large apples, peeled, cored, and grated |
| 1 | large egg white | | | |
| 1/2 | cup granulated sugar | | 1/2 | cup seedless raisins |
| 3 | tablespoons canola oil | | | grated zest of 1 lemon |
| 1/2 | teaspoon cinnamon | | 1/4 | cup brown sugar |

Preheat the oven to 350 degrees F.

Lightly coat an 11 by 7 by 2-inch nonstick baking pan with cooking spray.

In a medium bowl, crumble the matzo and cover with water; let stand for 10 minutes. Drain off any water that has not been absorbed, then mash.

In a small bowl, beat the eggs and egg white with the sugar until creamy. Beat in the canola oil, matzo, cinnamon, and salt. Fold in the apples, raisins, and lemon zest, then pour the mixture into the baking pan. Sprinkle the top with the brown sugar and bake until set and lightly browned, 30 to 35 minutes.

- More than half of the fat in this recipe is from potentially protective monounsaturated sources.
- The peel of citrus not only lends aroma and flavor, but also contains limonene, a phytochemical that may help your body dispose of carcinogens.
- Apples and raisins contain plant polyphenols that are potent antioxidants.

*Per serving:*

| calories | protein | carbohydrates | fat | cholesterol | dietary fiber | saturated fat |
|----------|---------|---------------|-----|-------------|---------------|---------------|
| 242 | 3 Gm | 45 Gm | 6 Gm | 27 mg | 2 Gm | 1 Gm |

**% of Calories**: 72% carbohydrate, 6% protein, 22% fat

**Major Sources of Potential Cancer Fighters**

**Phytochemicals**: plant polyphenols (flavonoids, phenolic acids), plant sterols, terpenes (limonene)

# ❧ *Broccoli and Tomato Salad* ❧

## 6 SERVINGS

- *Don't serve this salad only on holidays: it is a terrific course to any meal during any season.*

- *Serve warm or at room temperature; it's a portable vegetable serving you can bring to work, a picnic, or a party.*

| | |
|---|---|
| 1 large head of broccoli (about 2 pounds) | 1 tablespoon rice wine vinegar |
| 2 shallots (about 2 ounces), peeled and very thinly sliced | 1½ tablespoons extra virgin olive oil salt and freshly ground pepper |
| 2 medium tomatoes (about 10 ounces), diced | |

Bring 4 quarts of salted water to a boil.

Trim and blanch the broccoli. Separate the florets from the stems; break the florets into bite-size pieces and, using a vegetable peeler, peel the tough outer skin from the stems until you reach the tender green part. Slice the stems into 1/4-inch coins.

Add the coins to the boiling water and cook until slightly tender but still firm, about 4 minutes; add the florets. Check for doneness after 2 to 3 minutes: it should be easy to pierce both stem pieces and florets with a fork. Drain and transfer to a bowl of ice water. When cool, drain again and transfer to a large serving bowl.

Add the shallots, tomatoes, vinegar, and olive oil to the serving bowl and toss to combine with the broccoli. Season with salt and pepper and serve.

---

- Broccoli is a near-perfect vegetable; it is rich in beta-carotene, vitamin A, vitamin C, folate, and calcium. It is also a member of the cruciferous vegetable family, and contains cancer-fighting phytochemicals.
- Broccoli is a potentially good source of selenium.
- Tomatoes and tomato products are also rich in vitamin C and contain the carotenoid lycopene, a potent antioxidant.
- High in fiber—20% of the DV per serving.

---

*Per serving:*

| calories | protein | carbohydrates | fat | cholesterol | dietary fiber | saturated fat |
|---|---|---|---|---|---|---|
| 112 | 5 Gm | 12 Gm | 5 Gm | 0 mg | 5 Gm | 1 Gm |

**% of Calories**: 42% carbohydrate, 18% protein, 40% fat

### Major Sources of Potential Cancer Fighters

**Phytochemicals**: allium compounds, glucosinolates, plant polyphenols (flavonoids, phenolic acids), plant sterols, terpenes (carotenoids, monoterpenes)

**Rosh Hashanah Menu**

# ✔ *Roman-style Braised Beef* ✔ *and Vegetables over Polenta (Stracotto alla Romana con Polenta)*

Giuseppe Lattanzi, Va Bene, New York, New York

6 SERVINGS

• *This ragu, or thick meat sauce, is heavenly over polenta. Giuseppe also suggests serving it as a flavorful topping for fettuccine.*

## Stracotto

| | | | |
|---|---|---|---|
| 2 | pounds beef round or shoulder, trimmed of all fat and cut into 2-inch cubes | 3 | medium carrots (about 10 ounces), peeled and sliced 1/2 inch thick |
| | salt and pepper | 4 | bay leaves |
| 1 | tablespoon extra virgin olive oil | 2 | tablespoons flour |
| 1 | medium white onion (about 6 ounces), chopped | 1 | cup white wine |
| 4 | celery stalks (about 7 ounces), chopped | 1 | can (28 ounces) tomato puree |

## Polenta

| | | | |
|---|---|---|---|
| 3 | cups chicken stock (page 147 or 148), or low-sodium canned broth or water | 1 | tablespoon olive oil |
| 1/2 | teaspoon salt | 1 | cup stone-ground yellow cornmeal |

Season the meat with salt and pepper. Heat the oil in a large, heavy saucepan. When almost smoking, add half of the seasoned meat and sear over high heat until browned on all sides (you will get better browning by dividing the meat into two batches). Remove the meat and reserve on a large plate. Repeat the process with the second batch.

Add the onion, celery, carrots, and bay leaves to the saucepan and cook over medium-high heat, stirring frequently, until they become somewhat soft and are well browned, 8 to 10 minutes. Sprinkle the flour over the vegetables and stir until there are no lumps and flour is no longer visible. Add the wine, stirring constantly, and cook over high heat for 2 to 3 minutes, then add the tomato puree, 3/4 cup water and meat (and any juices that have been released on the plate), to the saucepan. Cook, covered, over medium-low heat for 2 hours; the meat should be very tender, breaking apart when pressed between two fingers. Adjust the seasoning with salt and pepper.

During the last 30 minutes of cooking, prepare the polenta. In a heavy-bottomed 2-quart saucepan, combine the chicken stock, salt, and olive oil and bring to a simmer. Slowly add the cornmeal, whisking constantly. Lower the heat and continue stirring with a wooden spoon until the mixture thickens, about 15 minutes.

Divide the polenta among 6 shallow soup bowls and spoon the beef over the top.

---

- Trimmed beef round is one of the leanest cuts of beef, containing only about 2 Gm of fat per ounce (similar to chicken and some types of fish). A higher ratio of the fat is saturated, so moderate how much lean beef you eat. When eaten braised or in a stew, portion sizes tend to be less than when steaks or fillets are prepared.
- Moderate intake of lean meat and fish is a good way to get selenium.
- Each serving provides more than 130% of the DV for vitamin A and 30% for vitamin C.
- High in fiber—more than 30% of the DV per serving.

---

*Per serving of Polenta:*

| calories | protein | carbohydrates | fat | cholesterol | dietary fiber | saturated fat |
|---|---|---|---|---|---|---|
| 90 | 2 Gm | 16 Gm | 3 Gm | 0 mg | 2 Gm | 0 Gm |

*Per serving of Stracotto alla Romana:*

| calories | protein | carbohydrates | fat | cholesterol | dietary fiber | saturated fat |
|---|---|---|---|---|---|---|
| 380 | 42 Gm | 20 Gm | 14 Gm | 73 mg | 4 Gm | 4 Gm |

*Per serving of Roman-style Braised Beef and Vegetables over Polenta:*

| calories | protein | carbohydrates | fat | cholesterol | dietary fiber | saturated fat |
|---|---|---|---|---|---|---|
| 480 | 44 Gm | 36 Gm | 17 Gm | 73 mg | 6 Gm | 4 Gm |

**% of Calories**: 31% carbohydrate, 32% protein, 31% fat, 6% alcohol

### Major Sources of Potential Cancer Fighters

**Phytochemicals**: allium compounds, plant polyphenols (flavonoids, phenolic acids), plant sterols, terpenes (carotenoids)

# ❦ *Red Snapper Livornese Style* ❦
## *(Dentice alla Livornese)*

Giuseppe Lattanzi, Va Bene, New York, New York

### 6 SERVINGS

- *A light, full-flavored second course for this Rosh Hashanah menu. Make it an easy main course for any evening by adding small boiled potatoes to the tomato sauce.*
- *Cod, grouper, halibut, or swordfish can be substituted for snapper.*

| | |
|---|---|
| 2 pounds plum tomatoes (about 10 each), peeled, seeded, and chopped | 2 tablespoons chopped fresh Italian parsley |
| 1/2 baguette, cut into thin rounds | 2 pounds red snapper fillets (6 5- to 6-ounce fillets), cleaned and bones removed |
| 6 garlic cloves, peeled and crushed | |
| 2 tablespoons extra virgin olive oil | salt and pepper |

To peel and seed the tomatoes, bring 2 quarts of water to a boil in a large pot. Cut the core from the tomatoes with a paring knife and plunge them into boiling water for 30 seconds. Remove with a slotted spoon and immediately immerse in ice water until cool. Use a knife to gently peel the skin, which should be discarded. Slice the tomatoes in half and gently squeeze to force out the seeds. Use your fingers to remove any remaining seeds. Discard the seeds, chop the tomatoes, and reserve.

Preheat the broiler.

Rub the baguette rounds with 2 cloves of crushed garlic and spread them out on a baking sheet. Place under the broiler until nicely toasted, 2 to 3 minutes. Set aside.

Heat the olive oil in a large skillet (at least 14 inches, preferably nonstick). Sauté the remaining 4 cloves garlic until it turns a light golden color, then add the parsley and cook for another minute. Add the tomatoes and simmer over moderate heat until the sauce thickens slightly, about 10 minutes.

Season the snapper fillets with salt and pepper and place in the skillet in a single layer. Cook for 10 minutes on a low simmer, covered, shaking the pan occasionally. Do not try to turn or move the fillets: red snapper is delicate and may break apart. Add a little bit of water, if necessary. Use a large slotted spatula to remove the fish from the pan. Transfer to large soup bowls, top with some tomato sauce, and serve with toasted baguette rounds.

- Snapper is a potentially good source of selenium.
- Tomatoes provide a substantial amount of vitamin C (40% of the DV per serving) and lycopene, a carotenoid that is a potent antioxidant.

*Per serving:*

| calories | protein | carbohydrates | fat | cholesterol | dietary fiber | saturated fat |
|----------|---------|---------------|-----|-------------|---------------|---------------|
| 302 | 41 Gm | 14 Gm | 8 Gm | 70 mg | 2 Gm | 1 Gm |

**% of Calories**: 20% carbohydrate, 56% protein, 24% fat

**Major Sources of Potential Cancer Fighters**

**Phytochemicals**: allium compounds, plant polyphenols (flavonoids, phenolic acids), plant sterols, terpenes (carotenoids, monoterpenes)

# ❧ *Risotto with Raisins* ❧
# *(Riso con L'Uvetta)*

Giuseppe Lattanzi, Va Bene, New York, New York

6 SERVINGS

- *Lower in fat than traditional risotto and slightly sweet for this festive holiday.*

| | | | | |
|---|---|---|---|---|
| 2 | tablespoons extra virgin olive oil | | | salt and pepper |
| 1 | small onion (about 3 ounces), finely diced | | 3 | cups hot chicken broth (page 147 or 148), low-sodium canned broth or water |
| 1 | cup Italian Arborio rice | | | |
| 1 | cup dry white wine | | 6 | feathery dill leaves, for garnish |
| 1/3 | cup seedless raisins | | | |

Heat 1 tablespoon of the olive oil in a large, heavy saucepan. Sauté the onion over medium heat until limp, 2 to 3 minutes; do not brown.

Add the rice and "toast" it in the saucepan for 1 minute while stirring with a wooden spoon. Add the white wine and simmer, stirring, until the wine has evaporated. Add the raisins, salt, and 1 cup of hot broth.

Continue to cook and stir frequently, uncovered, over medium-high heat. Add more broth, 1/3 cup at a time, as liquid is absorbed. After about 15 to 17 minutes rice will be al dente and the consistency should be loose, but not watery. Remove from the heat, adjust the seasoning, and stir in the remaining 1 tablespoon olive oil. Garnish with a sprig of fresh dill and serve immediately.

Raisins contain plant polyphenols that are potent antioxidants.

**Per serving:**

| calories | protein | carbohydrates | fat | cholesterol | dietary fiber | saturated fat |
|----------|---------|---------------|-----|-------------|---------------|---------------|
| 233 | 5 Gm | 36 Gm | 6 Gm | 5 mg | 2 Gm | 1 Gm |

**% of Calories:** 61% carbohydrate, 8% protein, 21% fat, 10% alcohol

**Major Sources of Potential Cancer Fighters**
**Phytochemicals:** allium compounds, plant polyphenols (flavonoids, phenolic acids)

# ❧ Grandma's Apples Wrapped ❧ in Phyllo (Mela della Nonna)

Giuseppe Lattanzi, Va Bene, New York, New York

6 SERVINGS

- *A homestyle dessert that tastes great.*
- *This crispy baked apple can be made in under 30 minutes.*

| | | | |
|---|---|---|---|
| 6 | Golden Delicious Apples (about 2 pounds), core removed and cone-shaped caps reserved | 2 | tablespoons brown sugar juice of 1/2 lemon |
| 1/3 | cup seedless golden raisins | 2 | tablespoons margarine, melted |
| 3 | tablespoons dark rum | 6 | sheets phyllo dough |
| | | 2 | tablespoons granulated sugar |

Preheat the oven to 375 degrees F.

Core the apples without punching a hole in the bottoms. Divide the raisins, rum, brown sugar, and lemon juice and pour into the center of each apple.

Mix the margarine and 2 tablespoons water in a small bowl. Spread out 6 phyllo pieces on a baking sheet. Brush them with the margarine-water mixture and sprinkle evenly with the granulated sugar. Fold the phyllo in half crosswise, so that you have 6 double-layered phyllo squares. Brush again and place an apple in the center of each one.

Pull up the sides of the phyllo, making neat folds as necessary to prevent bunching; push excess phyllo into the center of the apple. Brush the outer surface of the apples with the remaining margarine-water mixture and bake for 20 to 25 minutes, until the phyllo is golden brown and the apple is tender. Place the reserved caps over the center of the apples and serve immediately.

> Though apples do not contain substantial amounts of vitamins A or C, they are very good sources of fiber and contain protective plant polyphenols.

**Per serving:**

| calories | protein | carbohydrates | fat | cholesterol | dietary fiber | saturated fat |
|---|---|---|---|---|---|---|
| 259 | 2 Gm | 50 Gm | 5 Gm | 0 mg | 4 Gm | 1 Gm |

**% of Calories**: 74% carbohydrate, 3% protein, 18% fat, 5% alcohol

**Major Sources of Potential Cancer Fighters**
**Phytochemicals**: plant polyphenols (flavonoids, phenolic acids), plant sterols

## Thanksgiving Side Dishes

# ✔ Barley Stuffing with ✔ Dried Fruit and Sage

### 10 SERVINGS

• *A great blend of flavors, textures, and colors, this version of Thanksgiving stuffing has much less fat and much more fiber than traditional bread stuffing.*

2   cups dried pearl barley
4   cups chicken stock (page 147 or 148), or canned, low-sodium broth
2   bay leaves
1   tablespoon olive oil
2   shallots (about 3¹/₂ ounces), minced
4   small carrots (about 8 ounces), peeled and diced

3   celery stalks (about 6 ounces), diced
4   fresh sage leaves, chopped
1   cup mixed dried fruit (any combination of apricots, seedless raisins, currants, cranberries, or prunes cut into small pieces)
    salt and pepper

Rinse the barley and place in a saucepan with the chicken stock and bay leaves; bring to a boil. Reduce to a simmer and cook, covered, for 25 to 30 minutes, until the barley is tender and the stock has been absorbed.

In a 10-inch nonstick skillet, heat the olive oil and sauté the shallots for 1 to 2 minutes, then add the carrots and celery. Continue to cook on moderate heat (without browning) for 8 minutes, add the sage, and cook for 2 to 3 minutes more. Set aside.

Transfer the barley into a very large bowl and discard the bay leaves. Add the sautéed vegetables and dried fruit to the barley and toss to combine. Adjust the seasoning with salt and pepper. Transfer to a serving bowl or stuff in the cavity of a turkey when cool.

---

- Each serving provides more than 30% of the DV for vitamin C, and enough carotenoids to supply almost 200% of the DV for vitamin A.
- Barley is a potentially good source of selenium.
- High in fiber—almost 50% of the DV per serving.

---

**Per serving:**

| calories | protein | carbohydrates | fat | cholesterol | dietary fiber | saturated fat |
|----------|---------|---------------|-----|-------------|---------------|---------------|
| 282 | 9 Gm | 56 Gm | 4 Gm | 0 mg | 12 Gm | 1 Gm |

**% of Calories:** 76% carbohydrate, 12% protein, 12% fat

**Major Sources of Potential Cancer Fighters**

**Phytochemicals:** allium compounds, plant polyphenols (flavonoids, phenolic acids), plant sterols, protease inhibitors, terpenes (carotenoids, monoterpenes)

---

## ❧ Citrus Cranberry Sauce ❧

### 10 SERVINGS

- *This easy-to-prepare relish has just the right contrast of sweet and tart flavors.*
- *The perfect spread to replace mayonnaise on leftover turkey sandwiches.*

| | | |
|---|---|---|
| 12 | ounces fresh cranberries | grated zest of 1 orange |
| 1/2 | cup packed brown sugar | grated zest of 1 lime |
| 1 | cup fresh orange juice | |

In a medium saucepan, combine all ingredients. Bring to a boil, then lower to a simmer and cook until the cranberries burst open, about 10 minutes. Let the sauce cool and refrigerate.

---

- Cranberries contain ellagic acid, a phytochemical that may help boost enzymes that rid the body of cancer-causing substances.
- Cranberries also have a substantial amount of vitamin C—30% of the DV per serving (canned has about 75% less than fresh).
- The peel or zest of citrus fruit contains limonene, a phytochemical that may help increase the production of cancer-fighting enzymes that get rid of carcinogens.

---

*Per serving:*

| calories | protein | carbohydrates | fat | cholesterol | dietary fiber | saturated fat |
|----------|---------|---------------|-----|-------------|---------------|---------------|
| 70 | 1 Gm | 17 Gm | 0 Gm | 0 mg | 2 Gm | 1 Gm |

**% of Calories**: 97% carbohydrate, 3% protein, 0% fat

**Major Sources of Potential Cancer Fighters**
**Phytochemicals**: plant polyphenols (flavonoids, phenolic acids), plant sterols, terpenes (carotenoids, limonene)

---

# ❧ *Root Vegetable Mashed Potatoes* ❧

## 10 SERVINGS

- *This blend of autumn root vegetables is nutrient rich and contains only half the fat and calories of traditional mashed potatoes.*

1 medium rutabaga (about 1¹/₂ pounds), peeled and coarsely cut into 1-inch chunks

3 medium turnips (about 1 pound), peeled and coarsely cut into 1¹/₂-inch chunks

4 large white potatoes (about 2¹/₂ pounds), peeled and coarsely cut into 1¹/₂-inch chunks

¹/₃ teaspoon salt
2 cups 2% milk, warm
2 tablespoons olive oil
   salt and pepper

Place the rutabaga, turnips, and potatoes into a large saucepan, cover with cold water, and add the salt. Bring to a boil, then reduce the heat to medium and simmer until the vegetables are tender when pierced with a knife, about 20 minutes.

Drain the boiled vegetables and transfer them to a large bowl.

Heat the milk on the stovetop in a small saucepan or in the microwave. Using an electric mixer, begin pureeing the potatoes while drizzling warm milk into the bowl (use only as much milk as needed to make the puree creamy and light). Beat in the olive oil and season with salt and pepper. Serve hot.

---

- Potatoes and rutabagas are both rich in vitamin C; this recipe provides more than 60% of the DV per serving.
- Rutabagas and turnips belong to the cancer-protective cruciferous family of vegetables.
- A good source of fiber 13% of the DV.

---

**Per serving:**

| calories | protein | carbohydrates | fat | cholesterol | dietary fiber | saturated fat |
|----------|---------|---------------|-----|-------------|---------------|---------------|
| 174 | 5 Gm | 30 Gm | 4 Gm | 10 mg | 3 Gm | 1 Gm |

**% of Calories**: 69% carbohydrate, 11% protein, 21% fat

### Major Sources of Potential Cancer Fighters

**Phytochemicals** allium compounds, glucosinolates, plant polyphenols (flavonoids, phenolic acids)

---

# ❧ Sautéed Swiss Chard with Red Onions ❧

## 10 SERVINGS

- *The sweetness of red onions balances the slight bitterness of Swiss chard. The flavors blend well with traditional Thanksgiving menu items, as well as game or Marinated Pork Tenderloin, page 251.*
- *Serve tossed with pasta (such as penne or fusilli) and diced tomatoes.*

3 pounds Swiss chard (about 2 large bunches, red, if available), stems removed and reserved, leaves torn into bite-size pieces

2 tablespoons olive oil
10 garlic cloves, peeled and halved
2 medium red onions (about 12 ounces), chopped
salt and pepper

Cut out the tough, triangular inner core of each leaf of Swiss chard, and slice into 1/4- to 1/2-inch slices. Rinse the leaves and stems separately and reserve.

Heat 1 tablespoon of olive oil in a large nonstick skillet and add the garlic, cooking until the garlic turns golden brown; don't let the garlic get too brown or it will be bitter. Remove the garlic and set aside. Reserve the oil in the skillet.

Add the remaining tablespoon of olive oil and the chopped onions to the skillet, and sauté until tender, about 5 minutes. Add the chopped stems from the Swiss chard and continue to cook over moderate heat, stirring frequently, until the stems are very tender, 15 to 20 minutes. Add the Swiss chard leaves, season with salt and pepper, and cover. Cook for 10 minutes, stirring often; you may need to add 1/2 cup of chicken stock or water to keep the leaves moist.

Transfer to a serving bowl and top with the crispy garlic.

---

- Swiss chard is a good source of beta-carotene, providing more than 40% of the DV for vitamin A per serving of this recipe. It is also a good source of vitamin C, providing more than 70% of the DV per serving.
- Garlic is a member of the allium compounds or onion family of vegetables and contains phytochemicals that may help increase enzymes that dispose of carcinogens.
- A good source of fiber.

---

**Per serving:**

| calories | protein | carbohydrates | fat | cholesterol | dietary fiber | saturated fat |
|---|---|---|---|---|---|---|
| 65 | 3 Gm | 9 Gm | 3 Gm | 0 mg | 3 Gm | <1 Gm |

**% of Calories**: 48% carbohydrates, 16% protein, 36% fat

**Major Sources of Potential Cancer Fighters**

**Phytochemicals**: allium compounds, plant polyphenols (flavonoids), plant sterols, terpenes (carotenoids)

---

## ❧ *Herb-roasted Shallots* ❧

10 SERVINGS

- *Roasting shallots brings out their natural sweetness.*
- *A terrific accompaniment to your Thanksgiving turkey and other savory sides; also works well with nonholiday menus that may include grilled or roasted meat, fish, or vegetables.*

| | | | |
|---|---|---|---|
| 1½ | pounds shallots, unpeeled, trimmed, root left intact | 3 | fresh rosemary sprigs |
| 1½ | tablespoons olive oil | 3 | fresh thyme sprigs |
| | | | salt and freshly ground pepper |

Preheat the oven to 425 degrees F.

Halve any large shallots so that they are all about the same size. In a large bowl, toss the shallots, olive oil, and herbs until well coated.

Spread the shallots in a single layer on a large, preferably nonstick, baking sheet or roasting pan, and season with salt and pepper. Roast for 20 to 25 minutes, until tender and golden brown. Transfer to a serving bowl and serve.

- Shallots belong to the onion family and contain allium compounds that may bolster cancer-fighting enzymes.
- Rosemary contains carnosol, which is a potent antioxidant and may also boost enzymes that rid the body of carcinogens.

***Per serving:***

| calories | protein | carbohydrates | fat | cholesterol | dietary fiber | saturated fat |
|---|---|---|---|---|---|---|
| 68 | 2 Gm | 12 Gm | 2 Gm | 0 mg | 1 Gm | 0 Gm |

**% of Calories:** 64% carbohydrate, 10% protein, 26% fat

**Major Sources of Potential Cancer Fighters**

**Phytochemicals:** allium compounds, plant polyphenols (flavonoids), terpenes (carnosol)

# Skillet Sweet Potato Pie

8 SERVINGS

• *This deliciously spiced pie can be made with sweet potato or pumpkin puree, and contains about 75% less fat than traditional pumpkin pie.*

**Crust**

| | | | |
|---|---|---|---|
| 12 | ginger snap cookies | 1 | tablespoon orange juice |
| 1 | teaspoon melted butter | | |

*Filling*

| | | | |
|---|---|---|---|
| 2 | medium sweet potatoes or 1¹/₂ cups pumpkin puree | 1 | tablespoon flour |
| 2 | eggs | ¹/₂ | teaspoon ground nutmeg |
| ¹/₂ | cup granulated sugar | ¹/₂ | teaspoon ground cloves |
| ¹/₄ | cup brown sugar | 2 | teaspoons ground cinnamon |
| 1¹/₂ | cups evaporated skim milk | ¹/₂ | teaspoon ground ginger |
| | | ¹/₄ | teaspoon salt |

Preheat the oven to 350 degrees F.

Bake the sweet potatoes for 1 hour to 1 hour and 15 minutes, until tender when pierced with a knife. Remove from the oven and let them cool to room temperature. Peel away the skin from the potatoes, and scoop the flesh into a medium bowl; beat until smooth. (You should have 1¹/₂ cups puree.) Increase the oven temperature to 375 degrees F.

While the potatoes bake, prepare the crust. Place the ginger snaps in the bowl of a food processor and pulse, turning the machine on and off, until coarsely ground. Drizzle in the butter and orange juice and pulse again for 2 to 3 seconds, just to combine.

Spray a 10-inch nonstick skillet with cooking spray (or rub with a small amount of canola oil). Transfer the crust to the skillet and evenly spread across the bottom to 1 inch up the sides. Place the skillet in the oven for 4 minutes. Remove and set aside.

In another medium bowl, beat the eggs with the granulated and brown sugars until creamy. Add the evaporated skim milk, mixing well. Pour into a large bowl with the flour, nutmeg, cloves, cinnamon, ginger, and salt and beat until thoroughly combined. Pour the pie mixture into the skillet with the baked crust and bake for 40 to 45 minutes, until set. Remove from the oven and let cool. Refrigerate for at least 2 hours before serving.

Remove the pie from the skillet by loosening the sides: gently run a rubber spatula between the edge of the pie and the skillet. Carefully slide the pie out of the skillet onto a serving plate.

---

- Sweet potatoes provide enough carotenoids to supply 110% of the DV for vitamin A. They also contain substantial amounts of vitamin C, providing more than 20% of the DV.
- Nutmeg contains monoterpenes that may function as an antioxidant and help boost cancer-fighting enzymes.

---

**Per serving:**

| calories | protein | carbohydrates | fat | cholesterol | dietary fiber | saturated fat |
|---|---|---|---|---|---|---|
| 235 | 7 Gm | 46 Gm | 3 Gm | 56 mg | 2 Gm | 1 Gm |

**% of Calories**: 77% carbohydrate, 11% protein, 12% fat

> **Major Sources of Potential Cancer Fighters**
> **Phytochemicals**: plant polyphenols (flavonoids), plant sterols, terpenes (carotenoids, monoterpenes, triterpenes)

## Christmas Menu

### ❧ *Carrot Soup with Chives* ❧

Alain Sailhac, Dean of Culinary Studies, The French Culinary Institute, New York, New York

8 SERVINGS

• *For creamy texture without the fat, Alain Sailhac recommends vegetable puree soups and sauces. After vegetables soften with cooking, they can be pureed and strained to make them velvety smooth. The small amount of rice in this recipe acts as a thickening agent. In many recipes a starch, such as rice or potato, can replace a high-fat roux (equal proportions of butter and flour).*

• *For a nice presentation, garnish each with a large, butterflied shrimp that has been sautéed and lightly browned.*

| | |
|---|---|
| 1 tablespoon canola oil | 8 cups chicken stock (page 147 or 148), low-sodium canned broth, or water |
| 1 teaspoon unsalted butter | 1/4 cup uncooked rice |
| 2 pounds carrots, peeled and chopped | 1 1/2 cups 2% milk or lite soy milk |
| 1 medium onion (about 5 ounces), chopped | salt and pepper |
| 2 large leeks, cleaned, white part only (about 5 ounces), sliced | 2 tablespoons snipped chives |

Heat the oil and butter in a large saucepan and sauté the carrots, onion, and leeks until they become tender. Adjust the heat so that they do not brown. Add the chicken stock and rice and bring to a boil. Reduce the heat so that the mixture simmers; cover the pot and cook until the rice is soft and the carrots are tender enough to be easily crushed between two fingers, about 40 minutes. Stir from time to time to make sure the vegetables do not stick to the bottom of the saucepan and burn.

Puree the soup in batches in a blender or food processor. If the soup is too thick, add a little more stock or water (don't thin the soup too much—milk will be added).

Using a rubber spatula, push as much liquid as possible through a medium strainer into a clean saucepan. Add the milk and bring the soup to a low simmer. Adjust the seasoning with salt and pepper.

Ladle into warm soup bowls and garnish with a pinch of chopped chives in the center.

---

- Carrots provide the majority of beta-carotene: per serving this recipe provides more than 300% of the DV for vitamin A.
- A good source of fiber.

---

**Per serving:**

| calories | protein | carbohydrates | fat | cholesterol | dietary fiber | saturated fat |
|---|---|---|---|---|---|---|
| 183 | 9 Gm | 26 Gm | 5 Gm | 6 mg | 4 Gm | 2 Gm |

**% of Calories**: 55% carbohydrate, 20% protein, 25% fat

**Major Sources of Potential Cancer Fighters**

**Phytochemicals**: allium compounds, plant polyphenols (flavonoids, phenolic acids), terpenes (carotenoids, monoterpenes)

---

# ❧ *Duck with Ginger and* ❧ *Cassis Sauce and Sautéed Celeriac*

Alain Sailhac, Dean of Culinary Studies, The French Culinary Institute, New York, New York

8 SERVINGS

- *Duck makes any holiday menu even more special, and when the breast is used (without the skin) the amount of fat is not much greater than that of chicken. This recipe is simple to prepare and the flavorful sauce is loaded with cancer-protective nutrients and phytochemicals.*
- *Serve with Mushroom-filled Potato Cakes, page 328.*

## Ginger and Cassis Sauce

| | | | | |
|---|---|---|---|---|
| 3 | tablespoons sugar | | 1/2 | cup fresh orange juice |
| | grated zest of 1 orange | | 1/4 | cup lemon juice |
| | grated zest of 1 lemon | | 1 | cup Madeira wine |
| 1 | tablespoon green peppercorns, well drained | | 1 | tablespoon minced fresh ginger |
| | | | 2 | tablespoons ginger preserves |
| | | | 2 | tablespoons black currant jelly |

1/2 cup demi-glace of veal or duck
    (see Notes)

1/4 cup black currants
    salt

### Duck

8 duck breasts (5 ounces each,
    2 1/2 pounds), skinned and
    trimmed of all fat

    salt and pepper
4 teaspoons olive oil

### Sautéed Celeriac

2 celeriac (celery root), peeled
    and cut into 1/2-inch cubes
    (see Notes)
1 tablespoon butter

1 teaspoon sugar
    salt
2 tablespoons chopped parsley

To make the ginger and cassis sauce, in a heavy saucepan, caramelize the sugar: heat the sugar over medium-high heat until crystals begin to melt. Continue cooking until the sugar turns a rich amber brown, being careful not to let it burn. Remove from the heat, add the orange and lemon zest, and stir for 2 minutes.

Add the peppercorns, orange and lemon juice, and Madeira. Bring to a boil, reduce the heat slightly, and maintain a full, but not rolling, boil to reduce the sauce by half, about 10 minutes. Add the ginger, ginger preserves, black currant jelly, and demi-glace and cook, simmering, for 15 minutes, then add black currants and cook until the sauce becomes syrupy. Season with salt to taste. Reheat when needed. Cook at a low simmer for 2 minutes before serving.

To make the duck, season the breasts with salt and pepper. Heat 2 teaspoons of olive oil in a large nonstick sauté pan. Place 4 pieces of duck, breast side down, in the pan and cook for 4 minutes, until well seared. Turn over and cook for 3 to 4 minutes more, depending on the thickness of the breast. Transfer to a plate and cover loosely to keep warm. Repeat the process with the remaining oil and breasts. (Better browning will be achieved if you cook the duck breasts in two batches rather than all at once.)

To make the sautéed celeriac, place the cubes of celery root in a sauté pan with butter and 3/4 cup water, then sprinkle with sugar and season with salt. Bring to a boil, then reduce the heat to a simmer. Cook, covered, until the vegetables are tender when pierced with a fork, about 8 minutes. Add more water, if necessary, to continue cooking and prevent sticking and burning. Stir in the chopped parsley.

Place wedges of Mushroom-filled Potato Cakes (page 329) on one side of the plate with their tips pointing toward the center of the plate and crossing. Place a small mound of sautéed celery root in the center. Cut each duck breast into 4 to 5 slices lengthwise and fan out over the mound of celery root. Spoon the ginger and cassis sauce around the duck and the plates.

*Notes:* Demi-glace is the reduction of a brown stock, such as chicken, veal, or duck. Its flavor becomes very rich and concentrated, and it is used as a base for many other sauces. Demi-glace can be purchased at most gourmet specialty stores.

Celeriac or celery root has a flavor that is a cross between celery and parsley. It can be found at many supermarkets and green markets during the winter months.

---

- Each serving provides more than 150% of the DV for vitamin C and 25% for folate.
- A good source of fiber.

---

*Per serving of Duck with Ginger and Cassis Sauce and Sautéed Celeriac:*

| calories | protein | carbohydrates | fat | cholesterol | dietary fiber | saturated fat |
|---|---|---|---|---|---|---|
| 380 | 31 Gm | 35 Gm | 11 Gm | 114 mg | 3 Gm | 4 Gm |

**% of Calories**: 37% carbohydrate, 32% protein, 26% fat, 5% alcohol

**Major Sources of Potential Cancer Fighters**

**Phytochemicals:** allium compounds, plant polyphenols (flavonoids, phenolic acids), terpenes (carotenoids, limonene; triterpenes)

*Per serving of Duck with Ginger and Cassis Sauce:*

| calories | protein | carbohydrates | fat | cholesterol | dietary fiber | saturated fat |
|---|---|---|---|---|---|---|
| 322 | 29 Gm | 25 Gm | 9 Gm | 111 mg | 1 Gm | 2 Gm |

*Per serving of Sautéed Celeriac:*

| calories | protein | carbohydrates | fat | cholesterol | dietary fiber | saturated fat |
|---|---|---|---|---|---|---|
| 58 | 2 Gm | 10 Gm | 2 Gm | 3 mg | 2 Gm | 2 Gm |

# ❧ *Mushroom-filled Potato Cakes* ❧

Alain Sailhac, Dean of Culinary Studies, The French Culinary Institute, New York, New York

8 SERVINGS

• *Alain managed to transform his delicious, buttery recipe into an equally wonderful healthy version. The potato cakes become so crispy it seems impossible that they are so low in fat. Alain credits the tasty result to careful heat control and use of a good-quality nonstick skillet.*

| | |
|---|---|
| 1 teaspoon canola oil | 3 long potatoes (about 1¹/₂ pounds, |
| 1 teaspoon butter | preferably a starchy type such |
| 5 cups domestic or wild mushrooms | as russet), peeled and very |
| (about 12 ounces, trimmed, | thinly sliced lengthwise |
| rinsed, well dried, and sliced | (see Note) |
| 2 small shallots, minced | 1 tablespoon olive oil |
| 1 fresh rosemary sprig | salt and pepper |
| 2 sage leaves, chopped | 8 fresh thyme sprigs for garnish |
| leaves from 3 to 4 thyme sprigs | |

Heat the canola oil and butter in a nonstick skillet and add the sliced mushrooms. Sauté for about 5 minutes. When the water evaporates, add the shallots and cook for another 2 to 3 minutes. Add the herbs, toss to combine, and turn off the heat. Remove the rosemary sprig and set aside.

In a medium bowl, toss the potato slices with the olive oil.

If you have 2 8-inch nonstick skillets, prepare 2 potato cakes at the same time and repeat the process one more time. Otherwise, repeat the following method 4 times:

Place 1 long, large slice of potato in the center of each pan. Fan other slices out lengthwise so that they overlap the center slice and each other and fall slightly over the edge of the sauté pan. Season the potatoes with salt and pepper. Over medium heat, begin cooking the potato slices. After 3 to 4 minutes, place one-quarter of the mushroom mixture into the center of each pan and spread out evenly over the potatoes. When the potato slices become somewhat malleable, fold them inward so that a disk shape forms. If there are any gaps (in the center or between potato slices), "patch" them with any extra potato slices that seem to fit well. Sauté on medium-low heat, flipping the cake occasionally (or carefully turning with a spatula) so that the potato cooks and browns but does not burn. It will take 20 to 25 minutes. Be sure both sides of the potato cake are seasoned. Remove from the pan and place on a clean baking sheet.

Slice each cake into 4 wedges and serve with Duck with Ginger and Cassis Sauce and Sautéed Celeriac, page 326. Place a fresh thyme sprig over each wedge to garnish.

Potato cakes can be prepared up to 1 hour in advance and reheated quickly in a 400 degree F oven.

*Note:* Use a mandoline to thinly slice the potatoes. A kitchen tool made of stainless steel or plastic, it is usually sold with a variety of blades for thin slicing and julienning and french fry cutting. A mandoline is essential to cut uniform, thin slices for this recipe. Inexpensive, good-quality plastic mandolines are available at most culinary stores.

---

- Mushrooms contribute selenium as well as other minerals.
- Potatoes are terrific sources of vitamin C: each serving of this recipe provides 25% of the DV.
- Sage, thyme, and rosemary all have phytochemicals that are potent antioxidants.

---

*Per serving:*

| calories | protein | carbohydrates | fat | cholesterol | dietary fiber | saturated fat |
|----------|---------|---------------|-----|-------------|---------------|---------------|
| 92 | 2 Gm | 15 Gm | 3 Gm | 1 mg | 2 Gm | 1 Gm |

**% of Calories**: 62% carbohydrate, 10% protein, 28% fat

### Major Sources of Potential Cancer Fighters
**Phytochemicals**: plant polyphenols (flavonoids, phenolic acids), terpenes (monoterpenes)

---

# ❧ *Traditional Christmas Roll* ❧ (*Bûche de Nöel*)

Alain Sailhac, Dean of Culinary Studies,
The French Culinary Institute, New York, New York

12 SERVINGS

- *With delicious Italian meringue and fruit filling replacing buttercream frosting, the fat content of this traditional French Christmas dessert is very low.*

### Sponge Cake

| | | | |
|---|---|---|---|
| 4 | large egg yolks | 4 | large egg whites |
| 1/2 | cup sugar | 1/2 | cup plus 2 tablespoons flour, sifted |

### Filling

| | | | |
|---|---|---|---|
| 1/3 | cup black currant jam | 1 | cup fresh strawberries |
| 1 | pint fresh raspberries | 2 | tablespoons sugar |

### Meringue

| | | | |
|---|---|---|---|
| 3 | large egg whites | 1 | teaspoon vanilla extract |
| 3/4 | cup sugar | | |

To prepare the sponge cake, preheat the oven to 400 degrees F. Line a 15¼ by 10½ by 1-inch baking sheet with parchment paper or wax paper (if using wax paper, dust it lightly with sugar).

In a large bowl, beat the egg yolks with 1 tablespoon of sugar.

Using a kitchen mixer or handheld electric mixer, whip the egg whites with ¼ cup of the sugar. Gradually add the remaining sugar and whip until firm, glossy peaks form, about 5 minutes. Do not overbeat so that the peaks become dry. Fold the egg whites into the yolks using a rubber spatula. Fold the flour into the eggs to combine; do not beat.

Spread the cake batter out on a baking sheet, rotating it so that the batter is evenly spread. Bake for 9 to 10 minutes, until the cake pulls away from the sides and springs back when touched.

Trim ¼ inch from all sides of the cake. While the sponge cake is still warm, carefully remove it from the pan (it will be easier to roll if filled when still warm). Peel away the parchment or wax paper and place the cake on a large, clean baking sheet. Evenly spread berry filling (see below) on the sponge cake and begin to roll it tightly starting with the lengthwise end. Let cool.

Prepare the filling while the sponge cake bakes. Put all ingredients in a medium non-stick skillet. Simmer until the berry mixture thickens, about 8 minutes. Remove from the heat and set aside.

To make the meringue, in a mixer, whip the egg whites with ¼ cup of the sugar. Gradually add the remaining sugar and whip until firm, glossy peaks form, about 5 minutes. At the last moment add the vanilla extract. Transfer three-quarters of the meringue to a pastry bag fitted with a slanted tip.

Completely cover the cake with meringue by running long, even strips down the top, sides, and ends of the cake. Change to a round pastry tip and refill the pastry bag with the remaining meringue. Make decorative "mushrooms" on the cake by pressing the pastry bag once to form the "stem" and, without moving the bag, squeezing again to form the "cap." Scatter mushrooms on top of the cake.

Increase the oven temperature to 450 degrees F and bake until the meringue is lightly browned, about 5 minutes. Watch it carefully so that it doesn't burn. Slice with a serrated knife and serve.

---

The berry fruit filling replaces the classic buttercream filling and provides vitamin C, as well as carotenoids and protective plant polyphenols.

---

**Per serving:**

| calories | protein | carbohydrates | fat | cholesterol | dietary fiber | saturated fat |
|---|---|---|---|---|---|---|
| 360 | 4 Gm | 75 Gm | 2 Gm | 75 mg | 2 Gm | 1 Gm |

**% of Calories**: 90% carbohydrate, 5% protein, 5% fat

**Major Sources of Potential Cancer Fighters**

**Phytochemicals**: plant polyphenols (flavonoids, phenolic acids)

# One-Week Sample Menus

The sample menus that follow show that a healthy diet need not be boring or difficult to follow. It is possible to accommodate food preferences and availability, as well as lifestyle, and still maintain recommendations to lower the risk of cancer and other diseases.

Here are a few guidelines for using the sample menus:

**1.** Keep in mind that these menus serve as flexible examples. Note the moderate portion sizes of high-protein foods; the use of soy products as an alternative protein source; the number of servings and variety of types of fruits and vegetables; the limited amounts of added fats (butter, oils, salad dressings, mayonnaise, and other high-fat spreads) and processed foods; and the use and variety of whole grains and legumes.

**2.** These menus provide the following daily *average* for nutrients:

1,800 calories, 90 grams protein, 40 grams fat per day
% calories equals 20% protein, 60% carbohydrate, 20% fat
30 to 35 grams dietary fiber per day
4 to 6 vegetable servings plus 2 to 3 fruit servings daily

**3.** If the calorie level of this plan is too much to maintain a healthy weight, adjust the portion sizes of *all* foods down proportionally. If you require more calories to maintain your desired body weight, try to boost calories with high-nutrient items, such as fruit, whole grains, and legumes, rather than meat, alcohol, and sweets.

**4.** Beverages other than green tea are not included in sample menus. Refer to page 55 for some healthy drink ideas.

**5.** These menus list serving sizes for adults. With minor adaptations in portion sizes, the menus are appropriate guides for teenagers and children, and unless medically contraindicated, fat intake can be more liberal. Soy products, such as soy milk and soy cheese, are used extensively as dairy substitutes because they have cancer-fighting phytochemicals, low levels of fat, and no saturated fat. Because many soy milk products do not contain the equivalent amount of calcium as their dairy counterparts, you will need to read labels to verify that your soy product selection contributes to your calcium needs. Refer to page 72 to see what your daily calcium requirements are and see the list of Selected Calcium-Rich Foods on page 74.

**6.** If you do not care for a particular menu item, try to substitute a nutritionally similar item.

- Substitute tuna, bass, swordfish or bluefish for the omega-3–rich salmon on the menu for Saturday's lunch.
- For high-protein items, substitute the equivalent amount of another lean protein source.
- When substituting fruits or vegetables, be sure you are selecting not only a vegetable you like, but one that is nutrient rich. For example, if you are replacing broccoli, try to stick with the cruciferous family (broccoli, Brussels sprouts, cabbage, cauliflower, turnips, rutabagas, collard greens, kale), or replace an orange with another citrus fruit, such as a grapefruit.
- If you do not like yogurt, substitute any low-fat or nonfat dairy item.
- Replace one breakfast cereal with another that is similar in amounts of fiber, fat, and sugar.
- For starches, such as pasta, an equivalent amount (weight) of potatoes, rice, whole grains, or legumes may be substituted. Try to make sure the substituted item does not have high amounts of added fat.

# ONE-WEEK MENU FOR CANCER PREVENTION

## Monday

### Breakfast
1 cup green tea
³/4 cup Shredded Wheat mixed with
¹/4 cup All Bran cereal
³/4 cup 1% lite soy milk
¹/2 cup sliced strawberries
4 ounces orange juice

### Lunch
Roast turkey sandwich (2 to 3 ounces
turkey) on wheat bread with
lettuce, tomato, and mustard
1 serving (5 ounces) Broccoli and
Tomato Salad (page 311)

### Afternoon Snack
Small handful of Brazil nuts
1 orange

### Dinner
Chicken Cacciatore (page 245)
1 whole wheat dinner roll
Tossed green salad with
1 tablespoon vinaigrette

### Evening Snack
1 cup fresh raspberries or
any other seasonal berry
¹/2 cup vanilla yogurt or a soy-based yogurt

## Tuesday

### Breakfast
1 cup green tea
¹/2 sesame bagel with 2 tablespoons
low-fat cream cheese or tofu cream cheese
¹/2 red grapefruit

### Lunch
1 serving Healthy Tuna Salad
(page 161) on 2 slices rye bread
with lettuce and tomato
1.5-ounce bag pretzels

**Afternoon Snack**
1 apple
1 handful of low-fat wheat crackers
1 tablespoon tahini

**Dinner**
7 ounces cooked pasta with Tomato-Basil
Sauce
1 serving Sautéed Spinach
with Garlic (page 179)

**Evening Snack**
Strawberry Soup (page 283)

## Wednesday

**Breakfast**
1 cup green tea
1 small bran muffin
1/2 cup fruit salad
1/2 cup 1% cottage cheese

**Lunch**
1 cup Black Bean Soup (page 132)
Grilled, poached, or roasted chicken
breast sandwich (3 to 4 ounces chicken)
on wheat bread with lettuce, tomato,
and reduced-fat mayonnaise or
tofu-based mayonnaise

**Afternoon Snack**
2 plums
2 small biscotti cookies

**Dinner**
1 serving Sicilian style
Cauliflower Soup (page 134)
1 veggie burger (preferably soy)
on whole wheat roll with lettuce,
tomato, and red onion slices
1 sweet potato

**Evening Snack**
1 Creamy Mocha Chocolate and Raspberry "Parfait" (page 290)

## *Thursday*

**Breakfast**
1 cup green tea
1 cup Raisin Bran cereal
3/4 cup 1% lite soy milk
4 ounces orange juice

**Lunch**
1 slice pizza
small tossed salad with lettuce,
tomato, and shredded carrot
1 tablespoon olive oil–vinegar vinaigrette
1 cup cubed cantaloupe

**Afternoon Snack**
1 peach

**Dinner**
1 Scrambled Egg Burrito (page 202)
1 cup steamed broccoli
1 slice whole wheat toast

**Evening Snack**
2 oatmeal raisin cookies
1 cup lite vanilla soy milk

## *Friday*

**Breakfast**
1 cup green tea
3/4 cup oatmeal topped with
1/4 cup All Bran
1/4 cup raisins
1/3 cup 1% lite soy milk
1/2 red grapefruit

**Lunch**
I piece skinless, roasted chicken breast
(4 to 5 ounces)
1/2 cup corn or 1 ear corn on the cob
1 baked potato or 1/2 cup mashed potatoes

**Afternoon Snack**
1 handful of low-fat wheat crackers
1 pear

**Japanese Dinner Out**
1 serving miso soup
1 serving seaweed salad
2 California Rolls
4 pieces sushi (2 tuna, 1 salmon, 1 shrimp)
12 ounces green tea

**Evening Snack**
$1/2$ cup green tea ice cream

---

## Saturday

**Breakfast**
1 cup green tea
1 cup low-fat yogurt or soy yogurt
topped with handful of low-fat granola
$1/3$ cantaloupe

**Lunch**
1 cup vegetable barley soup
1 serving Warm Salmon Salad
with Capers, p. 168

**Afternoon Snack**
1 small bag of pretzels

**Dinner**
1 serving Mexican
Lasagne (page 204)
tossed green salad (*dark* leaves)
with olive oil–vinegar dressing

**Evening Snack**
1 serving Peach and Blueberry Crisp (page 286)
$1/2$ cup vanilla frozen yogurt

---

## Sunday

**Breakfast**
12 ounces green tea
1 soft-boiled egg
2 slices multigrain bread, toasted
2 tablespoons fruit spread
4 ounces tomato juice

**Lunch**
Caesar salad with grilled chicken
with 2 tablespoons Caesar Dressing
(page 151); order dressing on
the side if dining out

**Dinner**
1 serving Marinated Pork
Tenderloin (page 251)
baked sweet potato or 1 serving
Smashed Orange-scented Sweet
Potatoes (page 251)
1 serving Sweet and Sour
Cabbage (page 181)
1 whole wheat dinner roll

**Evening Snack**
1 serving Apple Strudel (page 296)

# Restaurant Dining

Restaurants that make health claims or include nutritional descriptions on their menus must support these claims in compliance with the Nutrition Labeling and Education Act of 1990 (NLEA). Restaurants that include such comments as "low-fat," "reduced-calorie," "heart healthy," or "fat-free" must be able to demonstrate that their menu claims are consistent with the claim definitions established under NLEA.

Dining out does not need to be the downfall to an otherwise good day of healthy eating. Here are some general suggestions for menu selections to keep fruit and vegetable intake high and fat intake low.

*Select menu items that are prepared in the following manner:*

baked
braised
broiled
en papillote (sealed in paper or foil and cooked via steam, concentrating flavor)
grilled
poached
roasted
sautéed (request that minimal fat be used in cooking)
seared
steamed
stewed

*Consider menu items with these descriptions:*

au jus (served in its own juices—often better than a stock-based sauce)

coulis (served with a strained fruit or vegetable sauce)

marinara (spicy tomato sauce that is usually moderate in fat)

pilaf (simple and healthy whether rice or another type of grain)

Provençal (cooked in the style of southwest France; will include any combination of the following: tomatoes, garlic, onions, capers, anchovies, olives, eggplant, olive oil, and fresh herbs, such as rosemary, thyme, marjoram, oregano, tarragon, or sage)

ragout (a classic, thick, well-seasoned stew of meat or fish; many restaurants incorporate vegetables or prepare vegetable ragouts)

salsa (usually raw vegetables and/or fruits combined with a minimal amount of fat to form a topping, dip, or sauce)

Look for entrées served with vegetable accompaniments or select vegetable side dishes.

*Limit selection of menu items that use these cooking methods:*

barbecued (The sauce is not inherently unhealthy, but the types and cuts of meat that are typically cooked in this style are usually high in fat. If you know the barbecued item is lean, then it is okay.)

blackened

charbroiled

charcoal-grilled

deep-fried

fried

pan-fried

smoked

*Limit menu items that have these descriptions:*

almondine (cooked in a style with almonds, and usually a lot of butter as well)

au gratin

batter-dipped

béarnaise (a classic French sauce made with a reduction of wine, vinegar, shallots, and tarragon and finished with egg yolks and butter)

béchamel (a basic French white sauce made by stirring milk into equal parts of butter and flour) beurre (includes butter, probably a lot of it)

breaded (unless oven-baked, the next step is frying; even if the breaded item is sautéed, the bread coating acts as a sponge for fat)

creamy (unless otherwise indicated as healthy)

crispy

croquette (whether made of potato or fish, these oval cylinders are usually deep-fried)

en croute (usually signifies food is wrapped in buttery puff pastry)

escalloped (cooking style that generally includes butter and cream)

flaky

fritters

hollandaise (a rich, buttery emulsion sauce typically served with egg dishes, fish, or vegetables)

Newburg (usually includes chopped shellfish, cream, eggs, and butter)

parmigiana (indicates use of Parmesan cheese, which is not necessarily a problem; however, food served alla parmigiana is also typically dredged in flour, eggs, and bread crumbs then fried or sautéed in a lot of oil, and finally smothered in Parmesan and mozzarella cheese)

scampi (unless you request minimal butter and oil, expect a lot)

Here are some tips for ethnic menus. Keep in mind that the lists serve to provide guidance, but they are not exhaustive. You are likely to encounter many foods that do not appear on these lists. In these situations, follow the general menu selection guidelines provided above.

## *Italian*

CHOOSE:

antipasti ( healthy examples include roasted peppers, tomatoes, and bean salads)

calamari, sautéed or grilled

cacciatore (usually chicken or fish and vegetables stewed in a tomato sauce)

cioppino (tomato-based fish stew)

grilled or roasted chicken or fish, simply prepared

minestrone soup or other vegetable or bean soups

mussels served in a marinara or a white wine sauce

pasta e fagioli (a flavorful bean and pasta soup)

pasta with clam sauce (request only a moderate amount of olive oil be used)

pasta with tomato and basil or marinara sauce

pasta with vegetables

risotto (This Italian rice with vegetables, fish, or meat *can* be a healthy balance of carbohydrates and protein as well as a good base for vegetables. The final step of preparation, when a substantial amount of butter or olive oil is stirred in, can be the downfall. Request that this step be omitted.)

vegetable-filled ravioli

vegetable sides

wood-burning ovens, almost anything made in: pizza, fish, meat, and especially vegetables

### LIMIT OR AVOID:

"alla carbonara" (sauce includes eggs, cream, bacon, and Parmesan cheese)

"alla parmigiana."

cheese-filled baked pastas, such as manicotti, ziti, lasagne, or ravioli

fettuccine Alfredo and other pastas with cream

fried calamari

veal marsala (can be okay, but depends on sauce—often butter is used to emulsify sauce)

veal piccata (can be okay, but depends on sauce—often butter is used to emulsify sauce)

## Asian (Japanese, Chinese, Thai)

### CHOOSE:

California rolls

chicken, shrimp, or vegetable chow mein

hot and sour soup

Hunan shrimp, chicken, or tofu

miso soup

rice, steamed brown or white

seaweed salads

shabu shabu (beef cooked in a hot broth at the table; usually lean beef is sliced paper thin, helping with portion control)

shrimp or chicken with garlic sauce

shrimp with vegetables

spiced beet salad

steamed or broiled fish

steamed vegetable dumplings

steamed vegetables with rice and side sauces, such as garlic, black bean, or brown

stir-fried vegetables or vegetable-chicken or vegetable-fish combinations

sushi hand rolls

sushi or sashimi

sweet and sour shrimp

Szechuan shrimp, chicken, or tofu

teriyaki chicken, fish, or beef with vegetables

Thai chicken

Thai salad

vegetable curries prepared without coconut milk

wonton soup

yakitori (a Japanese term meaning "grilled fowl," usually small pieces of marinated chicken that are grilled)

yosenabe, (a one-pot meal usually consisting of a combination of chicken, fish, shellfish, and vegetables in a broth)

## LIMIT OR AVOID:

beef with cashews

coconut soups

curries or soups prepared with coconut milk

egg rolls

fried rice or anything that says crispy or fried

fried tofu

General Tso's chicken

Kung pao chicken

lo mein, beef, chicken, or pork

moo-shu pork

noodles, sautéed or fried

Peking duck

sweet and sour pork

tempura

Thai rolls

whole fried fish

# *Indian*

CHOOSE:

aam chatni (mango chutney)
aloo bhaji (braised potatoes, tomatoes, and spices)
aloo ghobi (braised potatoes, cauliflower, onions, and spices)
aloo mattar gajar (spicy carrots, peas, and potatoes)
aloo paratha (potato-stuffed flat bread)
bainagn bharta (roasted eggplant with spices)
basmati rice
chapatis (whole wheat flatbread)
chicken or shrimp curry
curried or saffron rice
kachoomber (tomato salad)
kali dal (spicy black lentils)
kheere ka raita (cucumber and mint salad)
masoor dal (a red lentil stew)
murgh dhansak (chicken with vegetables and lentils)
rajma (translated as "royal beans," this traditional northern Indian dish is a combination of red beans, onions, garlic, tomatoes, and spices)
tandoori (select breads, chicken, and fish that have been cooked in the tandoori oven)
tomatar jingha (spicy shrimp cooked in tomatoes)
whole roasted fish

LIMIT OR AVOID:

anything fried
anything with a cream sauce
anything with ghee (clarified butter)
keema mattar (spicy ground beef with peas)
keema paratha (meat-stuffed flatbread)
pakoras (vegetable fritters)
poori (fried puffed whole wheat bread)
pork, beef, or lamb curries
samosas (meat- or vegetable-filled pastries)

# Mexican

**CHOOSE:**

beans, pinto or black
black bean soup
chicken, seafood, or vegetable tacos
fajitas
Mexican rice
refried beans (prepared with minimal or no fat)
tostados
vegetable, chicken, or shellfish burritos
vegetable chili

**LIMIT OR AVOID:**

added cheese, guacamole, and sour cream
beef burritos
cheese quesadillas
chiles rellenos
chimichangas
enchiladas
nachos
taco salads with deep-fried baskets
tortilla chips (unless they are baked)

## Fast Food or Franchise Restaurants

**CHOOSE:**

baked beans or rice and beans
baked potatoes (select vegetable toppings and order other toppings, such as cheese, chili, or sour cream, on the side so that you can spoon on only a small amount.
broiled, grilled, or roasted chicken (skin removed) or fish
broth-based or bean soups made without pork
grilled chicken salad (go light on the dressing)
grilled chicken sandwich (opt for lettuce, tomato, onion, and whatever other vegetable topping offered)
pita sandwiches or wraps with vegetables and low-fat dressing
roasted, boiled, or mashed potatoes (hold the gravy) rather than french fries
rice pilaf, brown rice, or Cajun rice

rotisserie or roasted chicken (without skin)

salad bars (Select fresh greens, chopped vegetables, low-fat salad dressings, beans, fruit salad, fresh bread, or breadsticks. Limit selections that are drenched in dressing or mayonnaise.)

thin-crusted pizza from wood-burning ovens, or even pizzeria-style pizza (Select vegetable toppings and blot any fat from the surface with a napkin. Request less cheese.)

turkey sandwich with mustard, lettuce, and tomato (select higher-fiber breads, such as rye, pumpernickel, whole wheat, or multigrain)

vegetable sides (Many fast food restaurants now offer vegetable side dishes, such as sautéed spinach, mashed potatoes or mashed sweet potatoes, corn, broccoli, okra, and fruit salad)

LIMIT OR AVOID:

almost everything else

Now that you know what to order, here are some quick tips to help keep dining out enjoyable and broaden your healthy selections.

- Eat slowly and enjoy all aspects of the dining experience.
- Fill up on vegetable first courses (antipasto, grilled vegetables, soups, crudites, etc.).
- Restaurants want to please you, so ask questions. Don't order food unless you are sure about what is in it and the preparation methods.
- Many restaurants are flexible with preparation methods. Request that the sautéed shrimp be grilled or the sautéed carrots be steamed.
- Look at all choices on the menu and be creative—make combinations to end up with a healthy entrée. For example, if one entrée is served with a healthy sauce or vegetable that appeals to you, request that this be added to or substituted for your choice.
- Go heavier on rice and vegetables and add meat as a topping (more like a condiment). When dining with a companion, order a vegetarian entrée and a meat- or fish-based selection. By dividing them, you and your dining partner will both be closer to appropriate portion sizes.
- Indulge in your favorite desserts occasionally, but limit your portion by sharing with a friend.

# CHAPTER 6

# Prevention: Lifestyle Modifications to Minimize Cancer Risk

**C**ancer is a serious public health problem. President Richard Nixon declared "war on cancer" in 1971 and since then vast amounts of resources, including time and money, have been spent to win this war. Research has focused primarily on finding a cure for cancer using medical advances. Unfortunately, no magic bullet has been discovered and we have not been the victors.

*An estimated 60 to 80 percent of all cancer could be prevented by simple lifestyle and behavior changes.* Some experts believe that the U.S. death rate from cancer could be decreased by as much as 50 percent if these changes were implemented. Prevention of cancer before it occurs is obviously better than trying to treat cancer after it has invaded the body. Cancer screening also plays an important role and can help identify cancer early when treatment is more successful.

Every day we read in the paper, see in the news, or hear on the radio that "something" causes cancer. All too often these are the results of preliminary studies that fail to be confirmed by other researchers. The proportion of cancer that can be attributed to known cancer-causing agents varies. An individual's perception of what causes cancer also varies. For instance, many people are convinced that food additives are a major cause of cancer, but in fact they are responsible for very few cancer deaths. On the other hand, the benefits of an anticancer diet, one that is high in fruits and vegetables, are well established, but many people fail to modify their diet. This might be because focusing on an outside reason as the cause of cancer is simpler than identifying and changing one's own behavior.

Many factors other than diet are associated with cancer. There are lifestyle changes you can make for a more "cancer healthy" way of life.

# Smoking

*Smoking accounts for a large proportion of all cancers and about 30 percent of all cancer deaths.* Cigarette smoking is the cause of lung, oral cavity, laryngeal, esophageal, bladder, kidney, and pancreatic cancer. Colon and cervical cancer may be related to smoking. Smoking has also been linked to prostate, rectum, stomach, and liver cancer, although the findings are not definitive. The risk of these cancers is increased in people who smoke longer, smoke more, and start at a younger age. In addition, one-quarter to one-third of all heart disease can be attributed to smoking.

It has been established that smoking causes cancer and also depletes the body of antioxidants, which are valuable cancer fighters. The benefits of quitting have been established: 90 percent of lung cancer and one-third of all cancer deaths could be eliminated.

Exposure to environmental tobacco smoke (that is, involuntary or passive smoke) is also a cause of lung cancer in nonsmokers. The increased risk could be as high as 50 percent. It has been estimated that a few thousand people will die each year due to exposure to passive smoke. Users of smokeless tobacco, pipes, and cigars are also at increased risk of developing tobacco-associated cancers.

## Ten Tips to Help You Stop Smoking

**1.** Learn more about the health consequences of smoking by calling the American Lung Association or visiting lung cancer patients at a cancer hospital.

**2.** Try a smoking-cessation program or support group.

**3.** If you have already tried to quit smoking and were not successful, try something new like the nicotine patch or gum.

**4.** Make a commitment and try quitting with a friend or relative.

**5.** Stay positive: smoking is addictive, it's not your fault!

**6.** Put a picture of a spouse, child, or loved one in your cigarette pack and look at it each time you "light up."

**7.** Try eating hard candies or gum to keep your mouth "occupied."

**8.** Don't nag or yell at the person who cannot quit smoking—it only makes the situation worse.

**9.** If you absolutely cannot quit, start cutting back the amount you smoke and don't drink alcohol, which can increase the negative effect of smoking.

**10.** Don't give up: it usually takes a couple of tries before you quit successfully.

# Obesity

The U.S. National Center for Health Statistics has estimated 31 percent of men and 35 percent of women are overweight. There have been hundreds of studies that show being overweight increases the risk of developing many types of cancer, including kidney, colon, ovarian, endometrial, gallbladder, cervical, prostate, rectal, and breast. Obesity is also a risk factor for other diseases, such as heart disease, stroke, and diabetes. Further support for the link between being overweight and cancer comes from recent observations that height is a risk factor for common cancers: breast, prostate, and colon. The increase in stature that is now being observed parallels the increase in cancer rates over time. It may be that tall stature, a marker of growth rates, is the result of "overnutrition" or excess calories during childhood and adolescence.

Diet and excess calorie intake may directly influence obesity. It is not clear how obesity contributes to the development of cancer, but it is believed that being overweight is related to other risk factors, such as high-fat diets, high-calorie intake, inactivity, being menopausal, adverse hormone levels, and insulin resistance. *Maintaining an ideal body weight is a lifestyle change that everyone can adopt that will help prevent cancer.*

## Ten Tips to Help You Maintain an Ideal Weight

**1.** Refer to pages 19 to 20 for weight recommendations and calorie requirements.

**2.** A healthy diet and regular exercise are the two most important factors in weight loss and maintenance.

**3.** Be sure you are hungry before you eat.

**4.** A low-fat diet may make it easier to cut calories and eat lots of fruits, vegetables, and grains.

**5.** Pay attention to "fat-free" foods—they still contain calories and can make you gain weight if you overindulge.

**6.** Moderate your intake of alcohol; it contains "empty" calories and may make it hard for your body to control appetite.

**7.** Stress, boredom, and emotions can contribute to overeating and poor nutrition. Watch for those hard-to-handle situations and develop more beneficial stress fighters.

**8.** Make a commitment to lose weight and seek nutritional counseling if necessary.

**9.** Stay positive and be realistic about how much time it will take to lose weight.

**10.** There is no quick fix.

# Physical Activity/Exercise

*Individuals who exercise are at reduced risk of developing colon cancer and possibly breast and prostate cancer.* The evidence supporting the exercise–colon cancer link is strong and convincing. With respect to breast and prostate cancer the results are less conclusive. Increasing our physical activity levels is important from a cancer-prevention standpoint, because colon, breast, and prostate cancers are some of the most prevalent cancers in the United States. Inactivity probably accounts for about 5 percent of all cancer deaths.

It is not fully understood how exercise might protect against cancer, but it may increase the immune function, affect hormone and insulin levels, or shorten the stool's transit time through the intestine (reducing exposure to carcinogens). Generally, physically active people are not overweight and this would also help to decrease risk because obesity is related to many cancers.

The American population has become sedentary, but the benefits of exercise are tremendous. Television, VCRs, and computer games have replaced a walk or bike ride. Exercise that has the most benefit for reducing cancer risk is probably that done at moderate to vigorous levels. The Centers for Disease Control and Prevention (CDC) and the American College of Sports Medicine have recently revised their recommendations for physical activity. They suggest that every adult accumulate thirty minutes or more of moderate-intensity physical activity on most, preferably all, days of the week. Physical activity can be intermittent, such as walking fifteen minutes in the morning and fifteen minutes at lunchtime, as long as it is at least moderately intense. Also, flexibility and strength exercises are recommended. Here are some examples of moderate activity level:

> walking briskly at 3 to 4 mph
> biking at speeds up to 10 mph
> playing Ping-Pong, golfing (carrying or pulling clubs)
> fishing (casting from shore)
> canoeing at 2 to 4 mph
> vacuuming, weeding, mowing
> house painting

## Ten Tips to Help You Start Exercising

**1.** Be sure to consult your physician before starting an exercise program.
**2.** Figure out the best time to exercise and schedule an appointment to do it.
**3.** Work out with a friend; you'll be less likely to skip a day.

**4.** Have a variety of activities, both indoor and outdoor, so that bad weather doesn't get in the way.

**5.** Try walking. It's easy, fun, and you can do it almost anywhere and anytime.

**6.** Exercise while you are doing other things; for example, ride a stationary bike while watching the news.

**7.** Physical activity reduces stress and can lift your spirits. If you are in a bad mood, try exercising: everything usually looks better afterward.

**8.** Try to squeeze an exercise session in between other commitments.

**9.** Take advantage of friends and family for child care when visiting and go for a walk or run.

**10.** Stay positive, set realistic goals, and reward yourself often!

## Workouts of Moderate Intensity*

basketball (playing a game) for 15 to 20 minutes
basketball (shooting baskets) for 30 minutes
bicycling 5 miles in 30 minutes
bicycling 4 miles in 15 minutes
dancing fast (social) for 30 minutes
gardening for 30 to 45 minutes
jumping rope for 15 minutes
playing touch football for 30 to 45 minutes
playing volleyball for 45 minutes
pushing a stroller 1 1/2 miles for 30 minutes
raking leaves for 30 minutes
running 1 1/2 miles in 15 minutes (10-minute mile)
shoveling snow for 15 minutes
stairwalking for 15 minutes
swimming laps for 20 minutes
walking 1 3/4 miles in 35 minutes (20-minute mile)
walking 2 miles in 30 minutes (15-minute mile)
washing and waxing a car for 45 to 60 minutes
washing windows or floors for 45 to 60 minutes
water aerobics for 30 minutes
wheelchair basketball for 20 minutes
wheeling self in wheelchair for 30 to 40 minutes

*U.S. Department of Health and Human Services: Centers for Disease Control and Prevention: A Report of the Surgeon General: Physical Activity and Health 1996.

# Hormones

Hormones, including oral contraceptives and estrogen replacement therapy, have been linked to certain female cancers. These synthetic and natural hormones have regulatory effects on the menstrual cycle and pregnancy and probably increase the risk of some cancers by increasing cell division. Overall, these factors account for about 3 percent of observed cancer deaths.

Oral contraceptives are used to prevent pregnancy and have been associated with a small increased risk of breast cancer in women who are currently using them, probably before the age of forty-five. *Nevertheless, oral contraceptive use does not account for a large proportion of the observed breast cancer cases.* Oral contraceptives have also been shown to increase the risk of liver cancer. But liver cancer is a rare disease, especially in the United States, and does not account for a large proportion of cancer mortality.

A beneficial effect of oral contraceptives (the type that are combination pills containing estrogen and progestin) on ovarian and endometrial cancer has been consistently shown. Five or more years of use reduces the lifetime risk of developing these cancers by as much as 50 percent.

Estrogen replacement therapy is taken for menopausal symptoms, such as hot flashes and vaginal dryness, and in some instances to retard bone loss associated with osteoporosis and prevention of cardiovascular disease. *In long-term users (five to ten years or more) estrogen appears to increase the risk of breast cancer. Short-term use to relieve menopausal symptoms probably does not increase risk.*

In the 1970s, estrogen replacement therapy was shown to increase the risk for endometrial cancer in women who were long-term users. Subsequently, these estrogen preparations were prescribed in conjunction with opposed hormones (called progestins), which offset the risk. It has been suggested that estrogen replacement therapy may protect against colon cancer, but this remains to be confirmed. Preliminary studies have shown a potential beneficial effect of estrogen replacement therapy on risk of Alzheimer's disease. This is an interesting area for continued research. Discuss the risks and benefits associated with estrogen use with a physician.

Factors related to hormone levels increase the risk for some cancers while decreasing the risk for others. Pregnancy (as well as bearing more than one child) appears to protect against breast, endometrial, and ovarian cancer. Breast-feeding may be beneficial for breast and ovarian cancer (probably by decreasing the number of monthly ovulations and related cell divisions). Early age at onset of menstruation and late age at menopause increase the risk of both breast and endometrial cancer, while late age at first pregnancy increases the risk for breast cancer. These increased risks are most likely related to increasing cumulative exposure to estrogens.

It is important to know and understand the hormonal factors that might increase your risk of developing cancer. Adherence to cancer screening guidelines (page 357) and modification of risk factors are even more important.

# Occupation

Occupational exposures account for less than 5 percent of all fatal cancers, mainly lung and bladder. Workplace exposure to chemicals and carcinogens can be high, although the absolute number of people exposed tends to be small. Substances identified as human carcinogens include asbestos, formaldehyde, benzene, diesel exhaust, arsenic, vinyl chloride, and radon, to name just a few. However, tobacco smoke is by far the strongest contributor to occupational-associated cancers.

Fortunately, in the United States, the Occupational Safety and Health Act (1970) brought potential occupational hazards to the forefront of attention for both employers and employees. Since the identification of cancer-causing chemicals, there has been strict control and regulation of the amount of exposure in the workplace. This will likely prevent or reduce the risk of occupational-associated cancers in the future.

Although the number of people who work with or near chemicals is limited, everyone should be aware of chemical exposures at the workplace and their safety profile. Efforts should be made to minimize exposure.

## Five Tips for Minimizing Occupational Exposures

**1.** Be informed. Ask your employer or human resources manager about chemicals or substances that you are exposed to and any potential hazards; by law they must provide this information.

**2.** Always wear the appropriate protective clothing, gloves, and eyeglasses.

**3.** Follow safety rules carefully.

**4.** If you are exposed to chemicals at the workplace, ask your employer about the possibility of job rotation.

**5.** Be sure to quit smoking if exposed to workplace chemicals.

# Radiation

One of the most common misconceptions is that radiation causes a large proportion of all cancer. Although radiation exposure is a known cause of cancer, it has been estimated that only 2 percent of all cancers can be attributed to radiation and most of this is from natural sources, such as radon, cosmic rays, and ultraviolet radiation (sunlight). All of us are exposed to this "background" radiation each day.

## Ionizing Radiation

Radon is a radioactive gas that is emitted from the earth and is colorless and odorless. In high doses it can cause lung cancer. Most of the radon-induced lung and upper respiratory cancer is seen in underground miners, who are exposed to high levels. Furthermore, it has been shown that exposure to *both* smoking and radon increases the cancer risk far more than exposure to either one alone. Everyone should know that smoking is hazardous to your health, but it is even riskier in workers exposed to radon. Radon can also accumulate in buildings or homes, but most homes have extremely low levels and radon is usually found in the basement. Studies have not supported the theory that many cancers can be attributed to radon in the home. Simple home test kits are available to measure radon levels at home.

Radiation exposure and the potential cancer risk from medical X rays have been studied extensively. It appears that therapeutic radiation (radiotherapy in very large doses to treat a certain condition) does increase the risk for some cancers, such as thyroid, breast, and leukemia. However, diagnostic X rays (such as those X rays taken for breast cancer screening—mammography) emit a very low dose of radiation similar to that of dental X rays and the immediate benefits for medical use far outweigh any risks. For example, it has been estimated that mammographic X rays probably cause less than 1 percent of all breast cancers. This would increase a woman's lifetime risk of developing breast cancer from 9.09 percent (which is the average) to 9.18 percent (with mammography screening).

An increased risk of cancer has been observed in individuals exposed to X-ray sources at the workplace, such as radiologists. All workers should take precautionary measures, such as using protective shields. It is important to know your medical history and exposure to this type of therapeutic radiation. Adherence to cancer screening guidelines is even more important in people exposed to therapeutic radiation.

The media have devoted a lot of attention to "cancer clusters" and there has been an effort to explain increased rates of cancer observed in defined geographical areas. It has been proposed that people living near nuclear power plants have increased risk of developing cancer. Nuclear *accidents*, such as the one at Chernobyl in 1986, prove that radiation from nuclear materials can cause cancer. However, overall studies have failed to confirm the claim that leukemia rates are higher in people living near nuclear power plants in the absence of any nuclear accident.

## Sunlight (Ultraviolet Radiation)

*The majority of radiation-induced cancer is caused by the ultraviolet rays from the sun that damage the skin cells.* More than 90 percent of skin cancer is caused by sun exposure. The majority of all skin cancers can be prevented by "sun-smart" strategies:

**1.** Avoid or minimize sun exposure, especially during the hours of 10 A.M. to 3 P.M.

**2.** Use a sunscreen, with an SPF of 15 or above.

**3.** Protect exposed parts of the body with clothing.

**4.** Be especially careful to protect children from sunburns.

**5.** Sun causes wrinkles and makes you look old before your time.

**6.** Eliminate sunbathing so that you'll have a lot more time for other fun activities!

**7.** Try some of the new self-tanning creams, available at cosmetic counters.

**8.** Check any skin growths. A mole or spot that changes in size, shape, or color should be immediately checked by a physician. Most skin cancers are curable when detected early; an important aspect of skin cancer prevention is screening.

**9.** See a physician for regular skin cancer screening, especially if you have fair skin.

**10.** No amount of suntanning is safe. Even "indoor" suntanning in sunbeds or with sunlamps is unsafe.

## Electromagnetic Radiation (Nonionizing Radiation)

Electromagnetic field (EMF) exposure refers to the magnetic fields from power lines and electromagnetic radiation from cellular telephones, video display terminals, and electrical household appliances. These are either extremely low frequency fields (power lines and electrical household appliances) or radio-frequency radiation (cellular telephones, microwaves, and other "wireless" devices). The frequency is lower than ionizing radiation or ultraviolet radiation. The amount of radiation emitted from electromagnetic radiation does not have the "energy" to induce a cancer-causing mutation.

Because of the intense public interest in the health effects of EMF exposure, many scientific groups and regulatory agencies have examined the effects on disease, particularly cancer. There have been some studies that suggest there may be an effect on childhood leukemia (these often make news headlines), but these studies have been criticized for methodological limitations and the overall evidence is weak. Because we do not have the technology necessary to study the effects of EMF exposure, and it is not logistically feasible to measure EMF exposure from such common sources as power lines, household appliances, and other electronic devices, long-term EMF exposure cannot be measured accurately. Although there is a possibility of negative health effects from EMF exposure, at this time the evidence is weak and does not support electromagnetic radiation as a significant cause of cancer or any other disease.

# Environmental Pollution

We are all exposed to environmental pollutants daily, but fortunately the level of these exposures is low and they do not appear to cause a significant increase in cancer risk. The overall contribution of environmental pollution, both air and water pollution, to cancer rates is small (probably accounting for only 2 percent of cancer mortality). Smoking and diet play a much larger role in explaining cancer risk.

Probably the most significant form of air pollution is tobacco smoke, and the effect is not only on smokers but on nonsmokers as well. Air pollution also includes combustion products from industrial emissions, motor vehicle emissions, and heating units and airborne asbestos and radon particles. After observations that city dwellers have increased rates of cancer as compared to rural dwellers, it was suggested that urban air pollution is responsible for a large proportion of lung cancer. In fact, studies have suggested that only a small amount (less than 1 percent) of lung cancer can be attributed to urban air pollution. The effect of air pollution on risk is increased in those individuals who are smokers. City dwellers who may be exposed to a substantial amount of pollution can minimize outdoor activities during times when traffic volume is heavy and pollution is at its highest.

Pesticides such as DDT, combustion by-products, and industrial products can be passed along into the food chain and can accumulate in the body. It has been suggested that pesticides could be the cause of some forms of cancer. However, the current available evidence is inconclusive and does not support a causal role of these compounds as a cause of cancer.

Drinking water may contain known and suspected carcinogens, such as industrial chemicals that seep into the water supply or by-products of the purification process (chlorination). Asbestos, nitrates, radon, pesticides, and metals have all been identified in water supplies, but the levels are extremely low and usually do not present a problem in the United States. The Environmental Protection Agency has rigorous guidelines for hazardous waste disposal, and in the United States water supplies are monitored for many carcinogens. Your drinking water can be tested; an alternative is to use filtered or bottled water.

Most pesticides (99.99 percent) in the American diet are naturally occurring, produced by plants themselves as a defense mechanism against insects, fungi, and predators. They present little danger to our food supply. However, some natural substances and chemical substances have been shown to be carcinogenic in animal tests, but there are many uncertainties when relying on animal cancer tests for human prediction. Regulatory agencies use animal studies to formulate policy, and we often do not have human data available. Furthermore, the results from animals studies can be blatantly wrong. For instance, smoke and alcohol, two very potent carcinogens in humans, were not detected as cancer-causing agents in animals for quite some time.

Synthetic (man-made) pesticides used in coloring or preservation have not been shown to be carcinogenic in animal studies. However, a conservative approach would include limiting our exposure to man-made pesticides. This can be done by thoroughly washing produce or buying organically grown products.

Meat and animal products treated with hormones and/or antibiotics have received considerable attention. To date, no link to cancer has been shown. However, aflatoxin, a potent toxin that may be produced when crops are improperly stored, can interact with hepatitis B virus and cause liver cancer. The United States has federal regulations that limit the amount of aflatoxin that can be present in crops.

# Infections and Viruses

Viruses are infectious agents, some of which have the ability to cause cancer. They can invade and alter cells in the body to induce or increase the susceptibility to cancer. However, the immune system works effectively against most infectious agents so that serious disease does not occur. Viruses contribute to about 5 percent of cancer deaths. Here are the viruses associated with cancer:

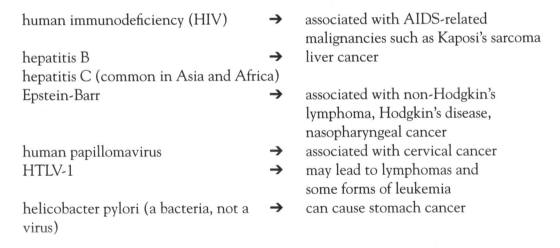

| | | |
|---|---|---|
| human immunodeficiency (HIV) | → | associated with AIDS-related malignancies such as Kaposi's sarcoma |
| hepatitis B | → | liver cancer |
| hepatitis C (common in Asia and Africa) | | |
| Epstein-Barr | → | associated with non-Hodgkin's lymphoma, Hodgkin's disease, nasopharyngeal cancer |
| human papillomavirus | → | associated with cervical cancer |
| HTLV-1 | → | may lead to lymphomas and some forms of leukemia |
| helicobacter pylori (a bacteria, not a virus) | → | can cause stomach cancer |

The overall prevalence of these infections is higher in developing countries than in the United States. Strategies for prevention include avoiding blood exposures, regular Pap screening for women, and vaccination. Improved screening of blood products and implementation of disposable syringes will help decrease the prevalence of some viruses. The blood supply is currently screened for HIV, hepatitis B and C, and HTLV-1. If you believe you are at risk, discuss precautions, testing, and vaccination with your doctor.

# Heredity

The study of hereditary cancers is a relatively new field of research made possible by the technological advances of molecular biology and cancer genetics. Even prior to these advances, observations of cancer clusters within families had been observed.

Overall, having a family history of a particular cancer increases your risk for developing that same cancer by about twofold. However, it is not inevitable that you will develop cancer if a family member has the disease. Also, individuals may be susceptible to environmental carcinogens because of their genetic makeup. This increases the role of nongenetic factors in causing cancer.

Most cancers are caused by environmental factors, primarily diet and smoking, or a combination of heredity and environment. Heredity probably accounts for only 5 percent of all cancer mortalities. Know your family history! Increased cancer screening as well as lifestyle and behavior changes are important for individuals with a family history of cancer.

# Medical Drugs

Cancer treatment often includes therapy in the form of drugs and radiation. Some chemotherapy drugs and radioactive drugs used in the treatment of cancer and other conditions increase a person's risk of a second malignancy. Immunosuppressive drugs, used in organ transplantation, also increase the risk of cancer because they suppress the immune system, making it vulnerable to precancerous and cancerous cells. It is important to remember that these drugs, although they do carry some increased risk, have been used successfully to cure many people. Anabolic steroids and painkillers that contain phenacetin are also human carcinogens. The amount of overall cancer caused by these drugs is extremely small, probably less than 1 percent.

# Stress

Stress has been implicated anecdotally as a cause of cancer; however, there is no scientific evidence to support this. Nor have increased stress levels been shown to decrease survival of patients with cancer. Stress has been associated with other conditions, such as gastrointestinal disorders, infection, hypertension, fatigue, insomnia, impotence, backaches, and headaches. Stress can depress the immune system, and we do know that a healthy immune system is important in fighting cancer. It should be noted that decreasing stress levels will increase the quality of life, which is important for everyone, especially those individuals who are undergoing cancer therapy.

## Ten Tips for Keeping Stress to a Minimum

**1.** Have a support system. Vent your frustrations to friends and relatives.

**2.** Exercise—it's a great stress buster. Take ten deep breaths or a walk around the block—it really helps!

**3.** Try not to overeat or drink alcoholic beverages in response to stress; overeating and overimbibing just lead to more stress.

**4.** Try to remove the source of stress if possible or remove yourself from the stressful situation.

**5.** Try relaxation/meditation techniques or take a stress management class.

**6.** Adopt a pet. They are great stress relievers.

**7.** Engage in a pleasurable hobby or activity.

**8.** Don't take life too seriously—accept what you can't change.

**9.** Try not to be a perfectionist and overachiever: set reasonable goals and priorities.

**10.** If you feel under intense, continuing stress, seek professional counseling. We all need help at certain times in our lives.

# Screening

The prevention strategies highlighted above coupled with screening can make a significant impact on cancer mortality. Screening is the process whereby medical professionals look for disease in people without cancer symptoms. Early detection of cancer can generally ensure a better prognosis because the cancer is diagnosed in a treatable stage before it has the opportunity to spread to other vital organs.

Many cancer screening tests are available. Strang Cancer Prevention Center guidelines for screening are as follows:

### Strang Cancer Prevention Center Screening Guidelines for Women*

| Test/Procedure | Age | Frequency |
|---|---|---|
| Complete cancer checkup | 20–39 | Every 3 years |
| | 40 and over | Every year |
| Clinical breast exam | 20 and over | Every year |
| Breast self-exam | 20 and over | Every month |
| Pap test | 18 and over | Every year |
| Pelvic exam | 18 and over | Every year |
| Mammography | 40 | Initial baseline screen |
| | 40–49 | Every 1–2 years |
| | 50 and over | Every year |

Endometrial tissue sample†

| | | |
|---|---|---|
| Digital rectal exam | 40 and over | Every year |
| Stool occult blood test | 50 and over | Every year |
| Flexible sigmoidoscopy | 50 and over | Every 3–5 years |

*These are guidelines, not rules, and apply only to individuals who do not have symptoms. If you have symptoms, discuss them with your doctor. If you have a personal or family history of any of these cancers, your doctor should discuss your individualized screening recommendations with you. A complete cancer-related checkup should also include examination of the skin, mouth, thyroid, lymph nodes, and ovaries. Health counseling should include smoking cessation, weight and exercise management, and nutritional counseling.

†At menopause if at increased risk for endometrial cancer (those who have a history of infertility, obesity, abnormal uterine bleeding, unopposed estrogen use, or tamoxifen therapy).

## Strang Cancer Prevention Center Screening Guidelines for Men*

| Test/Procedure | Age | Frequency |
|---|---|---|
| Complete cancer checkup | 20–39 | Every 3 years |
| | 40 and over | Every year |
| Testicular self-exam | 20–40 | Monthly |
| Digital rectal exam | 40 and over | Every year |
| Stool occult blood test | 50 and over | Every year |
| Flexible sigmoidoscopy | 50 and over | Every 3–5 years |
| Prostate-specific antigen | 50 and over | Every year |

*These are guidelines, not rules, and apply only to individuals who do not have symptoms. If you have symptoms, discuss them with your doctor. If you have a personal or family history of any of these cancers, your doctor should discuss your individualized screening recommendations with you. A complete cancer-related checkup should also include examination of the skin, mouth, thyroid, and lymph nodes. Health counseling should include smoking cessation, weight and exercise management, and nutritional counseling.

# Nutrition and Cancer Information Resources and Cancer Facts

For those interested in more detailed and current information about cancer research and treatment, we have included here contact numbers for several prominent national information centers. We have also provided some of the latest statistics about cancer, as well as more information about how cancer studies are researched.

## Nutrition and Cancer Information Resources

For more information on nutrition, contact:

American Dietetic Association: (800) 877-1600; http://www.eatright.org
American Dietetic Association Nutrition Hotline: (800) 366-1655
Environmental Nutrition Newsletter: (800) 829-5384
Flax Council of Canada: (800) 817-9894; http://www.flaxcouncil.ca
Harvard Health Letter: (800) 829-9045; http://www.med.harvard.edu/publications/
    Health Publications
International Food Information Council: (202) 296-6540; http://ificinfo.health.org
Nutrition Action Newsletter: fax (202) 265-4954; http://www.cspinet.org
Olive Oil Hotline: (800) 232-6548
The Soy Connection Newsletter: (800) TALK-SOY
Tufts University Health & Nutrition Letter: (800) 274-7581

For more information on cancer, contact:

American Cancer Society: (800) ACS-2345; http://www.cancer.org
American Institute for Cancer Research: (800) 843-8114; http://www.aicr.org
International Cancer Information Center; http://www.icic.nci.nih.gov.
Oncolink; http://www.oncolink.upenn.edu
Strang Cancer Prevention Center—Anne Fisher Nutrition Center: (800) 692-6566;
    http://www.strang.org
The National Cancer Institute: (800) 4-CANCER; http://www.nci.nih.gov.

## Proportion of Cancer Deaths Attributable to Specific Risk Factors

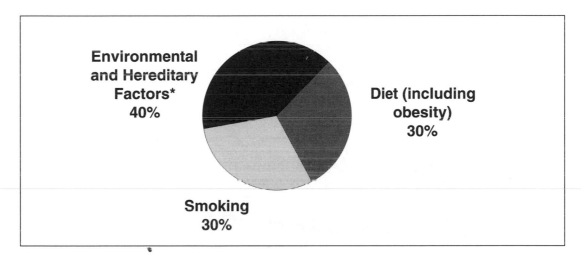

**Environmental and Hereditary Factors\* 40%**

**Diet (including obesity) 30%**

**Smoking 30%**

*Environmental and Hereditary Factors:
Inactivity: 5%
Infections and Viruses: 5%
Heredity: 5%
Occupation: 5%
Alcohol: 3%

Hormones: 3%
Environmental Pollution: 2%
Radiation (including sun exposure): 2%
Medical Drugs and Procedures: 1%
Food Additives (salt): 1%
Other: 8%

## Cancer Mortality Males

**Age-Adjusted Cancer Death Rates,\* Males by Site, U.S. 1930–1993**

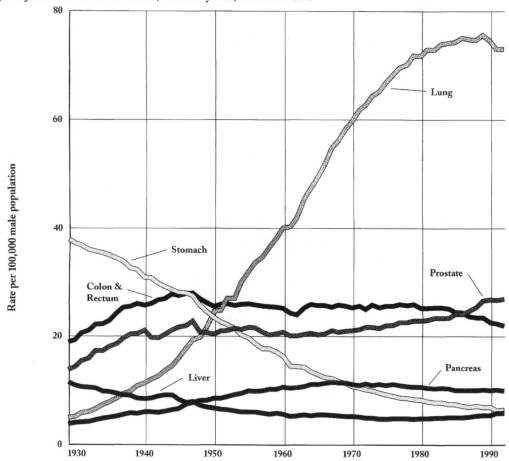

\*Rates are per 100,000 and are age-adjusted to the 1970 U.S. standard population.

**Note**: Due to changes in ICD coding, numerator information has changed over time. Rates for cancers of the liver, lung, and colon and rectum are affected by these coding changes. Denominator information for years 1930–1959 and 1991–1993 is based on intercensal population estimates, while denominator information for the years 1960–1989 is based on postcensal recalculation of estimates. Rate estimates for 1968–1989 are most likely of a better quality.

Source: Vital Statistics of the United States, 1993.

©1997, American Cancer Society, Inc.

## Cancer Mortality Females

**Age-Adjusted Cancer Death Rates,* Females by Site, U.S. 1930–1993**

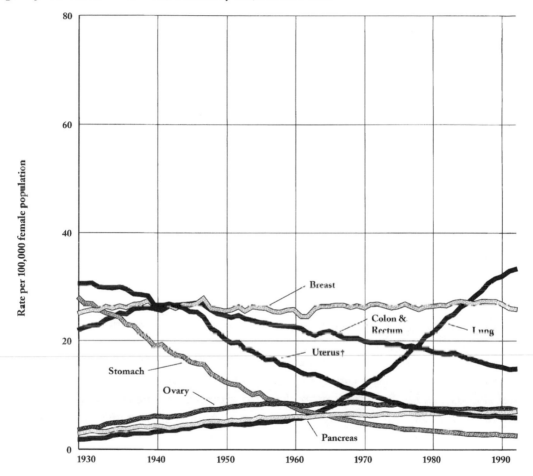

*Rates are per 100,000 and are age-adjusted to the 1970 U.S. standard population. †Uterine cancer death rates are for cervix and corpus combined.

**Note:** Due to changes in ICD coding, numerator information has changed over time. Rates for cancer of the uterus, ovary, lung, and colon and rectum are affected by these coding changes. Denominator information for the years 1930–1959 and 1991–1993 is based on intercensal population estimates, while denominator information for the years 1960–1989 is based on postcensal recalculation of estimates. Rate estimates for 1968–1989 are most likely of a better quality.

Source: Vital Statistics of the United States, 1993.

©1997, American Cancer Society, Inc.

# How Cancer Rates & Risk Factors Are Studied

Epidemiologists try to find a connection between particular foods, nutrients, or vitamins and cancer using different methods. Ecologic or correlational studies compare the dietary habits and cancer rates of countries or groups of people. Measuring dietary intake is usually done using per capita consumption of the country or group, which is inherently inaccurate. These studies do not take into account other factors, such as lifestyle habits, that might influence why a particular group got cancer. These other factors are called potential "confounders." For example, it has been observed that in countries with high rates of colon cancer, there is also a high consumption of red meat as compared to countries with low rates of colon cancer. Populations who have high consumption of red meat also tend to consume less fiber, fruits, and vegetables and tend to exercise less.

Ecologic or correlational studies are further hampered by the fact that a general diet cannot be directly linked to the person who got cancer. Only the diet and cancer rates of the population as a whole can be assessed. The interpretation of results from these studies is limited because of these flaws. However, much of the early data showing a link between diet and cancer was based on these types of studies. The findings were important because they gave some of the first "clues" to the link between diet and cancer.

Cohort studies, consisting of a large number of people, are considered one of the best study designs. Study subjects provide information on their diet by completing a questionnaire or interview. Participants also provide information on other confounding factors that may be related to diet and cancer. The individuals are then followed for many years to see if cancer develops. Repeated assessments (i.e., yearly) of diet can be obtained during this follow-up time period that will help to give a more precise measure of "true" dietary intake. Information on cancer occurrence can be obtained using a questionnaire completed by the study subject, state cancer registries, death certificates, or medical records. Investigators then compare the diets of those who developed cancer to those who did not using mathematical methods called statistics. A large number of individuals are needed for this type of study and the duration of follow-up is long because cancer takes many years to develop. One of the major limitations of this design is the potential for biased or incorrect results if many of the people initially enrolled cannot be located and their cancer status is unknown.

In another type of study design called a case control study, persons with cancer are identified using state cancer registries, death records, or hospital records. Individuals identified as having cancer (called cases) are asked to complete a questionnaire or are interviewed, and information is obtained on diet before the diagnosis and other risk factors for the disease. Subjects without disease (called controls) who are similar to the cases are recruited for the study and the same information is obtained. Statistical methods are then used to compare the diets of these two groups (case versus controls).

Case control studies require fewer numbers of people and the time needed to complete the study is shorter, as compared to the previously described cohort study. However, case control studies have the potential to give biased or inaccurate results because cases with cancer may have predetermined notions about the cause of their disease. They may "recall" their dietary patterns in a different way than nondiseased controls do, leading to recall bias. For instance, if people with esophageal cancer were asked about their fruit and vegetable intake over the past ten years, they may report their current diet, which is likely to have changed because of their illness. Because of their diagnosis, individuals might be aware of the benefits of eating fruits and vegetables and may over- or underestimate their intake. This is not a problem in a cohort study because information about diet is obtained well in advance of cancer diagnosis. When researchers select the control or comparison group, they might inadvertently choose a group (like very old subjects or health-conscious individuals) that is more or less likely to eat fruits and vegetables.

Intervention studies (also called randomized trials or experiments), if conducted properly, can best measure whether a particular factor is beneficial. They do not suffer from the same potential biases as other study designs. In these studies, subjects are randomly assigned to one of two groups. For example, depending on the focus of the study, one group might receive a vitamin supplement while the other group receives a placebo (inactive pill). Neither the study subjects nor the investigators know who gets the vitamin versus the placebo. Study participants are then followed for a designated time period and cancer occurrence ascertained.

The well-known studies on beta-carotene supplements and cancer are examples of intervention studies. People were randomly assigned to take beta-carotene, a vitamin thought to protect against some forms of cancer, or a placebo pill and then followed for the occurrence of cancer. Intervention studies are difficult to conduct for several reasons: first, it is hard to get people to comply; second, the amount of time between the diet change and the expected modification of cancer risk is uncertain; third, the amount of change needed to affect cancer risk is probably unknown; and fourth, the kinds of people who agree to be in a study tend to be healthier individuals and it may be that the dietary change only works in people who are at high risk for the cancer. The logistics of conducting this type of study make it extremely expensive. Due to ethical considerations, intervention studies are not done on factors thought to be harmful. Nevertheless, even though there are many hurdles to overcome when conducting epidemiologic research, well-conducted studies have been done and valuable information obtained about the role diet plays in cancer prevention.

# ↓ REFERENCES ↓

*Cancer Facts & Figures—1997*. American Cancer Society. 1997;1–2.

*Cancer Prevention*. American Cancer Society. 1997:1–2; http://www.cancer.org/prevent.html.

Position of The American Dietetic Association: Enrichment and fortification of foods and dietary supplements. The American Dietetic Association. 1997:1–8; http://www.eatright.org/aenrich-dietsupple.html.

Position of The American Dietetic Association: Food irradiation. The American Dietetic Association. 1997:1–8; http://www.eatright.org/airradi.html.

Position of The American Dietetic Association: Health implications of dietary fiber. The American Dietetic Association. 1996:1–5; http://www.eatright.org/adiet-fiber.html.

Position of The American Dietetic Association: Phytochemicals and functional foods. The American Dietetic Association. 1997:1–9; http://www.eatright.org/aphyto-chemicals.html.

Position of The American Dietetic Association: Use of nutritive and non-nutritive sweeteners. *Journal of the American Dietetic Association* 1993; 93:816.

Position of The American Dietetic Association: Vegetarian diets. The American Dietetic Association. 1997:1–6; http://www.eatright.org/avegdiets.html.

Position of The American Dietetic Association: Vitamin and mineral supplementation. The American Dietetic Association: Vitamin and mineral supplementation. The American Dietetic Association. 1996:1–13; http://www.eatright.org/asupple.html.

Adlercreutz, H. Phytoestrogens: Epidemiology and a possible role in cancer protection. *Environmental Health Perspectives* 1995; 103:103–112.

A food pharmacy: A potpourri of naturally occurring substances that may fight disease. *Eating Well* March–April 1992:41.

Ames, B.N. What are the major carcinogens in the etiology of human cancer? Environmental pollution, natural carcinogens, and the causes of human cancer: Six errors. *Important Advances in Oncology* 1989; 237–247.

Ames, B.N., Gold, L.S., Willett, W.C. The causes and prevention of cancer. *Proceedings of the National Academy of Sciences* 1995; 92:5258–5265.

Aruoma, O.L., Halliwell, B., Aeschbach, R., et al. Antioxidant and pro-oxidant properties of active rosemary constituents: carnosol and carnosic acid. *Xenobiotica* 1992; 22:257–268.

Baker, T.R., Piver, M.S. Etiology, biology, and epidemiology of ovarian cancer. *Seminars in Surgical Oncology* 1994; 10:242–248.

Barnes, S., Peterson, G., Grubbs, C., Setchell, K. Potential role of dietary isoflavones in the prevention of cancer. *In* Jacobs, M.M., ed. *Diet and Cancer: Markers, Prevention, and Treatment.* New York: Plenum Press, 1994.

Bergan, J.C., Brown, P.T. Nutritional status of "new" vegetarians. *Journal of the American Dietetic Association* 1980; 76:151–155.

Berkowitz, K.F. Is your coffee habit grounds for health concerns? *Environmental Nutrition* 1994; 17(2):1–6.

Bloch, A., Thomson, C.A. Position of The American Dietetic Association: Phytochemicals and functional foods. *Journal of the American Dietetic Association* 1995; 95:493–496.

Blondell, J.M. The anticarcinogenic effect of magnesium. *Medical Hypotheses* 1980; 6:863–871.

Bray, G.A., Ryan, D.H., eds. *Vitamins and Cancer Prevention.* Pennington Center Nutrition Series. Baton Rouge, La.: State University Press, 1993.

Caloric levels adapted from USDA's Food Guide Pyramid, U.S. Department of Agriculture, Human Nutrition Information Service, April 1992.

Cancer Causes and Control. 1996; 7:3–180.

Caragay, A.B. Cancer-preventative foods and ingredients. *Food Technology* 1992; 46:65–68.

Clairborne, C., Ryan, L.T., Donovan, M.D., eds. *The Professional Chef's Techniques of Healthy Cooking/The Culinary Institute of America.* New York: Van Nostrand Reinhold, 1993.

Clark, L.C., Combs, G.F. Jr., Turnbull, B.W., et al. Effects of selenium supplementation for cancer prevention in patients with carcinoma of the skin. *Journal of the American Medical Association* 1996; 276: 1957–1963.

Colditz, G.A. A prospective assessment of moderate alcohol intake and major chronic diseases. *Annals of Epidemiology* 1990; 1:167–177.

Colditz, G.A., Egan, K.M., Stampfer, M.J. Hormone replacement therapy and risk of breast cancer: Results from epidemiologic studies. *American Journal of Obstetrics and Gynecology* 1993; 168:1473–1480.

Correa, P. Human Gastric Carcinogenesis: A Multistep and Multifactorial Process—First American Cancer Society Award Lecture on Cancer Epidemiology and Prevention. *Cancer Research* 1992; 52:6735–6740.

Cramer, D.W., Harlow, B.L. Author's response to: "Progress in the nutritional epidemiology of ovary cancer." *American Journal of Epidemiology* 1991; 134:460–461.

Das, S. Vitamin E in the genesis and prevention of cancer: A review. *Acta Oncologica* 1994; 33:615–619.

Davis, D.L., Muir, C. Estimating avoidable causes of cancer. *Environmental Health Perspectives* 1995; 103(Suppl. 8):302–306.

Decker, E.A. The role of phenolics, conjugated linoleic acid, carnosine, and pyrroloquinoline quinone as nonessential dietary antioxidants. *Nutritional Reviews* 1995; 53:49–58.

De Jong, F.H., Oishi, K., Hayes, R.B., et al. Peripheral hormone levels in controls and patients with prostatic cancer or benign prostatic hyperplasia: Results from the Dutch-Japanese case-control study. *Cancer Research* 1991; 51:3445–3450.

Dietary Supplement—Health and Education Act of 1994. U.S. Food and Drug Administration, Center for Food Safety and Applied Nutrition. DSHEA-P.L.-103–471. 1996:1–4; http://vm.cfsan.fda.gov/~dms/dietsupp.html.

Di Mascio, P., Murphy, M.E., Sies, H. Antioxidant defense systems: the role of carotenoids, tocopherols, and thiols. *American Journal of Clinical Nutrition* 1991; 53:194S–200S.

Doll, R., Peto, R. The causes of cancer: quantitative estimates of avoidable risks of cancer in the United States today. *Journal of the National Cancer Institute* 1981; 66:1196–1308.

Gao, Y.T., McLaughlin, J.K., Blot, W.J., et al. Reduced risk of esophageal cancer associated with green tea consumption. *Journal of the National Cancer Institute* 1994; 86:855–858.

Garfinkel, L. Overweight and cancer. *Annals of Internal Medicine* 1985; 103:1034–1036.

Garfinkel, L., Boffetta, P., Stellman, S.D. Alcohol and breast cancer: A cohort study. *Preventive Medicine* 1988; 17:686–693.

Goodwin, T.W., Mercer, E.L. *Introduction to Plant Biochemistry*. Second Edition. Elmsford, N.Y.: Pergamon Press, 1983.

Hamilton, E.M.N., Whitney, E.N., Sizer, F.S. *Nutritional Concepts and controversies*. Fifth Edition. St. Paul, Minn.: West Publishing Company, 1991.

Harvard Report on Cancer Prevention, Volume 1: Causes of Human Cancer. *Cancer Causes and Control*. 1996; 7:3–58.

Havala, S., Dwyer, J. Position of The American Dietetic Association: Vegetarian diets. *Journal of the American Dietetic Association* 1993; 93:1317–1319.

Helzlsouer, K.J., Block, G., Blumberg, J., et al. Summary of the Round Table Discussion on Strategies for Cancer Prevention: Diet, Food Additives, Supplements, and Drugs. *Cancer Research* 1994; 54(Suppl.):2044s–2051s.

Henson, D.E., Block, G., Levine, M. Ascorbic acid: Biologic functions and relation to cancer. *Journal of the National Cancer Institute* 1991; 83:547–550.

Herbert, V. Vitamin B-12: plant sources, requirements, assay. *In* Mutch, P.B., Johnston, P.K., eds. First International Congress on Vegetarian Nutrition. *American Journal of Clinical Nutrition* 1988; 48(3 Suppl.):852–858.

Herbst, S.T. *The New Food Lover's Companion.* Second Edition. Hauppauge, N.Y.: Barron's Educational Series, Inc., 1995.

Herman C., Adlercreutz, T. Goldin, B.R., et al. Soybean phytoestrogen intake and cancer risk. *Journal of Nutrition* 1995; 125(3 Suppl.):757s–770s.

Howe, G.R. Dietary fat and breast cancer risks: An epidemiologic perspective. *Cancer Supplement* 1994; 74:1078–1084.

Hrabak, D. A fish oil story: Omega-3's return to fight heart disease, cancer. *Environmental Nutrition* 1994; 17(7):1–4.

Hunter, D.J., Spiegelman, D., Adami, H.O., et al. Cohort studies of fat intake and the risk of breast cancer—a pooled analysis. *The New England Journal of Medicine* 1996; 334:356–361.

Husten, L. Understanding risk: tricky business. *Harvard Health Letter* 1994; 19(12):9–12.

International Olive Oil Council. Press Kit 1997.

Katahn, M. *The Tri-Color Diet.* New York: W.W. Norton & Company, Inc., 1996.

Kennedy, A.R. The evidence for soybean products as cancer preventive agents. *Journal of Nutrition* 1995; 125(3 Suppl.):733s–743s.

Kestin, M., Rouse, I., Correll, R., et al. Cardiovascular disease risk factors in free-living men: comparison of two prudent diets, one based on lactoovovegetarianism and the other allowing lean meat. *American Journal of Clinical Nutrition* 1989; 50:280–287.

Kuczmarski, R.J., Flegal, K.M., Campbell, S.M., et al. Increasing prevalence of overweight among U.S. adults. *Journal of the American Medical Association* 1994; 272:205–211.

Laidlaw, S.A., Swendseid, M.E., eds. *Vitamins and Cancer Prevention.* New York: Wiley-Liss, 1991.

Law, C., Ra'ad, D. Beta carotene's fall from grace draws mixed reactions. *Journal of the National Cancer Institute* 1996; 88:235–236.

Lew, E.A., Garfinkel, L. Variations in mortality by weight among 750,000 men and women. *Journal of Chronic Diseases* 1979; 32:563–576.

Mandatory Nutrition Labeling—Final Rule: One of a Series of FDA Regulations Implementing The Nutrition Labeling and Education Act of 1990. Food and Drug Administration. Washington, D.C.: January 6, 1993.

Margen, S. *The Wellness Encyclopedia of Food and Nutrition*. University of California at Berkeley Wellness Letter. Health Letter Associates, 1992.

Marsh, A., Sanchez, T., Michelsen, O., et al. Vegetarian lifestyle and bone mineral density. *American Journal of Clinical Nutrition* 1988; 48:837–841.

Matanoski, G.M., Elliot, E.A. Bladder cancer epidemiology. *Epidemiologic Reviews* 1981; 3:203–229.

Messina, M., Barnes, S. The role of soy products in reducing risk of cancer. *Journal of the National Cancer Institute* 1991; 83:541–546.

Mettlin, C.J. Invited Commentary: Progress in the nutritional epidemiology of ovary cancer. *American Journal of Epidemiology* 1991; 134:457–459.

Michels, K.B., Willett, W.C. Vitamins and cancer: A practical means of prevention? *In* DeVita, V.T., Hellman, S., Rosenberg, S.A., eds. *Important Advances in Oncology*. Philadelphia, Pa.: Lippincott Company, 1994.

Micozzi, M.S., Moon, T.E., eds. *Macronutrients: Investigating Their Role in Cancer*. New York: Marcel Dekker, Inc., 1992.

Mirvish, S.S. Effects of vitamins C and E on N-nitroso compound formation, carcinogenesis, and cancer. *Cancer* 1986; 58:1842–1850.

———. The etiology of gastric cancer: Intragastric nitrosamide formation and other theories. *Journal of the National Cancer Institute* 1983; 71:631–647.

Moon, R.C., Mehta, R.G. Anticarcinogenic effects of retinoids in animals. *Advances in Experimental Medical Biology* 1986; 206:399–411.

Napier, K. Fat is everyone's issue. *Harvard Health Letter* 1996; 21(8):1–3.

———. Green Revolution. *Harvard Health Letter* 1995; 20(6):9–12.

———. Too Many Vitamins? *Harvard Health Letter* 1996; 21(3):1–3.

National Institutes of Health, National Cancer Institute. *Cancer: Rates and Risks* 1996.

Nelson, R.L., Davis, F.G., Sutter, E., et al. Body iron stores and risk of colonic neoplasia. *Journal of the National Cancer Institute* 1994; 86:455–460.

Newmark, H.L. Plant phenolics as potential cancer prevention agents. *In* Back, N., Cohen, I.R., Kritchevsky, D., eds. *Dietary Phytochemicals in Cancer Prevention and Treatment*. New York: Plenum Press, 1996.

Nutritionist IV for Windows: Food Labeling Module 1995; First DataBank Division, The Hearst Corporation, 1111 Bayhill Drive, San Bruno, California 94066.

Parazzini, F., Franceschi, S., Vecchia, C.L., et al. The epidemiology of ovarian cancer. *Gynecologic Oncology* 1991; 43:9–23.

Pate, R.R., Pratt, M., Blair, S.N., et al. Physical activity and public health. *Journal of the American Medical Association* 1995; 273:402–407.

Pennington, J.A.T., ed. *Bowes & Church's Food Values of Portions Commonly Used*. Sixteenth Edition. Philadelphia, Pa.: J.B. Lippincott Company, 1994.

Phillips, R.L., Garfinkel, L., Kuzma, J.W., et al. Mortality among California Seventh-

Day Adventists for selected cancer sites. *Journal of the National Cancer Institute* 1980; 65:1097–1107.

Recommended Dietary Allowances. Subcommittee on the Tenth Edition of the RDAs, Food and Nutrition Board, Commission on Life Sciences, National Research Council. Washington, D.C.: National Academy Press, 1989.

Risch, H.A., Jain, M., Marrett, L.D., et al. Dietary fat intake and risk of epithelial ovarian cancer. *Journal of the National Cancer Institute* 1994; 86:1409–1415.

Robinson, C.H., Weigley, E.S., Mueller, D.H. *Robinson's Basic Nutrition and Diet Therapy*. Eighth Edition. Upper Saddle River, N.J.: Prentice-Hall, Inc., 1997.

Ross, R.K., Bernstein, L., Lobo, R.A., et al. 5-alpha-reductase activity and risk of prostate cancer among Japanese and U.S. white and black males. *The Lancet* 1992; 339:887–889.

Rothman, K.J. *Modern Epidemiology*. Boston: Little, Brown and Company, 1986.

Ruddon R.W., ed. *Cancer Biology*. New York: Oxford University Press, 1995.

Sauber, C.M. The meaning of the word organic. *Harvard Health Letter* 1994; 19(6): 4–5.

Scientists spotlight phytoestrogens for better health. *Tufts University Diet and Nutrition Letter* 1995; 12:1–5.

Serdula, M.K., Coates, R.J., Byerst, et al. Fruit and vegetable intake among adults in 16 states: Results of a brief telephone survey. *American Journal of Public Health* 1995; 85: 236–239.

Shamsuddin, A.M. Inositol phosphates have novel anticancer function. *Journal of Nutrition* 1995; 125(3 Suppl.):725s–732s.

Shils, M.E. Nutrition and diet in cancer management. In Shils M.E., et al, eds. *Modern Nutrition in Health and Disease*. Malvern, Pa.: Lea and Febiger, 1994.

Shottenfeld, D. Principles and applications of cancer prevention. In Shottenfeld D., Fraumeni J.F. Jr., eds. *Cancer Epidemiology and Prevention*. New York: Oxford University Press, 1996.

Shu, X.O., Gao, Y.T., Yuan, J.M., et al. Dietary factors and epithelial ovarian cancer. *British Journal of Cancer* 1989; 59:92–96.

Simopoulos, A.P., Herbert, V., Jacobson, B. *Genetic Nutrition: Designing a Diet Based on Your Family Medical History*. New York: Macmillan Publishing Company, 1993.

Singh, M., Lu, J., Briggs, S.P., et al. Effect of excess dietary iron on the promotion stage of 1-methyl-1-nitrosourea-induced mammary carcinogenesis: pathogenetic characteristics and distribution of iron. *Carcinogenesis* 1994; 15:1567–1570.

Slattery, M.L., Schuman, K.L., West, D.W., et al. Nutrient intake and ovarian cancer. *American Journal of Epidemiology* 1989; 130:497–502.

Steinmetz, K.A., Potter, J.D. Vegetables, fruit, and cancer. II. Mechanisms. *Cancer Causes and Control* 1991; 2:427–441.

————. Vegetables, fruit, and cancer prevention: A review. *Jouranl of the American Dietetic Association* 1996; 96:1027–1038.

Stevens, R.G., Beasley, R.P., Blumberg, B.S. Iron-binding proteins and risk of cancer in Taiwan. *Journal of the National Cancer Institute* 1986; 76:605–610.

Sugimura, T., Shigeaki, S. Mutagens-carcinogens in foods. *Cancer Research* 1983; 43 (Suppl.):2415s–2421s.

Surh, Y.J., Lee, S.S. Capsaicin in Hot Chili Pepper: Carcinogen, co-carcinogen or anti-carcinogen? *Food Chemistry and Toxicology* 1996; 34:313–316.

Taubes, G. Epidemiology faces its limits. *Science* 1995; 269:164–169.

Nutrition Labeling and Education Act of 1990 (NLEA).

Trichopoulos, D., Li, F.P., Hunter, D.J. What causes cancer? *Scientific American* September 1996; 80–87.

Tzonou, A., Hsieh, C.C., Polychronopoulou, A., et al. Diet and ovarian cancer: A case-control study in Greece. *International Journal of Cancer* 1993; 55:411–414.

Vecchia, C.L. Nutritional factors and cancers of the breast, endometrium and ovary. *European Journal of Cancer and Clinical Oncology* 1989; 25(12):1945–1951.

Vecchia, C.L., Negri, E., Franceschi S., et al. Alcohol and epithelial ovarian cancer. *Journal of Clinical Epidemiology* 1992; 45:1025–1030.

Verhoeven, D.T.H., Goldbohm, R.A., van Poppel, G., et al. Epidemiological studies on brassica vegetables and cancer risk. *Cancer Epidemiology, Biomarkers & Prevention* 1996; 5:733–748.

Watson, R.R., Mufti, S.I., eds. *Nutrition and Cancer Prevention*. New York: CRC Press, 1996.

Wattenberg, L.W. Inhibition of carcinogenesis by minor dietary constituents. *Cancer Research* 1992; 52(Suppl.):2085s–2091s.

Weigley, E.S., Mueller, D.H., Robinson, C.H. Robinson's Basic Nutrition and Diet Therapy. Eighth edition. Upper Saddle River, N.J.: Prentice-Hall, Inc. Simon & Schuster, 1997.

Welland, D. As caffeine controversy rages on, what's a coffee lover to do? *Environmental Nutrition* 1996; 19:1–6.

Werbach, M.R. Illnesses and the effects of nutrients, toxic metals and food sensitivities: Cancer. In *Nutritional Influences on Illness*. Tarzana, Calif.: Third Line Press, 1993.

Willet, W.C. Diet and health: What should we eat? *Science* 1994; 264:532–537.

————. Diet, nutrition, and avoidable cancer. *Environmental Health Perspectives* 1995; 103(Suppl. 8):165–170.

————. Micronutrients and cancer risk. *American Journal of Clinical Nutrition* 1994; 59(5 Suppl.):1162s–1165s.

————. *Overview of Nutritional Epidemiology*. In MacMahon B., ed. *Nutritional Epidemiology*. New York: Oxford University Press, 1990.

————. Polyunsaturated fat and the risk of cancer. *British Medical Journal* 1995; 311:1239–1240.

————. Selenium, vitamin E, fiber, and the incidence of human cancer. *Advances in Experimental Medical Biology* 1986; 206:27–34.

————. The discipline of epidemiology. *Science* 1995; 269:1325–1326.

Willett, W.C., Colditz, G.A., Mueller, N.E. Strategies for minimizing cancer risk. *Scientific American* September 1996; 88–95.

Yamane, T., Takahashi, T., Kuwata, K., et al. Inhibition of *N*-methyl-*N*-nitro-*N*-nitrosoguanidine-induced carcinogenesis by (-)- epigallocatechin gallate in the rat glandular stomach. *Cancer Research* 1995: 55:2081–2084.

Yang, C.S., Wang, Z.Y. Tea and cancer. *Journal of the National Cancer Institute* 1993; 85:1038–1049.

Young, V.R. Soy protein in relation to human protein and amino acid nutrition. *Journal of the American Dietetic Association* 1991; 91:828–835.

Zemel, M. Calcium utilization: effect of varying level and source of dietary protein. *American Journal of Clinical Nutrition* 1988; 48:880.

Zhang, L., Cooney, R.V., Bertram, J.S. Carotenoids up-regulate *Connexin 43* gene expression independent of their provitamin A or antioxidant properties. *Cancer Research* 1992; 52:5707–5712.

Zheng, W., Doyle, T.J., Kushi, L.H., et al. Tea consumption and cancer incidence in a prospective cohort study of postmenopausal women. *American Journal of Epidemiology* 1996; 144:175–182.

Ziegler, R.G. Does beta-carotene explain why reduced cancer risk is associated with vegetable and fruit intake? *Cancer Research* 1992; 52(7 Suppl.):2060s–2066s.

# ❖ ABOUT THE CONTRIBUTORS ❖

The authors would like to thank the many extraordinary chefs who have contributed their recipes to this volume, all of whom combine a passionate interest in great taste with foods that are healthful and delicious. The chefs' names appear with the recipes they've created. All chefs were invited to provide a biographical sketch.

## Miles Angelo

Miles credits much of his foundation in modern Southwestern cuisine to his early kitchen experience at Sedlar at Abiquiu in Santa Monica, California, under Chef John Rivera. He defined his own place in Southwestern cuisine as the executive chef at New York City's Arizona 206. In Portobello Mushroom–Stuffed Chiles Rellenos, Miles combined flavors from the Far East and the Caribbean with indigenous Southwestern ingredients, such as corn, chiles, squashes, and beans, to make a perfectly balanced celebration of tastes, textures, and colors. Now at the Caribou Club in Aspen, Colorado, Miles creates modern American food while still drawing on Southwestern influences. Using the fresh ingredients and game of the Rocky Mountains, his seasonal menus demonstrate the perfect marriage of tradition with contemporary touches.

## Francesco Antonucci

Born in the beautiful Veneto region of Italy, Chef Antonucci brings us Venetian flavors combined with contemporary infusions and sophistication. After a long career as an acclaimed executive chef at El Touls in Italy, Valentino in Santa Monica, California, DDI Bistro in Trump Tower, and Alo Alo restaurant in New York City, Chef Antonucci teamed up with designer and partner Adam Tihany and opened the original Remi restaurant in New York City. Since 1990, he and Tihany have opened Remi in Santa Monica, California; Mexico City, Mexico; and Tel Aviv, Israel. He has consistently received both praise and awards from food critics and organizations. Most important, his customers' patronage speaks volumes about the quality and appeal of his cuisine. Chef Antonucci shares with us superb recipes that are both healthful and flavorful.

## Lidia Bastianich

Combining their names, Lidia and Felice, husband and wife opened New York City's Felidia in 1981. This was followed by the more recent openings of Becco and Frico. Born in Trieste, at the juncture of Italy and the former Yugoslavia, Lidia grew up surrounded by the delicacies of the Adriatic Sea and fresh ingredients of the region. She also had a grandmother who taught her the secrets of Italian cooking. Her book *La Cucina di Lidia* (Doubleday, 1990) weaves history, tradition, and warm memories of her homeland into each recipe. In 1994, Lidia decided to share her home-style ingredients with the rest of the country and created a mail-order company. Her catalog, *Il Cibo di Lidia*, offers a wide selection of fresh Italian ingredients and food products. Lidia shares her knowledge of the history of Italian cuisine and the anthropology of food by lecturing and editing *The New York Times Magazine* insert titled "Celebration of Italy."

## Robert Bennett

Robert Bennett and his pastry staff of seven create more than 600 desserts a week at Philadelphia's most celebrated restaurant, Le Bec Fin. Robert studied at the New England Culinary Institute and stayed on after graduation as a pastry instructor. After three semesters of teaching, he accepted a four-month consulting position at the Jumby Bay Resort in Antigua, West Indies. In 1987, he took a position as one of four pastry chefs at Le Bec Fin, and quickly worked his way up to the position of executive pastry chef. During the last ten years at Le Bec Fin, he has become actively involved in local pastry organizations, founding the Philadelphia Pastry Society, and has also been recently appointed to the board of directors of the North American Pastry Chefs Association.

## Daniel Boulud

Daniel Boulud is one of the most decorated chefs in the world. *Brilliant* and *innovative* are two words frequently used in describing the creations of this chef from Lyons, France. After working in the kitchens of the French masters Georges Blanc, Roger Vergé, and Michel Guérad, Chef Boulud earned accolades and four stars from the *New York Times* during his six years as executive chef at New York City's Le Cirque. In 1992, he left Le Cirque to open Restaurant Daniel. By 1994, he once again received four stars from the *New York Times*. Both food critics and customers assert that Daniel is the best classic French restaurant in New York, and one of the best in the world.

## Anthony Bourdain

Anthony Bourdain is both a writer and a chef. Bryan Miller, a former food critic for the *New York Times*, says, "Bourdain serves up food and felonies with delectable élan." His satirical thrillers include *Bone in the Throat* (Villard Books, 1995) and *Gone Bamboo* (Villard Books, 1996). Both have received acclaim from literary and food critics. Bourdain has cooked at some of New York City's finest restaurants, including the Rainbow Room. He is currently the chef at Ed Sullivan Restaurant next to the famous theater. Here Anthony presents American style food with a flair.

## Frank Brigtsen

After seven years of training in classic Creole cooking under internationally acclaimed chef Paul Prudhomme, Frank, with his wife and partner Marna, opened Brigtsen's. In March 1996, Brigtsen's celebrated its tenth anniversary. The following are just a few of the awards and recognition they have received during this time: one of the "Top Ten New Chefs," in 1988, *Food & Wine*; "Top Cajun Restaurant," *Zagat Survey*; and "Chef of the Year," New Orleans chapter of Chefs in America. As a chef Frank is "hands-on," personally visiting fish markets and vegetable stands and writing daily menus by hand. He is "on-site" every evening to oversee the preparation of such signature dishes as Rabbit Tenderloin on a Tasso Parmesan Grits Cake with Creole Mustard Sauce and Blackened Yellowfin Tuna with Smoked Corn Sauce and Red Bean Salsa.

## David Burke

Chef David Burke has worked in some of the finest kitchens in the United States and Europe, including The River Cafe, a restaurant where many of America's premier chefs have launched their careers. He has a gift for translating classic French cuisine into unique American presentations. Presently Burke oversees cuisine at New York's

Park Avenue Cafe and Maloney & Porcelli and Chicago's Mrs. Park's Tavern and Park Avenue Cafe. He is also involved with retail and wholesale distribution of specialty food items that are available under the Park Avenue Cafe label. His culinary excellence has been recognized by the following awards: First Auggie Award (named for Auguste Escoffier), 1996; Robert Mondavi Culinary Award of Excellence, 1996; and Nippon Award of Excellence, 1988.

### Adam Busby

Adam Busby reaped critical acclaim and industry recognition during his celebrated tenure in the Pacific Northwest kitchens of Bishops, Star Anise, and his own venture, Cascabel. At these restaurants, Adam drew upon the abundance of ingredients available in the Pacific Northwest to create progressive new American cuisine influenced by classical French technique. In 1997, he joined the Dubrulle French Culinary School in Vancouver, B.C., to direct their new Advanced Culinary Program. Here, Adam designed and teaches classes for those who have completed Dubrulle's Professional Culinary Diploma Program or are in the food industry.

### Cesare Casella

Born in beautiful Lucca, a walled medieval city in Tuscany, Cesare Casella grew up around food. His family has long owned Restaurant Vipore, a seventeenth-century farmhouse that has been converted to a restaurant. Following graduation from professional culinary training, Cesare became chef at Vipore, earning accolades and three fork ratings in both the Michelin and Veronelli guides to dining.

His love of using aromatic herbs to create simple, flavorful cuisine led him to create one of the largest world-class herb gardens in Italy. This emphasis on simplicity and freshness is not only the cornerstone of his cooking, but also his ideas about healthy eating. He finds Strang nutrition guidelines easy to follow: "The principles of Strang's nutrition program are not only common sense, but tradition to me." This intuitive balance of eating, learned early on by Cesare, is reflected in his seasonal menus, which include a wide range of choices and adaptations to accommodate both palate and diet preferences.

### Michael Chiarello

Michael Chiarello takes the splendid ingredients of northern California farms and produces award-winning Italian food at the stylish Tra Vigna restaurant, located in the heart of Napa Valley. Under his direction, Tra Vigna makes its own breads, salami, prosciutto, cheeses, and cured olives, and sells them to other local restaurants. Michael Chiarello has opened four other restaurants since 1994: Bump and Ajax Tavern in Aspen, Colorado, Caffé Museo in the San Francisco Museum of Modern Art, and Tomatina, a casual pizza and pasta restaurant adjacent to Tra Vigna. His company, Consorzio Foods, uses local ingredients to produce specialty mustards, flavored oils and vinegars, and vinaigrettes. Chef Chiarello hopes these retail ingredients help people cook with the same creative force he does: "Our philosophy is convenience without compromise," says Chiarello.

## Scott Cohen

In 1994, Scott Cohen was awarded the Bronze Medal of the French Vatel Club, honoring him as one of the nation's outstanding young chefs. The road to such recognition began after his high school graduation, when he enrolled in the Culinary Institute of America. He then worked at the Mansion at Turtle Creek in Dallas, the Carlyle Hotel, in New York City, and as sous-chef to the late Andre Gaillard at New York's La Reserve. His training with Gaillard and an apprenticeship at the famed Moulin de Mougins provided him with a solid foundation in classical French cooking. After earning accolades at the restaurant at the Stanhope Hotel, Scott moved on to the Ocean Grill in New York City and has provided us with a sampling of his nautical creations.

## Roberto Donna

Having made his commitment to the culinary arts at the age of thirteen, Roberto Donna completed four years of training in his native Italy, followed by experiences in England, France, and Switzerland. He is chef and owner of the famous Galileo in Washington, D.C., and owns four other restaurants emphasizing simplicity and freshness. Signature menu items include such specialties as Tomato Risotto with Monkfish and Eggplant and Braised Beef Angolotti in a Barolo Wine Sauce, served with a small onion tart. In 1996, Roberto won the prestigious James Beard Foundation Award for "Best Chef—Mid-Atlantic Region."

## Dean Fearing

At the renowned Mansion on Turtle Creek in Dallas, Texas, Chef Dean Fearing merges native ingredients of the Southwest with flavors from around the world to create his own signature Southwestern menu. Fearing was classically trained at the Culinary Institute of America and began his career at Maisonette in Cincinnati, Ohio. He is inspired by memories of simple backyard barbecues, which he elevates to sophisticated and colorful cuisine, incorporating a variety of home-grown vegetables, herbs, and game. The author of two cookbooks, *The Mansion on Turtle Creek Cookbook* and *Dean Fearing's*

*Southwest Cuisine: Blending Asia and the Americas*, Chef Fearing does not hesitate to "give away" one of his secrets. Says Fearing, "I can always create another one."

## Diane Forley

Diane Forley is the chef and proprietor of New York City's Verbena. Her interest in food began at an early age with a strong influence from the rich cultural heritage of her family, whose roots spread from Eastern Europe to the Mediterranean, the Middle East, and South America. She has trained with chefs here and in France and has worked at notable places, such as Adrienne's (in Maxim's Hotel) and The River Cafe and Park Avenue Cafe in New York City. While pastry chef at the Gotham Bar and Grill, she demonstrated her skills and expertise in pastry arts. Chef Forley's cultural experiences, extensive travels, and avid interests in nutrition and the history of food are the basis for her contemporary American cuisine.

## Maria Helm

Maria Helm began cooking professionally at age sixteen. After graduating from Union College, where she obtained a liberal arts degree, Maria attended the California Culinary Academy and the Konditeri Tivoli Pastry School in Denmark. After a seven-year stint as pastry chef, then executive chef, at the San Francisco Bay Area's The Sherman House restaurant, Maria became executive chef of PlumpJack Cafe in 1995. Here she has received critical praise, including *Food & Wine's* "Top 10 New Chefs" in 1996. She uses reductions of herb-infused natural juices to prepare sauces that enhance rather than mask the flavors of other ingredients. Her cuisine is a combination of simplicity and sophistication and she serves it with the spectacular wines of northern California.

## Erasmo "Razz" Kamnitzer

Native to Venezuela, Razz started his culinary career at age seventeen as the assistant manager of the Vegetarian Buffet in Caracas, where he was exposed to "healthy cooking." Since that time his career has taken him around the world, and he has cultivated these influences into exotic and well-balanced cuisine. In addition to years of on-the-job training, he attended the National Hotel School of Lausanne in Switzerland and the Culinary Institute of America. Since moving to Arizona in 1980, Razz has owned and operated several restaurants, including Auberge Du Canal, and has performed as chef de cuisine of Etienne's Different Pointe of View at the Pointe Hilton at Tapatio Cliffs, Phoenix. Razz's cuisine features herbs, edible flowers, and local fruits and vegetables.

Razz was kind enough to provide a delicious, versatile recipe with ingredients that can be found by those of us who don't live near the desert.

## Katy Keck

Katy began cooking at five years old, using an Easy Bake oven, and eventually won the blue ribbon in the butter cake division at the local 4-H fair. But cooking became a serious career option only after completion of her MBA at the University of Chicago and a successful career in marketing and finance on Wall Street. When Katy won the grand prize in the Flavors of France contest for her Marie Brizard chocolate torte recipe, the prize was an apprenticeship at Le Grand Monarue in Chartres, France. She followed this up by interning at three other Michelin-starred restaurants. On returning to the United States, she created Savoir Faire Foods, a consulting business specializing in recipe and new product development and marketing, food and demo styling, and culinary special events. In 1993, Katy and partner Richard Barber opened New World Grill at the Worldwide Plaza in New York City. Her menu is a mix of styles—Asian, French, and Southwestern to name a few—and represents a healthful approach to eating out. In 1996, Katy was honored as one of seven national finalists in the *Gourmet Magazine* Evian Healthy Menu Awards.

## Gray Kunz

Gray Kunz began his career by following his older brother, a chef, into the kitchen at the age of sixteen. After his classical European culinary training and experience, he moved on to become executive chef at Plume, one of Hong Kong's most renowned restaurants. Here he broadened his knowledge of Eastern cuisine and then came to New York, where he has been recognized as one of the top chefs in the world. Kunz has been described as a "culinary genius" for his ability to infuse Asian touches into modern French cuisine without betraying the characteristics of classical French techniques: he is masterful at marrying ingredients to create a harmonious explosion of flavors without one overpowering another. Since 1991, Kunz has been the executive chef at Lespinasse, the highly acclaimed restaurant at New York's St. Regis Hotel, which has received many accolades under his supervision.

## Giuseppe Lattanzi

The Roman-Jewish Lattanzi family has been in the restaurant business in New York for more than twenty-five years. The Lattanzi siblings' New York restaurants include Lattanzi Ristorante, Erminia, Porta Portese, Chelsea, Sumo, Paper Moon, Tevere, and

Va Bene. Giuseppe oversees Va Bene, an elegant, upscale, kosher Italian restaurant. He prides himself on providing classical Roman cuisine in adherence with kosher dietary laws. Giuseppe has provided a traditional Italian Rosh Hashanah menu that is rich in cancer-protective nutrients.

## Casadio Luca

Casadio Luca was born in Emilia-Romagna, the culinary heart of Italy. When studying at the renowned National Hotel School of Lausanne in Switzerland, he apprenticed at five different Michelin three-star restaurants in Italy and France. Since 1995, Casadio has been an executive chef for Bice Ristorante. The Bice organization is an institution among Italian restaurants. Started in Milan in 1906, Bice has always maintained top-quality food and service while evolving, modernizing, and continuing to set trends in Italian cuisine. Bice restaurants can be found in major cities throughout the world: Buenos Aires, Hong Kong, São Paulo, Sydney, and Tokyo, to name a few. Casadio upholds the long tradition of culinary excellence at the exquisite New York location.

## Barbara Lynch

Hard work and immense talent have brought Barbara Lynch to the top of America's culinary scene. While growing up in the housing projects of South Boston, Barbara worked 3 jobs to help her family with expenses. A high-school home-economics instructor inspired and encouraged her interest in cooking, and she has not looked back since. Barbara credits her 6-year combined culinary experience with Michela Larson (Michela's and Rialto) and Todd English (Olives and Figs) for fostering her interest and talent in Italian-style cooking. Her own studies of Italian tradition and cuisine and numerous trips to many of the regions of Italy have further developed her signature style. Over the last few years Barbara has been featured in articles in *The Boston Globe, The Boston Herald, Boston Magazine, Food & Wine, Eating Well,* and *Bon Appetit,* and in 1996 was named among *Food & Wine*'s "Top 10 New Chefs." Recently Barbara opened her own restaurant, No. 9 Park, in Boston.

## Zarela Martinez

Born and raised in Mexico, Zarela Martinez is without a doubt the first lady of Mexican cooking in America. Zarela has brought the tradition, intense flavors, and sophistication of true Mexican cooking to New York City, without a hint of Tex-Mex. At the popular, critically acclaimed Zarela Restaurant you can experience the warmth of her cooking. Zarela shares her traditions and recipes with the rest of the world in *Food from*

*My Heart* (Macmillan–Simon & Schuster, 1992). This autobiography-cookbook was nominated for the prestigious James Beard award as "Best International Cookbook of the Year." The ease of preparation and nutritious content of most of her recipes made our selection a difficult, but enjoyable process.

## Robert McGrath

During Robert McGrath's fifteen years in the culinary industry he has worked as executive chef of Arrowwood Resort in Westchester, New York; chef de cuisine at the Four Seasons Hotel in Austin, Texas; and chef-owner of "Sierra" restaurant in Houston, Texas. Since 1993, Robert has been the chef de cuisine at Window on the Green, The Phoenician Resort's Southwestern-inspired restaurant. In this spectacular setting the culinary magic he creates has earned him the following awards and recognitions: the James Beard Foundation's "America's Best Chef—Southwest," 1994, 1995; *Food & Wine*'s "The Ten Best New Chefs in America," 1988; and Evian's "Healthy Menu Awards National Winner," 1993, 1994. Robert's skill in maximizing flavor while still cooking healthy is evident in the recipes he has contributed to this book.

## Michael Mina

Michael Mina began cooking at the age of fifteen as a prep cook in a small French restaurant in Washington State. Following graduation, he attended the prestigious Culinary Institute of America where he met Charles Palmer, chef/co-owner of Aureole in New York City. Throughout culinary school, and for some time afterward, Mina worked at Aureole, learning all kitchen positions. In 1991, Michael was offered the chef de cuisine position for the opening of Aqua in San Francisco. The rave reviews haven't stopped since; Aqua is a nationally renowned restaurant and Michael has received such awards as his recent James Beard Foundation nomination as "Rising Chef of the Year." In 1995, the owner of Aqua, Charles Condy, opened another Bay Area restaurant, Charles Nob Hill, where Michael is also executive chef.

## Nick Morfogen

Having grown up in the restaurant business, Nick admits that cooking was a duty rather than a passion. Training with the late Gilbert La Coze at New York City's Le Bernadin changed his view. After Nick graduated from the Culinary Institute of America in 1987, Gilbert offered him a position and showed him endless creative possibilities. Other strong influences include working with Daniel Boulud at Le Cirque and as sous-chef to Michael Chiarello at Tra Vigne. In 1994, Nick and Michael became partners in the Ajax

Tavern in Aspen, Colorado. As the executive chef Nick created an American-style menu with Mediterranean influences. In 1997, Nick moved on to Maxaluna in Boca Raton, Florida. Here he has further defined his flair for Mediterranian cooking; focusing on the soulful flavors of Tuscany. He has received glowing reviews from food critics and customers, and in 1996 was named one of the "Top 10 New Chefs in America" by *Food & Wine*.

## Wayne Nish

At the age of thirty-two, Wayne left a successful career in the printing industry to pursue his passion for cooking. After attending The New York Restaurant School, he took his first kitchen job in Barry Wine's top-rated Quilted Giraffe in 1984. It was here that experimentation in post–nouvelle cuisine hit high notes and influenced many young cooks. Many of those cooks, Wayne Nish included, are a big influence in the culinary world today. After leaving The Quilted Giraffe, he became executive chef of La Colombe d'Or. Here Wayne created personal interpretations of Provençal cuisine that, four months after his arrival, earned a three-star review in the *New York Times*. In 1990, Wayne opened up his own restaurant with his partner, Joseph Scalice. March Restaurant has earned two three-star reviews from the *New York Times*, four stars from *Forbes* magazine, and a 27 out of 30 food rating in the *Zagat Survey*.

## Michael Otsuka

Michael developed an interest in cooking at the side of his mother and grandmother. He assisted them in preparing the recipes of his Austrian-Jewish and Japanese backgrounds. His professional experience began at the Seventh Street Bistro, where he worked as an apprentice to Joachim Splichal. Michael joined Joachim in his next restaurant, Max au Triangle in Beverly Hills. Here he was quickly promoted to sous-chef. To round out his culinary background, Michael spent a few years working in Michelin-starred restaurants and hotels in France and Belgium, most notably at the Hotel Negresco in Nice. In 1995, Michael became executive chef at Patina, where he was recognized by the James Beard Foundation, receiving a nomination for "Rising Star Chef." He is currently chef at Chasen's in Beverly Hills, California.

## Jacques Pépin

As the author of more than fifteen cookbooks, of which more than half provide healthy recipes, finding two recipes that contain cancer-fighting foods was not difficult for Jacques Pépin. In addition to being a renowned author, Jacques is a teacher and culinary consultant. Like Julia Child, he has taught many Americans the art of French cuisine via television. Jacques has also developed and perfected healthy cooking techniques, sharing them with his reading and viewing audiences. His other forums for culinary instruction include a graduate curriculum in gastronomy, which he oversees at Boston University, and his role as Dean of Special Studies at New York's French Culinary Institute. At The French Culinary Institute Jacques coaches and inspires future chefs through regular culinary demonstrations and student consultations.

### Marta Pulini

Marta Pulini began her cooking career in the most important kitchen in Italy—her mother's. Here she learned regional cooking and family recipes that had been passed down through the generations. After marrying and moving to the food capital of Italy, the region of Emilia-Romagna, Chef Pulini created PUMA, a very successful catering business and later opened La Brasserie in Modena, Italy. Since her move to New York City in 1989, Chef Pulini has been at the helm of some of New York's finest Italian kitchens. They include Bice in New York and Paris and Le Madri in New York. Marta is now the corporate chef for Toscorp., a company with Italian restaurants throughout the United States. Marta gives frequent seminars on Italian cooking and teaches food lovers how to use the best Italian ingredients. She published her first English cookbook, *The Art of Regional Cooking* (Sterling Publishers), in 1995. Chef Pulini believes healthy eating can be easy by avoiding extremes, eating in moderation, and utilizing the freshest ingredients.

### Tom Pustizzi

Tom Pustizzi began his cooking career while at college. Quickly he found that he was more interested in and enthusiastic about cooking than his studies. He has since worked his way up the culinary ladder to his present position of Sous Chef at the Dilworthtown Inn in West Chester, Pennsylvania. The art, architecture, and food at this lovely country inn represent the rich local history. For the last six years Chef Pustizzi has been creating award-winning cuisine at this historic landmark.

### Michael Romano

Union Square Café's chef and partner is a native New Yorker with strong family ties in Italy. Michael takes advantage of Union Square Café's fortunate location—next-door to the city's largest greenmarket. Farm-fresh ingredients of the season, grown by local producers, dominate the Union Square's menu. Romano has forged a unique personal style of contemporary food with French and Italian influences. His straightforward food presentations incorporate robustly flavored, soundly imaginative ingredient combinations. Michael Romano is justifiably considered one of the nation's most talented, trend-setting chefs. Chef Romano and his partner, Danny Meyer, have pioneered an exciting new breed of restaurant where excellent food and wine are paired with warm hospitality and outstanding value. Together they coauthored *Union Square Café Cookbook* (Harper-Collins, 1994).

## Alain Sailhac

Born close to the Italian-French border in Millau, France, Alain Sailhac grew up surrounded by the fragrances and fresh ingredients of Provence. The influence is evident in his cooking. Alain allows ingredients to speak for themselves, combining them in such a manner so that they complement rather than mask one another. After more than forty years in the culinary arts, during which he gained four stars for New York's Le Cygne and three stars for the world-famous Le Cirque, Alain Sailhac joined The French Culinary Institute. As the Dean of Culinary Arts, he develops the student curriculum, selects first-rate faculty, attracts accomplished guest lecturers, and acts as an inspirational student adviser. He also oversees the seasonal menu for L'Ecole, The French Culinary Institute's on-site restaurant.

## Martin Saylor

After studying cuisine at the Cordon Bleu in France and the Culinary Institute of America, Martin Saylor served in the U.S. Navy. As principal chef to both the Commander of the Seventh Fleet and Deputy Commander in Chief of U.S. Forces in Europe, he traveled extensively throughout Asia and Europe. Although known for his American-inspired cuisine with bold and well-defined flavors, the influences of his travels are subtly apparent. Following his naval service, he was chef to then Secretary of the Treasury James A. Baker III. Now we can all enjoy his creative cooking at the celebrated Lafayette at the Hay-Adams Hotel in Washington D.C.

## Gianni Scappin

Gianni Scappin grew up at Trattoria alla Pesa, his family's restaurant, located in the beautiful Veneto region of Italy. At age fifteen he attended the renowned Recoaro Terme Culinary Institute. The curriculum included an extensive externship program, which took him to kitchens all over Italy. When he arrived in New York in 1983, Gianni became executive chef of the highly successful restaurant Castellano. His four-year stint of blending modern flair with traditional Italian cuisine primed Gianni for his next adventure, opening restaurants in New York, Atlanta, and Washington, D.C. for the Bice Organization. He followed this with four years at New York's Le Madri. Under his guidance Le Madri was twice among the top two Italian restaurants in New York in Gault Millau's "Best of New York." Gianni is now the executive chef at New York's Maximillian, and is also working with the mother of actor/director Stanley Tucci on a cookbook which will include recipes from the film *Big Night*.

## Dieter Schorner

Born in Rehau, Germany, Dieter Schorner began his career in pastry as an apprentice at the age of fifteen. After studying at Coba Institute in Basel, Switzerland, he went on to work at some of the finest restaurants in Europe. At age twenty-seven he became the chef-pâtissier and chef confiseur at the acclaimed Savoy Hotel in London, England. Since arriving in the United States in 1968, Dieter has held executive pastry chef positions at such renowned restaurants as New York City's Le Cirque, Tavern on the Green, and La Côte Basque. In 1988, Dieter opened Pâtisserie Café Didier in Washington, D.C. This café has consistently received accolades, such as "best breakfast" in Washington, D.C., and in 1997, a 26 out of 30 food rating by *Zagat Guide*. Additionally, *Money Magazine* has rated Dieter's café as one of the best breakfast places in America. Dieter now shares his expertise and career achievements with students as the chairman of The French Culinary Institute's recently launched Classic Pastry Arts program.

## RoxSand Scocos

RoxSand is owner and executive chef at RoxSand's Restaurant & Bar in Phoenix, Arizona, and has won numerous awards: most recently she was nominated for "Best Chef—Southwest Region" for the second year in a row by the James Beard Foundation. Known for her fusion cuisine—the art of bridging a variety of cooking techniques and flavors—she focuses on the future of food in our society and understands the importance of food choices and health. RoxSand remarks, "Since both the health of our children and the environmental future of the planet are at stake, it is our duty as chefs to send an urgent message about sustainable food choices." She demonstrates this by including 100 percent organic products in her menu, when possible.

## Jimmy Sneed

Chef Jimmy Sneed's culinary initiation came at Le Cordon Bleu cooking school in Paris, where he had a job translating for American students. It was here that he was exposed to classic French cooking techniques and launched his culinary career. He returned to the States to begin six years in training with master chef Jean-Louis at the Watergate restaurant in Washington, D.C. With a firm grasp of French cooking, Sneed has been able to create "modern American cuisine" with a French flair. Now chef and proprietor at The Frog and the Redneck in Richmond, Virginia, Sneed serves fresh seasonal products from local growers with simple sophistication and a touch of savoir faire. In 1995, he earned a James Beard Foundation nomination for "Best Chef—Mid-Atlantic Region."

### Andre Soltner

In the 1960s, Master Chef Andre Soltner brought classic French haute cuisine to New York. During the next thirty years, as chef-proprietor of New York's Lutece, his commitment to traditional French cooking never wavered. Loyal patronage was gained through not only superb food, but also the impeccable service and charm that remained consistent in the dining room. Among his many awards and accolades are the Grande Medaille d'Or, Academie Culinaire de France, and the James Beard Foundation's Lifetime Achievement Award. Although semiretired, Andre shares his more than forty-seven years of cooking experience with aspiring chefs at The French Culinary Institute in New York. Here he is able to instill his firm belief that the classics are the foundations for culinary success.

### Jacques Torres

After completing his apprenticeship at La Frangipane, a small pastry shop near his hometown of Bandol, France, Jacques began the swift climb to his current status as one of the world's most acclaimed pastry chefs. In 1980, he began an eight-year working relationship with Jacques Maximin at the famous Hotel Negresco. During this period he traveled the globe and earned the degree of master pastry chef. In 1986, Jacques was awarded the prestigious Meilleur Ouvrier de France medal, the youngest chef to earn the distinction. One year after coming to the United States, in 1988, he joined New York's famous Le Cirque, where he still remains executive pastry chef. Cooking for presidents, kings, and celebrities is part of every workday. Jacques is also dedicated to sharing his passion for the art of pastry; his training and teaching are ongoing in the kitchen of Le Cirque and, in 1996, he was appointed Dean of Pastry Arts for The French Culinary Institute. The rest of us can learn some of Jacques's techniques by tuning in to his new Public Television program *Dessert Circus with Jacques Torres*.

### Jerry Traunfeld

After many years of culinary experience, including four as the executive chef at The Alexis Hotel in Seattle, Washington, Jerry had the opportunity to combine his longtime passions for gardening and cooking: in 1990, he accepted the chef's position at The Herbfarm. This unique restaurant is surrounded by acres of kitchen gardens and serves only one exquisite, multicourse menu each night. Jerry has planned and prepared more than 250 seasonal menus using the magnificent ingredients of the Northwest and, of course, the abundance of fresh herbs that are at his fingertips. During his tenure The Herbfarm has received high ratings and numerous accolades.

## Charlie Trotter

Charlie Trotter began his culinary career in 1982. Since 1987, when he opened his elegant Chicago town house restaurant, Charlie Trotter's, he has soared to the top of America's culinary community. Charlie Trotter's restaurant is one of only a handful of U.S. restaurants to have earned five Mobil stars and five AAA diamonds and to have been inducted into the internationally renowned *Relais & Chateaux*. Charlie has also been named America's "Best Chef—Midwest" by the James Beard Foundation. As an innovator of cuisine, Chef Trotter expands on classic French traditions and uses the freshest possible ingredients and imagination to produce recipes that blend the flavors of the world. To our benefit, Chef Trotter's recipes utilize many fresh fruits and vegetables; his book *Charlie Trotter's Vegetables*, a narrative on vegetable cuisine in America, contains stunning photographs to accompany each recipe.

## Ming Tsai

Currently executive chef at Santacafé in Santa Fe, New Mexico, Ming Tsai began his cooking career at his family's Chinese restaurant as a teenager in Dayton, Ohio. This led him to Paris, where he studied at the Cordon Bleu. He then returned to the United States and obtained a master's degree in hotel administration from Cornell University. Chef Tsai has launched his career with a unique approach to fusion cooking by merging Southwestern and Asian cuisine. Ming Tsai has become a creative force in the culinary world, earning a *Zagat Guide* food rating of 27 out of 30 for Santacafé.

## Norman Van Aken

As the father of South Florida's New World Cuisine, Norman Van Aken has ushered in a concept of global cuisine and has led the way for many other successful chefs. Johnson & Wales University awarded him an honorary doctorate for his innovative career achievements. He currently cooks, consults, and lectures internationally on New World Cuisine while still overseeing his award-winning restaurant, NORMAN'S, in Coral Gables, Florida. His culinary philosophy is "to create a marriage of the raw and rustic with the classic and intellectual in a celebration of the various places we live." This is New World Cuisine. He also won the 1996 James Beard Perrier Joüet Award for "Best Chef—Southeast."

## Susan Weaver

During her fourteen years with the Four Seasons Hotel organization, Susan has accumulated such critical acclaim as winning a top-ten finalist spot in the Bocuse d'Or and becoming the only female finalist in the Prix Culinaire International Pierre Tattinger. In 1994, she was selected as the U.S.A. Hotel Chef of the Year. Her incredible career began when she was backpacking in Europe. During a period of time in which she worked as a dishwasher and vegetable peeler on the small island of Corsica, her passion for the kitchen was born. After returning to the United States, Susan worked and studied under the world-renowned chef Fernand Guitierrez, who provided her with the foundation of classic technique. At Fifty Seven in New York City's Four Seasons Hotel, Susan serves "alternative" cuisine (sophisticated and elegant, yet relatively low in fat, sodium, and cholesterol)—a style of cooking she helped pioneer almost a decade ago.

## Janos Wilder

Janos Wilder began cooking as a teenager and continued throughout college. Following graduation from the University of California at Berkeley, he pursued a career in the culinary arts. Janos worked in several restaurants in the Rocky Mountains, utilizing fresh herbs, trout from the mountain streams, forest mushrooms, buffalo, antelope, and even rattlesnake. While working in two Michelin-starred French kitchens in Bordeaux, he fine-tuned his technique in classical and nouvelle cuisine. In 1982, Janos moved to Tucson, Arizona, and combined French influences and Southwestern ingredients at Janos. The restaurant, a National Historic Landmark, has received numerous accolades.

## Charles Wiley

Charles Wiley, executive chef at The Boulders in Carefree, Arizona, is committed to cuisine which is low in fat and sodium with a robust and intense flavor derived from spices instead of butter or cream. Wiley's self-taught skills are the product of 23 years cooking experience, although he has studied formally under Madeline Kamman at the Beringer Vineyards School for American Chefs. Charles has been recognized by numerous awards and accolades including *Food & Wine*'s "Top 10 New Chefs" in 1994. In keeping with the desires of their "healthy clientele," Wiley strives to combine regional flavors and colorful presentation with healthy dining.

## William Yosses

After completing a graduate program in French literature at Rutgers University and a restaurant management curriculum at New York Technical College, William Yosses decided to further expand his language and culinary skills in France. Starting at La Foux in Paris, he began a work "tour" that eventually led to other reputable restaurants in Paris and the provinces. William credits Jean Pierre LeMasson, pastry chef at Perigord Park Restaurant, and Marc Janodet, pastry chef at Roger Verge's Moulin de Mougins, as mentors who gave him true apprenticeships and passion for the pastry arts. Since then William has worked as pastry chef at New York's Tavern on the Green, Montrachet, and now at Bouley.

# INDEX

· A NOTE ON THE TYPE ·

The typeface used in this book is a version of Goudy (Old Style), originally designed by Frederick W. Goudy (1865–1947), perhaps the best known and certainly one of the most prolific of American type designers, who created over a hundred typefaces—the actual number is unknown because a 1939 fire destroyed many of his drawings and "matrices" (molds from which type is cast). Initially a calligrapher, rather than a type cutter or printer, he represented a new breed of designer made possible by late-nineteenth-century technological advance; later on, in order to maintain artistic control, he supervised the production of matrices himself. He was also a tireless promoter of wider awareness of type, with the paradoxical result that the distinctive style of his influential output tends to be associated with his period and, though still a model of taste, can now seem somewhat dated.